10673373

Implementing
Mental
Health Promotion

Dedication

This book is dedicated to all who work for the improvement of mental health.

For Elsevier:

Commissioning Editor: **Steven Black**

Development Editor: **Catherine Jackson**

Project Manager: **Jane Dingwall**

Design: **Stewart Larking**

Illustrator: **Chartwell Illustrators**

Illustration buyer: **Merlyn Harvey**

Lanchester Library
WITHDRAWN

Implementing Mental Health Promotion

Margaret M. Barry PhD
Professor of Health Promotion and Public Health,
Department of Health Promotion, National University of
Ireland, Galway, Ireland

Rachel Jenkins MD FRCPsych
Director, WHO Collaborating Centre, Institute of
Psychiatry, King's College, London, UK

FOREWORD BY
Maurice B. Mittelmark BS MA PhD FACE
Professor, Department of Education and Health
Promotion, University of Bergen, Bergen, Norway;
President, International Union for Health Promotion
and Education

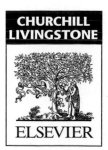

CHURCHILL
LIVINGSTONE

ELSEVIER

EDINBURGH LONDON NEW YORK OXFORD PHILADELPHIA ST LOUIS SYDNEY TORONTO 2007

CHURCHILL
LIVINGSTONE
ELSEVIER

© 2007, Elsevier Limited. All rights reserved.

First published 2007

No part of this publication may be reproduced, stored in a retrieval system, or transmitted in any form or by any means, electronic, mechanical, photocopying, recording or otherwise, without the prior permission of the Publishers. Permissions may be sought directly from Elsevier's Health Sciences Rights Department, 1600 John F. Kennedy Boulevard, Suite 1800, Philadelphia, PA 19103-2899, USA: phone: (+1) 215 239 3804; fax: (+1) 215 239 3805; or, e-mail: healthpermissions@elsevier.com. You may also complete your request on-line via the Elsevier homepage (http://www.elsevier.com), by selecting 'Support and contact' and then 'Copyright and Permission'.

ISBN-13: 978 0 443 10025 3
ISBN-10: 0 443 10025 X

British Library Cataloguing in Publication Data
A catalogue record for this book is available from the British Library.

Library of Congress Cataloging in Publication Data
A catalog record for this book is available from the Library of Congress.

Note
Knowledge and best practice in this field are constantly changing. As new research and experience broaden our knowledge, changes in practice, treatment and drug therapy may become necessary or appropriate. Readers are advised to check the most current information provided (i) on procedures featured or (ii) by the manufacturer of each product to be administered, to verify the recommended dose or formula, the method and duration of administration, and contraindications. It is the responsibility of the practitioner, relying on their own experience and knowledge of the patient, to make diagnoses, to determine dosages and the best treatment for each individual patient, and to take all appropriate safety precautions. To the fullest extent of the law, neither the Publisher nor the Authors assume any liability for any injury and/or damage to persons or property arising out of or related to any use of the material contained in this book.

The Publisher

ELSEVIER your source for books,
journals and multimedia
in the health sciences
www.elsevierhealth.com

The
Publisher's
policy is to use
**paper manufactured
from sustainable forests**

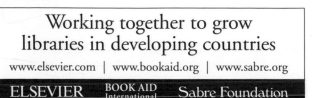

Working together to grow
libraries in developing countries

www.elsevier.com | www.bookaid.org | www.sabre.org

ELSEVIER   BOOK AID International   Sabre Foundation

Coventry University Library

Printed in China

Contents

Case Study Contributors

Kylee Bellingham BSSc MPsych MAPS
Formerly Project Manager, Depression Awareness Research Project, Mental Health Research Institute and Department of Psychiatry, University of Melbourne, Victoria, Australia

Zainab Farhan

Yvonne de Graaf MSc
National coordinator, Parenting Support Centre, Netherlands Institute for Care and Welfare, Utrecht, Netherlands

Ma. Asunción Lara MSc PhD
Head of Intervention Models Department, Ramón de la Fuente Institute of Psychiatry, San Lorenzo Huipulco, Mexico

Jo Mason MEd
National Coordinator, Strategic Planning, Mind Matters, Australia

Brenda Molloy RGN RM RPHN BA MSc
Director, Community Mothers Programme, Health Service Executive, Dublin, Ireland

Malik H Mubbashar MB FRCP FCPSPsych FRCPsych DPM
Professor and Vice Chancellor/Chief Executive, University of Health Sciences, Lahore, Pakistan

Kalliroi Papadopoulou PhD
Lecturer in Developmental Psychology, Department of Preschool Education, University of Athens, Greece

Eugene S Paykel MD FRCP FRCPsych FMedSci
Emeritus Professor of Psychiatry, University of Cambridge, England, UK

Richard H Price PhD
Barger Family Professor and Director, Interdisciplinary Program on Organizational Studies; Research Professor, Institute for Social Research, University of Michigan, Ann Arbor, USA

Bert Prinsen MSc
Project Manager, MIM Programme, Parenting Support Centre, Netherlands Institute for Care and Welfare, Utrecht, Netherlands

Louise Rowling MA MEd PhD
Associate Professor, Lecturer, University of Sydney, Australia

Khalid Saeed MB BCh MRCPsych
Senior Lecturer, Institute of Psychiatry, University of Rawalpindi, Rawalpindi, Pakistan

Anne Sheridan BSocSc CQSW
Mental Health Promotion Officer, Health Promotion Department, Health Service Executive West, Letterkenny, County Donegal, Ireland

Shona Sturgeon MSocSc (ClinSW)
President, World Federation for Mental Health; President, South African Federation for Mental Health; Senior Lecturer, Department of Social Development, University of Cape Town, South Africa

Suresh Sundram MBBS MMed FRANZCP PhD
Associate Professor; Head, Molecular Psychopharmacology, Mental Health Research Institute and Department of Psychiatry, University of Melbourne, Victoria, Australia

John Tsiantis MD DPM FRCPsych
Professor in Child Psychiatry, Athens University Medical School; Director, University Department of Child Psychiatry, Aghia Sophia Children's Hospital, Athens, Greece

Mieke Vergeer MSc
Implementation and dissemination, Parenting Support Centre, Netherlands Institute for Care and Welfare, Utrecht, Netherlands

Jukka Vuori PhD
Research Professor, Life Course and Work-theme; Vice Director, Finnish Institute of Occupational Health, Helsinki, Finland

Brian Waller
Formerly Director, Home-Start International, London, UK

Foreword

If asked to explain what the term 'health promotion' means, many if not most health professionals would respond by pointing to the importance of action to prevent, detect and treat emerging health problems. Professionals in the mental health arena experience daily encounters with patients whose problems include loneliness, apathy, sadness, helplessness and hopelessness, and whose diagnoses include depression, schizophrenia, social deviancy and anti-social behaviour, drug dependency and other self-destructive behaviour in all its guises. The emotions that accompany discourse about mental health are sadness, concern, worry and anger. No wonder that for many health professionals, 'health' is defined more by its absence than its presence.

Yet when ordinary people are asked to ponder what it means to be healthy, concerns about avoiding illness, disability and suffering are not necessarily the first thoughts that come to mind. As or more likely to be mentioned are the ability to participate in one's chosen form of life, to extract joy and meaning from doing so, and to experience satisfaction and zest with life despite its normal adversities. Even among people who are ill, with diagnoses and under care and treatment, quality of life has only partly to do with managing suffering. It has to do also with the experience of the highest level of mental, social and physical functioning possible under the circumstances, and with appreciation of the moments of satisfaction and joy that present themselves in almost everyone's lives regardless of their health situation.

So, there is a distinctly positive aspect to health in the minds of ordinary people, yet professional discourse about health tends to circle around the avoidance of misery rather than the stimulation of thriving lives. That this is so is not paradoxical – health professionals are trained intensively to restore the sick to the best level of health possible. It is therefore not too difficult to understand why, for many health professionals, the pursuit of happiness, satisfaction, joy, vitality and robustness may seem to have little to do with mental health promotion, and more to do with self-actualisation among the most fortunate and healthy of us. Similarly, the strengthening of social ties and social involvement may seem outside the sphere of concern with mental health per se. Intra-personal resources such as mastery, self-efficacy, hardiness and sense of coherence, while obvious resources to cope with the challenges of daily living, can appear to be off-subject when mental health concerns are at the centre of our attention.

Therein lies the special value of this volume, which explains clearly why and how mental health promotion aims to stimulate positive mental health and enhanced quality of life for all people, the well and the sick alike. The lesson that enhanced mental health is achievable by almost every person came to me

ix

with greatest force 30 years ago, when I worked as a research assistant for Professor Edwin Willems in the Behavioral Ecology Programme at the Texas Institute for Research and Rehabilitation, located in Houston.[1] We worked with spinal cord injured persons, many with severely limiting injuries, conducting studies to understand factors promoting recovery. Most of the patients were young men, the victims of their own audacity while motorcycling, diving, and competing with others in the one-and-a-thousand ways young men do. It is sadly ironic that in this way the most fit and active among us can suddenly be reduced to little or no movement and total dependency on others.

My job in the research team was to follow along with patients who volunteered for the study, recording in great detail their daily experiences in the various settings of the rehabilitation hospital – sleeping ward, treatment rooms, visitors lounge, dining room, and so forth. We aimed to collect and record behavioural observations from the time of entering the hospital until discharge, weeks or even months thereafter. During the period of hospitalisation, almost all the patients improved in their ability to negotiate their environment, care for themselves, engage in socialisation and plan for the future. One of the clearest impressions I have from those days is how a sense of humour seemed to promote recovery, and how much fun the patients had, as they explored their ever expanding capabilities. Noisy laughter was not an uncommon sound in the hallways, as wheel chair races (not permitted, of course!) gave vent to competitive spirits that had not faded. Just as often as not, it was the patients who comforted their troubled and worried families and friends, who initiated joking with staff, and who instigated pranks which seems aimed especially at we poor research assistants.

At the rehabilitation hospital, spinal cord injuries were treated, and mental health was promoted. The process of injury recovery promoted the mental health of everyone concerned, patients, family and staff alike. However, the 'fact sheets' about the rehabilitation hospital did not then, and still do not mention mental health promotion as an explicit goal of the institution. It is a most interesting facet of mental health promotion that most of what goes on to promote mental health in a community is not identified as such. A successful school-based anti-bullying programme certainly promotes the mental health of students, families and teachers (not to mention school bus drivers!), but these positive outcomes may well be acknowledged only implicitly, if at all.

Thus, mental health promotion is mostly undertaken by people who do not claim to be mental health promoters, and most professionals who engage in purposive mental health promotion do so not under the title 'mental health promoter', but rather as teacher, social worker, physician, occupational therapist, politician, among other vocations. This helps further explain how mental health promotion can be associated more with disease and ill health than with positive coping and thriving. Mental health promotion is in a sense 'hidden' because it is part and parcel of so many other community endeavours.

That is not to say, however, that purposive mental health promotion is and should be lackadaisical, quite the contrary. In recent years the professional field

[1] See the classic reference on behavioral ecology: Willems, E. P., & Campbell, D. E. (1975). Behavioral ecology: A new approach to health status and health care. In B. Honikman (Ed.), *Responding to social change.* Stroudsburg, PA: Dowden, Hutchinson & Ross. Pp. 200–210.

of health promotion has grown to include specialisation in mental health promotion. Because health promotion in general has so much to do with enhancement of quality of life, it has been inevitable that mental health courses have been developed, alongside offerings that have been more typical – such as those related to health lifestyle, for example. Whether a health promoter specialising in mental health or not, all professionals whose work touches on mental health promotion need to be equipped with knowledge about what types of interventions work best in various community settings. The expanding body of research is accumulating knowledge about effective change processes that promote positive mental health and enhanced quality of life: processes at the levels of the individual and the social group, the settings level such as workplaces and schools, and at the community and higher level (social and political processes).

Margaret Barry and Rachel Jenkins have worked hard to summarise that body of knowledge, especially as it relates to taking *action*. Hence the title of this book 'Implementing Mental Health Promotion' and the book's organisation, around settings for action – home, community, school, workplace, primary health care and mental health services settings. The systemisation of the widely scattered literature that this book represents is a welcome addition to the too few other books having 'mental health promotion' in their titles, precisely because of its comprehensive treatment of principles for taking effective action, illustrated with examples of excellent practice.

Maurice B. Mittelmark
Bergen, June 29, 2006

Preface

The publication *Implementing Mental Health Promotion* was motivated by the current paucity of texts on mental health promotion and also by the fact that issues of programme implementation are typically not addressed in the majority of publications. This book is written for a broad range of readers, including practitioners, policy makers and researchers working in mental health, health promotion and public health. Health promoters and professionals working across a range of service settings including communities, schools, workplaces, primary care and mental health services, will gain useful insights into evidence-based practice and the practical steps that are needed to ensure successful programme implementation. This book informs policy makers and decision-makers on what is needed to be put in place in order to translate the evidence in mental health promotion into best practice and policy. The text also provides a useful resource for researchers, academics and students in integrating the literature on mental health promotion with practical examples of effective programme implementation and dissemination.

Implementing Mental Health Promotion focuses on the importance of programme implementation and its critical role in advancing research, practice and policy in mental health promotion. The different dimensions of programme implementation are explored and the key factors affecting quality of implementation are examined across a range of programmes and settings. The practical and research challenges of implementing mental health promotion programmes are examined, including the challenge of developing and adapting interventions for use in different cultural settings. Best practice programmes and case study examples are presented to demonstrate how high quality implementation can be ensured through the use of research-based, theoretically grounded and culturally appropriate interventions. Based on the existing literature and research, the key factors that can improve the quality of programme implementation are highlighted and recommendations for practice and policy are discussed.

Implementing Mental Health Promotion aims to provide a practical guide to the implementation of mental health promotion programmes with different population groups in key settings such as the home, school, community, workplace and health services. The text is written from a 'how-to' perspective, combining an exploration of current research with practical advice to support the planning and implementation of mental health promotion programmes. The book provides examples of effective programmes and initiatives illustrating the process of implementation. Case studies of practical aspects of project development and delivery from different countries are included in order to illustrate the real life application of programmes. This book demonstrates how information from research can be used to inform effective programme development and implementation.

In terms of the structure of the book, Chapters 1 and 2 provide an introductory overview of the field of mental health promotion and a strong theoretical and conceptual base for action is outlined. A selective review of the theoretical and evidence base for the effectiveness of mental health promotion is included in Chapter 1 and international developments are discussed. In Chapter 2, a generic template for action is outlined covering the key steps involved in the planning and implementation of programmes. Chapters 3 to 8 demonstrate the application of the generic template for action with a range of population groups (children, adolescents, adults and older people) across key settings including the home, school, workplace, community, primary care and mental health services. Each chapter introduces the rationale for mental health promotion in that setting and an overview of current research findings in the area; examples of evidence-based programmes and case studies on the application of exemplary and innovative programmes are included. The best practice programmes and case studies are selected from across low, middle and high-income countries. Based on the research and case studies reviewed, each chapter concludes by identifying generic principles of best practice in implementing mental health promotion programmes in that area.

It is important to acknowledge that the book does not address all relevant settings, nor indeed does it include all best practice programmes. However, we have tried to include a selective sample of programmes that will illustrate key principles of good practice in programme implementation. The majority of the best practice examples are from programmes conducted in high-income countries, as this is where research funding is most likely to be made available. However, we have also included programme examples and case studies from middle and low-income countries in order to address the particular implementation challenges when working in those settings.

Across the chapters we have taken a population level approach, including mental health promotion programmes for the general population, those deemed to be at higher risk and also people with mental health problems. In keeping with the principles of health promotion, this approach adopts the view that we all have mental health needs and that positive mental health can be promoted for all, including those experiencing mental disorders.

Implementing Mental Health Promotion primarily addresses the implementation of discrete programmes, as this is where most evidence has been collated to date. However, we are mindful that mental health promotion embraces a much broader range of activities than defined programmes and that it includes policy change and the impact of broader macro level interventions. At this point, we have tried to bring together in one place a selection of the documented successful programmes and the factors that have been identified as making them work.

In bringing together the literature from research, practice and policy, *Implementing Mental Health Promotion* aims to advance the knowledge and practice of implementing effective, feasible and sustainable mental health promotion programmes across diverse population groups and settings. We hope that you will find the book both useful and enjoyable and that it will stimulate the development and implementation of high quality programmes and initiatives that will promote mental health.

Acknowledgements

We wish to thank everybody who made publication of this book possible. In particular, we acknowledge the contribution of the case study authors, who managed to condense their experiences of programme implementation into 2,000 words. Thanks to Josephine O'Keeffee, Róisín Egenton and Kathryn Meade, who contributed to background research on the book and the drafting of chapter sections, and to Therese Costello and Colette Dempsey who helped with final editing and referencing. We also acknowledge the contribution of Linda Seymour and Elizabeth Gale of Mentality, UK for their comments on an earlier draft of Chapter 8.

A special thanks from Margaret to Dug for his invaluable support throughout and from Rachel to Ruth and Ben.

Introduction to Mental Health Promotion

1

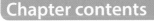
Introduction

This chapter provides an overview of current concepts and principles of mental health promotion and examines the conceptual frameworks and models for promoting positive mental health. The theoretical perspectives underpinning these frameworks are considered and the risk reduction and competence enhancement approaches to promoting mental health are outlined. An overview of international developments in terms of research, policy and practice developments is given, including the evidence concerning the effectiveness of mental health promotion programmes. The application of the growing knowledge and evidence base to current practice and policy is discussed. The chapter also considers the development of the necessary infrastructure to support effective policy and practice for promoting mental health and key requirements to advance development are outlined.

Mental Health Promotion

Mental health promotion is concerned with achieving positive mental health and quality of life. The focus of this multidisciplinary area of practice is on enhancing the strengths and competencies of individuals and communities, thereby promoting positive emotional and mental well-being. Mental health promotion focuses on promoting positive mental health among the general population and addresses the needs of those at risk from, or experiencing, mental health problems. The focus is, therefore, on the whole population and on strengthening protective factors and enhancing well-being and quality of life. Mental health promotion, while focusing on the positive aspects of mental health, has relevance across the entire spectrum of mental health interventions, including for people experiencing mental health problems and disorders. This includes creating supportive environments, reducing stigmatisation and discrimination and supporting the social and emotional well-being of service users and their families. The underlying principle of this approach is that mental health is an integral part of overall health and is, therefore, of relevance to all. Mental health is a positive concept which is embedded in the social, economic and cultural life of the community. Mental health promotion, therefore, focuses on improving the social, physical and economic environments that determine the mental health of populations and individuals. The delivery of such programmes requires the development of health and social policy, which extends beyond the clinical and treatment focus of current mental health service delivery to address the influence of broader social and environmental factors on mental health.

The Importance of Mental Health

Mental health is fundamental to good health and quality of life. Positive mental health is a resource for everyday life which enables us to manage our lives successfully. As a resource, mental health contributes to the functioning of individuals, families, communities and society. The need to address mental health as an integral part of improving overall health and well-being is increasingly recognised at the international level (US Department of Health and Human Services 1999, WHO 2001b, 2002). The concept of mental health cannot be separated from that of overall health, which was defined in the World Health Organization Constitution of 1946 (WHO 1946) as a state of complete physical, mental and social well-being and not merely the absence of disease or injury. More recent definitions have gone on to describe health as a resource for living and as a positive concept emphasising social and personal resources, as well as physical capacities (WHO 1986). Mental health contributes to the social, human and economic capital of society (Lehtinen et al 2005). The promotion of positive mental health is therefore important in its own right. The phrase 'there is no health without mental health' conveys clearly this positive sense of mental health. Mental health is intrinsic to good health and quality of life and as such is firmly placed within the broader public health and health promotion arena (Box 1.1).

> ## Box 1.1
>
> ### Key messages from the WHO summary report on promoting mental health: concepts, emerging evidence, practice (2004a)
>
> - there is no health without mental health
> - mental health is more than the absence of mental illness: it is vital to individuals, families and societies
> - mental health is determined by socioeconomic and environmental factors
> - mental health is linked to behaviour
> - mental health can be enhanced by effective public health interventions
> - collective action depends on shared values as much as the quality of scientific evidence
> - a climate that respects and protects basic civil, political, economic, social, and cultural rights is fundamental to the promotion of mental health
> - intersectoral linkage is the key for mental health promotion
> - mental health is everybody's business

Positive Concepts of Mental Health

The term mental health is often misunderstood and is frequently interpreted as referring to mental ill-health. Indeed many of our mental health services and mental health professionals are concerned with the treatment of mental disorders rather than with mental health per se. The concept of positive mental health is more than the absence of symptoms of mental disorder. Mental health is described by the WHO as 'a state of well-being in which the individual realises his or her own abilities, can cope with the normal stresses of life, can work productively, and is able to make a contribution to his or her community' (WHO 2001a:1). This description highlights the different aspects of positive mental health including subjective well-being and affective balance; the development of abilities to manage life, maximise one's potential, participate and contribute to society. Drawing on these different dimensions, the Victorian Health Foundation defined mental health as 'the embodiment of social, emotional and spiritual well-being. It provides individuals with the vitality necessary for active living, to achieve goals, and to interact with one another in ways that are respectful and just' (VicHealth1999:Research Summary 1). The former Health Education Authority in the UK, in their very useful publication on a quality framework for mental health promotion, also included in their definition of mental health, 'The emotional and spiritual resilience which enables us to enjoy life and to survive pain, disappointment and sadness' (HEA 1997:7). This highlights the important aspect of being able to use psychological stress as a development process; an opportunity for growth rather than hindering development. This very much relates to the concept of resilience which signifies the presence of personal capacities and resources that maintain or preserve good functioning in the face of adversity. These include capacities such as coping skills, problem-solving skills and optimistic thinking among others. Positive mental health, therefore, encompasses the abilities to develop psychologically, emotionally, intellectually, socially and spiritually. Jenkins et al (2001:8) draw together these different elements in their definition of mental health as 'a positive sense of well-being, a belief in our own worth and the dignity and worth of others, the ability to think, perceive and interpret, to manage life, to communicate, initiate, develop and sustain mutually satisfying personal relationships'. Mental health is characterised as a multidimensional construct, of universal relevance, since we all have mental health needs, and of concern to all sectors of society.

Mental ill-health is an umbrella term which encompasses a continuum from the most severe disorders to a variety of common mental health problems and mild symptoms of different intensity and duration. Mental disorders usually refer to a diagnosable clinical condition that significantly interferes with the individual's functioning and abilities. Mental disorders are defined by the existence of symptoms such as impaired mood, abnormal perceptions, thought processes and cognitions. Some of the major mental disorders include depression, psychosis and dementia. The term mental illness is also used to refer to mental disorders. Mental health problems include more common mental health complaints such as anxiety and depression, which may be less severe and of shorter duration than mental disorders. These problems may be experienced temporarily as a reaction to life stressors, but if left unattended may develop into more serious and chronic mental conditions. The distinction between the two is not well defined but usually the duration and intensity of the problems are the distinguishing characteristics.

The WHO (2004a) summary report, 'Promoting mental health: concepts, emerging evidence, practice', outlines the different ways in which positive mental health has been conceptualised. These include mental health as a positive emotion or affect, e.g. a subjective sense of well-being and feelings of happiness; a personality trait encompassing concepts of self-esteem and sense of control; and resilience in the face of adversity and the capacity to cope with life stressors. Marie Jahoda, in her 1958 book titled 'Current concepts of positive mental health' (one of the few publications addressing this topic), sought to define positive mental health in terms of a list of attributes, such as an efficient perception of reality, self knowledge, the exercise of voluntary control over behaviour, self-esteem and self-acceptance, the ability to form affectionate relationships and productivity. While many of these attributes feature in current definitions, there is a concern that these characteristics may be specific to culture, gender, time and place. For example, Kovess-Masfety et al (2005) point out that the definition of mental health is clearly influenced by the culture that defines it and may have different meanings depending on socioeconomic and political influences. Pilgrim and Rogers (1993) argue that mental health may be seen as being socially constructed and socially defined, and Weare (2000) points out that different professions, cultures and societies may have different ways of conceptualising the nature and determinants of mental health and ill-health. What we understand by positive mental health depends on our values, assumptions, the nature of society and our role within it (Caplan & Holland 1990, Tudor 1996).

Antonovsky's salutogenic model (1996) provides a useful theory within which to understand positive mental health as it focuses on coping and positive well-being rather than breakdown and the 'salutary' factors rather than risk factors. Antonovsky posited the construct of sense of coherence as being vital to positive health as it involves the capacity to comprehend and make sense of one's experiences and the ability to manage and respond flexibly to the inevitability of life stressors. Mental health is, therefore, conceptualised in positive rather than negative terms and is viewed as an intrinsic part of overall health and quality of life.

Determinants of Mental Health

Mental health is determined by multiple biological, psychological, social and environmental factors which interact in complex ways (Mrazek & Haggerty 1994). The determinants of mental health reside in the physical and psychological make up of the individual, their interpersonal and social surroundings and the external environmental and broader social influences. Demographic factors such as age, gender and ethnicity are important determinants of mental health. However, mental health promotion tends to focus on those modifiable determinants, which can be altered effectively in order to promote positive mental health and reduce the likelihood of mental ill-health. At the population level these include a range of psychosocial and environmental factors including living conditions, education, income, employment, access to community resources, social support and personal competencies.

The factors that determine mental health may be clustered into three key areas (HEA 1997, Lahtinen et al 1999, Lehtinen et al 1997):

1. structural level factors which include social, economic and cultural factors that are supportive of positive mental health. Healthy structures and environments such as good living environments, housing, employment, transport, education and a supportive political structure
2. community level factors including a positive sense of belonging, social support and a sense of citizenship and participation in society
3. individual level – the ability to deal with thoughts and feelings, to manage life, emotional resilience and the ability to cope with stressful or adverse circumstances.

These determinants translate into risk and protective factors that influence the mental health of individuals and population groups. Risk factors or vulnerability factors increase the likelihood that mental health problems and mental disorders will develop and may also increase the duration and severity when a mental disorder occurs. Exposure to multiple risk factors over time can have a cumulative effect (Kazdin & Kagan 1994). Protective factors enhance and protect positive mental health and reduce the likelihood that a disorder will develop. Protective factors enhance people's capacity to successfully cope with and enjoy life and mitigate the effects of negative life events. In relation to both risk and protective factors, it should be noted that the strength of association and evidence of causation varies considerably.

Albee (1982) characterised the incidence of mental health problems as an equation, with incidence being determined by the relationship between risk factors such as organic causes, stress and exploitation, and protective factors such as coping skills, self-esteem and support systems. Strengthening both sides of the equation, i.e. boosting protective factors and reducing risk factors, provides an effective approach to prevention and promotion. A useful depiction of key risk and protective factors for mental health is outlined in both the HEA (1997) mental health promotion quality framework document and the Commonwealth Department of Health and Aged Care (2000) publication, 'Promotion, prevention and early intervention for mental health'. MacDonald and O'Hara (1998) also provide a useful map of the factors that promote and demote mental health. Table 1.1 provides illustrative examples of risk and protective factors operating across the individual, social and structural levels.

Risk and protective factors operate at the level of the individual, the family, community and at the macro level of society as a whole. Therefore, an ecological perspective provides the most useful framework for addressing these factors and endorses the need for comprehensive mental health promotion programmes (Nelson et al 1999). Many of the determinants of mental health such as education, income, employment and socioeconomic status lie outside the health area and there is, therefore, a need for collaboration across different sectors in order to

Table 1.1 Examples of risk and protective factors for mental health

	Protective factors	Risk factors
Individual level	positive sense of self good coping skills attachment to family social skills good physical health	low self-esteem low self-efficacy poor coping skills insecure attachment in childhood physical and intellectual disability
Social level	positive experience of early attachment supportive caring parents/family good communication skills supportive social relationships sense of social belonging community participation	abuse and violence separation and loss peer rejection social isolation
Structural level	safe and secure living environment economic security employment positive educational experience access to support services	neighbourhood violence and crime poverty unemployment/economic insecurity homelessness school failure social or cultural discrimination lack of support services

address the wide range of risk and protective factors. Albee et al (1988) highlighted the influence of degrading and exploitative social conditions including poverty, poor working conditions, racism and sexism on mental health. 'The mental health of a population is determined by the extent to which the environments within which people live and work ensure that all people have access to the resources they need to achieve and maintain optimal health' (Building Australia's capacity to promote mental health 1997:25). Social and economic disadvantages limit access to resources as do low levels of education. This points to the need for change at the level of social systems and for different sectors working together in order to create more supportive environments through policy and organisational change. The full range of factors influencing mental health, including those at the broad social, organisational and structural levels, needs to be addressed. Current mental health promotion and prevention programmes have been criticised for being too individually focused, failing to address wider social factors, and being expert-driven rather than adopting a more participatory approach. Drew et al (2005) outline a human rights approach as a useful tool for identifying and addressing the determinants of mental health. A climate that protects basic civil, political, social, cultural and economic rights is fundamental to the promotion of mental health. They point out that the principles of equality and freedom from discrimination, which are integral to the international human rights framework, call for particular attention to the vulnerable, disadvantaged and marginalised groups in society. This approach underscores the need for social and policy changes as well as those that target individual skills and competencies. Many initiatives which influence mental health, such as improved housing, welfare, access to childcare, transport, etc., are not evaluated in terms of their impact on mental health. The development of these types of interventions and evaluation of their impact and effectiveness are important parts of a comprehensive and integrated approach to promoting health at the population level.

Meeting the Global Challenge of Promoting Population Level Mental Health

Mental health promotion has a key role to play in meeting the global challenge of promoting population level mental health. The WHO world health report (2001b) points to the fact that more than 450 million people suffer from mental disorders worldwide and one in four persons will develop a mental or behavioural disorder throughout their lifetime. The WHO and the World Bank report (Murray & Lopez 1996) has drawn attention to the rise in mental health problems as a major public health problem to be addressed in the 21st century. Five of the 10 leading causes of disability worldwide are psychiatric conditions (Hosman & Jané-Llopis 1999). It is predicted that by the year 2020, neuropsychiatric problems such as depression will constitute the biggest health problem in the developing world, and will be the second biggest cause of disease burden worldwide. Linked to the rise in depression are the increasing levels of suicidal behaviour, especially completed suicides, in many countries which are strongly associated with the presence of both diagnosed and undiagnosed mental health problems (Arsenault-Lapierre et al 2004). Mental and behavioural disorders are common and are present across all age groups, cultures and population groups.

The burden of mental disorders is substantial and it arises from individual suffering, disability, premature death, loss of economic productivity, poverty and family burden and leads to intergenerational cycles of disadvantage (Jenkins et al 2001). Marshall-Williams et al (2005) point to the fact that in the USA the estimated total annual cost of mental disorders is $147 billion, which exceeds the cost attributable to other health problems such as cancer, AIDS and respiratory disease. The aggregate cost of mental disorders is estimated to be between 2.5% and 4% of global gross national product (WHO 2003). Added to this, the hidden costs of mental disorders and health problems such as the impact on individuals, their families and communities, stigma and violations of human rights, may go unmeasured.

The existence of social inequalities in the distribution of common mental disorders, such as anxiety and depression, is now well documented (Fryers et al 2003). Patel (2005) provides an overview of the relationship between poverty and mental health. Citing recent reviews of community studies from low and middle income countries, Patel highlights that most studies reported an association between the risk of depression and indicators of low education and low socioeconomic status such as poor housing and low income. Melzer et al (2004) review the evidence from nine large-scale population-based studies carried out over the last 20 years, and they conclude that common mental disorders are significantly more frequent in socially disadvantaged populations. They report that the evidence is strongest when material indicators of social position, education or unemployment are used to define disadvantaged groups. Markers of social disadvantage, such as having poorer material circumstances (housing tenure and lack of car ownership), being unemployed or economically inactive and less education (having left school before the age of 16) were all found to be associated with higher prevalence rates of common mental disorders, after adjusting for gender and age. Patel (2005) argues that irrespective of the average per capita income of a society, those at the bottom end of the social hierarchy are at greatest risk of experiencing mental health problems, and this effect appears to be most pronounced in more unequal as well as poorer societies.

In addressing the global burden of mental ill-health, it is recognised that treatment approaches alone are not sufficient and that a more comprehensive population level approach is required. The WHO (2001b) advocates a comprehensive public health approach which places importance on mental health promotion and prevention as well as treatment and rehabilitation. The WHO Mental Health Global Action programme highlights the need for population level mental health. The WHO 'Prevention and promotion in mental health' report lays out clearly the rationale for adopting a mental health promotion approach and advocates that 'Priority should be given to prevention and promotion in the field of mental health to reduce the increasing burden of mental disorders' (2002:7). As pointed out by Hosman and Jané-Llopis (1999), the high prevalence and incidence of mental disorder and the associated mortality and social and economic costs for society make a strong case for the development of national and international mental health promotion policies. A number of key international organisations are playing an important role in stimulating collaborative action to promote the value placed on mental health at national and international levels.

International Developments

Mental health is moving onto the political agenda and there is a momentum behind international and national developments in terms of policy, research and practice (Marshall-Williams et al 2005). A number of key international organisations, such as the WHO, the World Federation for Mental Health and the International Union for Health Promotion and Education are playing an important role in stimulating collaborative action to promote the value placed on mental health promotion at national and international levels. Jenkins et al (2001) provide an interesting overview of a variety of EU and international initiatives aimed at enhancing the implementation of mental health promotion. At a European level these include: the European Network on Mental Health Policy established in 1995, the Key Concepts for European Mental Health Promotion in 1997, and EC Mental Health Indicators Project in 1999. The Implementing Mental Health Promotion Action (IMHPA) network published a policy for Europe in 2005 (Jané-Llopis & Anderson 2005), which calls for the development of comprehensive country-based action plans across EU member states, in particular paying attention to 10 action areas and five common principles (Box 1.2). The European WHO Ministerial conference held in Helsinki in 2005 brought together all

---

Box 1.2

Mental health promotion and mental disorder prevention: a policy for Europe
(Jané-Llopis & Anderson 2005)

10 action areas:
- support parenting and the early years of life
- promote mental health in schools
- promote workplace mental health
- support mentally healthy ageing
- address groups at risk for mental disorders
- prevent depression and suicide
- prevent violence and harmful substance use
- involve primary and secondary health care
- reduce disadvantage and prevent stigma
- link with other sectors

Five common principles:
- expand the knowledge base for mental health
- support effective implementation
- build capacity and train the workforce
- engage different actors
- evaluate policy and programme impact

52 countries in the WHO European region, and the conference's declaration and action plan will drive the policy agenda on mental health in Europe for the coming years. The action plan sets out the details of commitments and responsibilities of both the WHO and national governments. The European Commission published a Green Paper on 'Improving the mental health of the population. Towards a strategy on mental health for the European Union' in 2005 and a consultation process was undertaken concerning the need for a strategy at EU level and its possible priorities. A strategy on mental health for the EU is expected to be published by the end of 2006. These initiatives serve to strengthen mental health policy and practice, exchanging experiences and expertise and stimulating joint research and practice developments on a cross-European basis.

Particular recognition is given to the added value of concerted strategic action between countries in enhancing the value and visibility of mental health in Europe and internationally (Hosman 2000). There have been a number of significant international developments which have placed mental health promotion on the public and political agenda. These include the following initiatives:

1. The WHO has instituted a number of initiatives on increasing the global awareness and understanding of mental health promotion:
    *   the Nations for Mental Health programme
    *   the annual World Mental Health day every October, supported by the World Federation of Mental Health
    *   the WHO Mental Health Global Action programme and the WHO 'Prevention and promotion in mental health' document (2002)
    *   the WHO publications, 'Promoting mental health: concepts, emerging evidence, practice' (Herrman et al 2005, WHO 2004a) and 'Prevention of mental disorders: effective interventions and policy options' (Hosman et al 2006, WHO 2004b), which aim to clarify concepts of promotion and prevention, review the evidence of effectiveness and examine the public health policy and practice implications
    *   The joint publication of the World Federation for Mental Health and the WHO (Saxena & Garrison 2004) on 'Mental health promotion: case studies from countries' which show-cases a range of programmes from low-, middle- and high-income countries.
2. The World Conference series on the Promotion of Mental Health and Prevention of Mental and Behavioural Disorders organised by the World Federation for Mental Health and the Clifford Beers Foundation in collaboration with the Carter Centre and the WHO. The published proceedings from the 2000 inaugural conference in Atlanta, the 2002 conference in London and the 2004 conference in New Zealand are available from the World Federation for Mental Health (email: info@wfmh.com).
3. The International Union for Health Promotion and Education (IUHPE) has included mental health promotion as a priority area in the following initiatives:
    *   the Global Programme on Health Promotion Effectiveness (GPHPE), including the publication in 2005 on 'The evidence of mental health promotion effectiveness: strategies for action' (Jané-Llopis et al 2005)

- the influential mental health promotion chapter by Hosman and Jané-Llopis (1999) published in a report for the European Commission on 'The evidence of health promotion effectiveness: shaping public health in a new Europe' which targets policymakers and practitioners and has been translated into several languages worldwide
- the inclusion of mental health promotion as a major stream in the World Conference series on Health Promotion and Education since the Melbourne Conference in 2004 (www.iuhpe.org).

4. The establishment of a Global Consortium for the Advancement of Promotion and Prevention (GCAPP) in Mental Health, which seeks to act as a catalyst for building international consensus and synergy of action through effective collaboration and partnerships among relevant international organisations (secretariat email: info@wfmh.com).
5. The development of dedicated journals in the area such as the International Journal of Mental Health Promotion published by the Clifford Beers Foundation (www.cliffordbeersfoundation.co.uk) and the Journal of Public Mental Health published by Pavilion in association with the Mental Health Foundation (www.pavpub.com) in the UK.

Promoting Positive Mental Health: Theoretical Frameworks for Practice

As a multidisciplinary area, mental health promotion derives its theoretical base from a number of diverse disciplines. The development of this area needs to be underpinned by sound conceptual and theoretical frameworks which provide coherent models for designing, conducting and evaluating programmes. In considering these frameworks, it may be useful to make a distinction between the practice of mental health promotion and the prevention of mental disorders. These two areas, while clearly related and overlapping, are informed by different sets of principles and hence tend to operate within different conceptual frameworks. Mental health promotion focuses on positive mental health and its main aim is the building of strengths, competencies and resources. In contrast, the area of prevention concerns itself primarily with specific disorders and aims to reduce the incidences, prevalence or seriousness of targeted problems, i.e. mortality, morbidity and risk behaviour outcomes. Articulated as such, these two fields have different starting points and seek to impact on different outcomes. In practice, however, there is much common ground between the two areas, particularly with regard to primary prevention and mental health promotion programmes. The current conceptual frameworks and models informing both the mental health promotion and prevention areas will now be considered.

Prevention Frameworks

The most widely used prevention framework in the mental health area is that put forward by Caplan (1964). This framework distinguishes between three types of prevention:

1. primary prevention aimed at reducing the incidence of mental disorders of all types in a community
2. secondary prevention aimed at reducing the prevalence of disorders by reducing duration
3. tertiary prevention aimed at reducing the impairments which may result from disorders.

Caplan's framework proposes a continuum between prevention and treatment as part of a wider spectrum of activities designed to reduce the incidence and prevalence of disorder. However, this framework has been criticised for blurring the distinction between early treatment and prevention interventions.

A more recent prevention framework was put forward by Mrazek and Haggerty (1994) in the report entitled 'Reducing risks for mental disorders: frontiers for preventive intervention research'. This framework, originally depicted as a half circle, places prevention activities in the wider mental health intervention spectrum of prevention, treatment and maintenance (Fig. 1.1). Three main categories of prevention activities are identified:

* universal – targeting the general population
* selective – targeting high-risk groups
* indicated – targeting high-risk individuals or groups with minimal but detectable signs or symptoms of mental disorder.

While clearly articulating the different types of prevention, this framework does not include interventions focusing on promoting positive mental health, nor does it explicitly identify links across the different areas of prevention, treatment, maintenance and rehabilitation. However, it would appear that at least conceptually there is quite an overlap between universal prevention activities, as

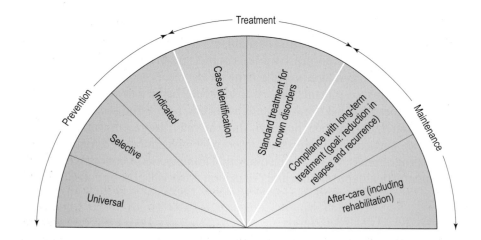

Figure 1.1 ● The mental health intervention spectrum for mental disorders (adapted from Mrazek & Haggerty 1994 and reprinted with permission of the National Academies Press)

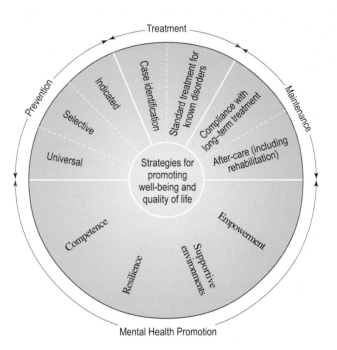

Figure 1.2 ● Modified mental health intervention spectrum (adapted from Barry 2001 and reprinted with permission of the International Journal of Mental Health Promotion)

outlined in the framework, and those of mental health promotion. Taking the lead from Mrazek's (1998) own suggestion that perhaps the second half of the circle depicting the mental health intervention spectrum consists of mental health promotion, the circle has been completed by Barry (2001) (Fig. 1.2) to include mental health promotion, indicating some core concepts by way of example (by no means meant to be exhaustive or exclusive). This amended circle depicts mental health promotion as the largest part of the circle given its universal relevance and indicates the unifying central area between the different interventions as that centred on strategies for promoting well-being and quality of life.

Promotion, prevention, treatment and rehabilitation programmes all have at their core the overall goal of promoting well-being and quality of life. While these intervention categories clearly differ in their target populations, programme objectives, content and process, they may share many core intervention components derived from underlying theoretical constructs. For example, there is an extensive literature on the potency of core constructs such as self-efficacy, sense of control, self-esteem, social support and resilience, which have been successfully applied across the spectrum of health and mental health interventions. Clearly, there is much opportunity for shared learning and development around the application of these constructs with different populations across the diverse areas of practice.

A Population Health Framework

An interesting population perspective on promoting mental health is outlined in the Australian discussion document 'Building capacity to promote the mental health of Australians' (Health Australia Project 1996). This model (Fig. 1.3) clearly shows the relevance of mental health promotion across populations ranging from healthy populations to those with mental disorders. The framework outlines the opportunities for mental health promotion across these different population groups and articulates the diverse aims and goals of mental health promotion strategies across the different areas of practice. These range from building resilience and promoting health for healthy populations to reducing risk and early identification for high-risk groups, to treatment and optimal care for those with mental disorders. This framework covers the spectrum of promotion, prevention, treatment and rehabilitation and, though not explicitly identified, holds open the possibility of links across the different areas of practice.

A Health Promotion Framework

Adopting a health promotion framework locates mental health within a holistic definition of health and, therefore, builds on the basic tenets of health promotion as outlined in the Ottawa Charter (WHO 1986) and subsequent WHO directives. The underlying principle of this approach is that mental health promotion is an integral part of overall health and is, therefore, of universal relevance to all. Health promotion was introduced by the WHO as a comprehensive new approach to bring

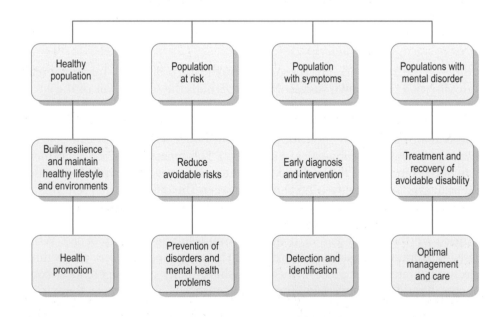

Figure 1.3 ● Opportunities for mental health promotion: a population perspective (adapted from 'Building capacity to promote the mental health of Australians', Health Australia Project 1996)

about social changes for improved health at the population level. Health promotion is based upon a social model of health and has been defined by the WHO (1986) as 'the process of enabling people to increase control over, and improve, their health'. Health promotion emerged as a dynamic force within the new public health, aimed at addressing the major determinants of health and thus contributing to the positive development of health at a population level. Health promotion has shifted the focus away from an individual, disease prevention approach towards the health actions and wider social determinants that keep people healthy.

Health promotion is rooted in a salutogenic view of health (Antonovsky 1996) and is aimed at whole populations across the life course and across settings. The salutogenic view means strengthening people's health potential. Health promotion focuses not only at the level of the individual but also on groups, communities, settings where people live their lives and on entire populations. Adopting a settings-based approach, health promotion emphasises that health is created within the settings where people live their lives and as such these everyday contexts or settings, such as the home, school, workplace, community, are where health can be promoted.

The principles of health promotion practice, as articulated in the Ottawa Charter for Health Promotion (WHO 1986), are based on an empowering, participative and collaborative process, which aims to increase control over health and its determinants. As described by Kickbusch (2003), the Ottawa Charter initiated a redefinition and repositioning of actors at the 'health' end of the disease–health continuum. This reorientation shifts the focus from the modification of individual risk factors or risk behaviours to addressing the context and meaning of health action and the protective factors that keep people healthy. The inextricable link between people and their environments forms the basis of this socioecological approach to health and provides a conceptual framework for practice.

The concept of health promotion is positive, dynamic and empowering and provides an attractive and useful framework to inform the conceptualisation and practice of promoting mental health. Based on this framework the following principles of mental health promotion may be articulated:

- involves the population as a whole in the context of their everyday life, rather than focusing on people at risk from specific mental disorders
- focuses on protective factors for enhancing well-being and quality of life
- addresses the social, physical and socioeconomic environments that determine the mental health of populations and individuals
- adopts complementary approaches and integrated strategies operating from the individual to socioenvironmental levels
- involves intersectoral action extending beyond the health sector
- based on public participation, engagement and empowerment.

The Ottawa Charter (WHO 1986) provides a socioecological framework for mental health promotion as it draws attention to a systems approach spanning individual, social and environmental factors that influence health: The Ottawa Charter outlined five key areas for action to promote health: to build healthy public policy, create supportive environments, strengthen community action, develop personal skills and reorient health services. Using this framework each of the five areas may be applied to promoting mental health.

1. Building healthy public policy puts mental health promotion on the agenda of all policy makers and calls for coordinated action across health, economic and social policies for improved mental health. Building healthy public policy includes diverse approaches such as investment in government and social policy, the implementation of legislation and regulations, organisational change and partnerships. This action area highlights the important influence of policies beyond the health sector on mental health, e.g. employment, housing, transport, education and childcare policies, and calls for increased attention to assessing the impact of such policies on the mental health of the whole population.

2. Creating supportive environments moves mental health beyond an individualistic focus to consider the influence of broader social, physical, cultural and economic environments. This action area emphasises the importance of the interaction between people and their environments and highlights the importance of mediating structures such as homes, schools, communities, workplaces and community settings as key contexts for creating and promoting positive mental health.

3. Strengthening community action focuses on the empowerment of communities through their active engagement and participation in identifying their needs, setting priorities and planning and implementing action to achieve better health and take control of their daily lives. Community development approaches strengthen public participation and lead to the empowerment of communities, and increased capacity to improve mental health at the community level.

4. Developing personal skills involves enabling personal and social development through providing information, education and enhancing life skills. Improving people's knowledge and understanding of positive mental health as an integral part of overall health forms an important part of this action area highlighting the need for improved mental health literacy. Developing personal skills such as self-awareness, improved self-esteem, sense of control and self-efficacy, relationship and communication skills, problem-solving and coping skills have all been shown to improve mental health and to facilitate people to exercise more control over their life and their environments.

5. Reorienting health services requires that mental health services embrace promotion and prevention activities as well as treatment and rehabilitation services. This calls for a health care system which contributes to the pursuit of health as well as the treatment of illness. In terms of mental health, this emphasises the important role of, for example, primary care and mental health services in promoting mental health across different population groups such as children, young mothers, people with chronic health problems and mental health service users and their families. Reorienting health services to promote mental health requires greater attention to the organisation and structure of health services and the training and education of health professionals.

The Ottawa Charter underscores the importance of synergistic action across these different levels highlighting the need for top-down policy approaches and bottom-up community action working together to achieve common goals. The five strategies from the Ottawa Charter have been shown to be effective tools in addressing a range of health issues (Mittelmark et al 2005). Reviews of health promotion interventions indicate that the most effective interventions employ multiple health promotion strategies (Box 1.3) and operate at multiple levels – structural, community/social group and individual – and include a combination of integrated actions to support each strategy (Hoffman & Jackson 2003, IUHPE 1999). Friedli (2001) argues that a strategic approach to mental health promotion should include a balance of developing individual coping skills, promoting social support and networks and addressing structural barriers to mental health in areas such as education, employment and housing.

Most reviews stress that health promotion interventions are only effective when they are made relevant to the context in which they are to be used. This includes awareness of the social, cultural, economic and political contexts and realities of particular population groups, settings and communities.

The Bangkok Charter for health promotion, which builds upon the values, principles and action strategies of health promotion established by the Ottawa Charter, calls for an integrated policy approach across sectors and settings, strong political action, broad participation and sustained advocacy in order to progress towards a healthier society (WHO 2005a:3). The Bangkok Charter highlights four key commitments, to make the promotion of health:

1. central to global development
2. a core responsibility for all of government
3. a key focus of communities and civil society
4. a requirement for good corporate practice.

Box 1.3

Key health promotion strategies identified in several reviews as being central to the effectiveness of interventions

(based on Jackson et al 2005)

- community participation and engagement in planning and decision making
- intersectoral collaboration and interorganisational partnerships at all levels, involving multiple sectors such as governmental and non-governmental organisations, groups and local stakeholders
- creating healthy settings, particularly focusing on the settings of schools, workplaces, cities and communities
- political commitment, funding and infrastructure for social policies

Such policies and commitments are also key to the promotion of global mental health.

The health promotion framework has been applied to the promotion of mental health by a number of writers (Barry 2001, Friedli 2001, HEA 1997, Joubert 2001, MacDonald & O'Hara 1998, Raeburn 2001, Secker 1998, Tudor 1996, Weare 2000) and more recently in the WHO publications on promoting mental health (Herrman et al 2005, WHO 2004a). The health promotion framework endorses the broad determinants of health and mental health. The UK Health Education Authority in their mental health promotion quality framework (HEA 1997) positions mental health promotion as an integral part of health promotion and advocates the same basic principles of practice. An example of a comprehensive strategy for mental health promotion is that developed by the Victorian Health Promotion Foundation in Australia (VicHealth 1999). A health promotion framework is used to guide its action on mental health promotion. Central to the framework is the focus on:

- three key determinants of mental health – social inclusion, freedom from discrimination and violence, economic participation
- the identification of priority population groups such as children, older people and indigenous communities
- areas and settings for action – community, workplace, etc.
- a description of anticipated benefits such as improved self-determination and control, reduced health inequalities and improved quality of life.

The VicHealth framework highlights the relationships between socioeconomic factors and mental health, and endorses the view that success in promoting mental health can only be achieved and sustained by the involvement and support of the whole community, and the development of partnerships between a range of agencies in the public, private and non-governmental sectors.

Clearly the different prevention and promotion frameworks inform different models of practice and are underpinned by different theoretical perspectives. The conceptual approaches to prevention and promotion will now be considered. In particular, the two interrelated approaches of the risk reduction model and the competence enhancement model will be outlined.

Current Conceptual Models

The Risk Reduction Model

Recent advances in the understanding of risk and protective factors for mental health problems form the basis of the risk reduction model. Indeed, the report by Mrazek and Haggerty (1994) endorsed the risk reduction model as the best theoretical model to guide preventive interventions at this time. This model is concerned with the reduction of risk factors for general as well as specific mental disorders and the enhancement of protective factors. Current research indicates the presence of generic risk and protective factors that are common to many disorders and dysfunctional states. Mrazek and Haggerty suggest that, rather than attempting to identify risk factors unique to specific mental disorders, 'there may be greater value in clarifying the role of those risk factors that appear to be common to many mental disorders, especially in view of the frequent comorbidity of these disorders (1994:182). Applied to prevention interventions, this model aims at reducing 'modifiable' risk factors and strengthening protective factors. The risk reduction model draws on the findings from aetiological and treatment research and adapts intervention techniques, for example, cognitive–behavioural or social learning approaches, to the area of prevention.

The report by Mrazek and Haggerty (1994), which reviewed 39 prevention programmes tested by randomised trials, concluded that there is strong evidence that preventive interventions can lead to a reduction of risk factors and enhancement of protective factors associated with the first onset of substance abuse and mental health problems. However, the report found that there was minimal evidence that mental disorders have been prevented through such risk reduction. Mrazek and Haggerty recommended that the most fruitful approach for preventive interventions may be to use a risk reduction model that includes the enhancement of protective factors and to aim at clusters or constellations of risks or protective factors. The goal of preventive interventions, therefore, becomes the reduction of risk rather than the prevention of disorders per se. An example of a successful prevention programme applying this approach is the JOBS intervention project (Caplan et al 1989, Price & Vinokur 1995, Vinokur & Schul 1997), which targets job loss as one of most consistent antecedents of depression and designs a preventive intervention targeting unemployed workers (see Ch. 6 for further details of this programme). The conceptual framework guiding the programme focuses largely on increasing protective factors through increasing sense of mastery and the enhancement of personal control and job search self-efficacy. The programme has produced impressive results including significantly better employment outcomes in terms of better quality and higher paying jobs, and also improved mental health through enhanced role and emotional functioning and reduced depressive symptoms. Commenting on the findings from the JOBS programme, Price (1998) points to the interweaving effects of the promotive and preventive aspects of the intervention which had preventive effects for those at high risk of depression and promotive effects for those at lower risk. The JOBS programme is, therefore, a good example of an intervention that operates on both risk and protective factors simultaneously. Clearly, from the outset this programme had a strong emphasis on protective factors, as self-efficacy and sense of control were identified as integral components of the intervention.

The Competence Enhancement Model

While the risk reduction model begins with a focus on reducing risks for mental disorders, the competence enhancement model focuses on enhancing competence and positive mental health. The competence approach signals a shift from an individual-centred, disorder-focused approach to one embracing an emphasis on psychological strengths and resilience. The goal, therefore, becomes enhancing potential rather than focusing on reducing disorders. This perspective is in keeping with the basic thrust of health promotion which clearly articulates that 'health promotion involves the population as a whole in the context of their everyday life, rather than focusing on people at risk for specific diseases' (WHO 1985:6). Mental health is, therefore, reconceptualised in positive rather than in negative terms. Mental health promotion programmes adopting a competence perspective are primarily concerned with building strengths and competencies and feelings of efficacy in diverse life areas (Weissberg et al 1991). An enhancement model assumes that, as an individual becomes more capable and competent, their psychological well-being improves. This approach builds on the theoretical base of areas such as lifespan developmental theory and the ecological perspective of community psychology.

Cowen (1991) argues for a comprehensive lifespan approach to the promotion of wellness, one that takes into account age, situation, group, and society-related determinants of, and impediments to, wellness. Based on current knowledge and theory, four key concepts are proposed to guide the pathway towards the promotion of psychological wellness:

1. competence – life skills and competencies such as social, academic and work competencies, that are critical for psychological well-being
2. resilience – the ability to survive and cope effectively with major life stressors
3. social system modification – changing social environments and systems so that they promote people's wellness
4. empowerment – enhancing people's perceived and actual control over their life.

These constructs are put forward by Cowen as providing the knowledge base to guide the formulation of programmes, policies and practices designed to promote psychological wellness. In developing this wellness perspective, an ecological perspective is employed that stresses the interdependence of the individual, the family, community and society. It, therefore, views mental health as both a community and individual resource. From this community psychology theoretical perspective, which draws on Lewin's (1951) person-in-context principle, mental health is conceptualised as the interaction over time, between persons and social settings and systems, including the structure of social support and social power (Orford 1992). This perspective clearly moves the concept of mental health beyond an individualistic focus to consider the influence of broader social, economic and political forces.

A key concept underpinning this ecological perspective is that of interdependence, i.e. the fact that behaviour is influenced by multiple interacting systems. Bronfenbrenner's (1979) model of nested systems provides a useful set of constructs to understand the nature of these different levels. Bronfenbrenner postulates a set of nested structures ranging from the micro, meso, exo and macro levels to indicate the ways in which systems operating at individual, family, community and broader societal levels interact with and mutually influence each other. This model points to the importance of the larger sociocultural and policy context within which individuals, group systems and social settings are embedded. The model underscores the important role of mediating structures such as schools, workplaces and communities as providing key contexts for social interventions operating from the micro to the macro levels.

As a multi-level construct, empowerment plays a key role in this framework as it is capable of operating at many different levels from the micro to the macro but particularly at the level of organisations and community. Empowerment may be defined as 'a social action process through which individuals, communities and organisations gain mastery over their lives in the context of changing their social and political environment to improve equity and quality of life' (Rappaport 1984, 1985, Wallerstein 1992). Embracing an empowerment philosophy of mental health requires that attention be focused away from an exclusive concern with individual factors to consider the interface between the individual and wider community and social forces. This points to a need to address poverty, economic and social disadvantage, social injustice and discrimination as key determinants of mental health. This approach, therefore, underscores the importance of social interventions addressing systems of socialisation, social support and control and operating at multiple levels of analysis.

Programmes focusing explicitly on competence enhancement appear to concentrate primarily on children and adolescents. A number of reviews of successful interventions (Durlak & Wells 1997, Hosman & Jané-Llopis 1999, Jané-Llopis et al 2005, Price et al 1988, Weissberg et al 1991) point to strong evidence that high-quality comprehensive programmes that focus on young people and their socialising environments produce long-lasting positive effects on mental, social and behavioural development. Durlak and Wells (1997) carried out a meta-analysis review of 177 evaluation studies of primary prevention and mental health promotion programmes for children and adolescents. The findings from this review indicate that most programmes examined achieve significant positive effects, reporting mean effect sizes of between 0.24 and 0.93. In practical terms, they report that the average participant in the intervention programmes surpassed the performance of between 59–82% of those in control groups. The positive programme effects were found to be long lasting and to impact on functioning across multiple domains. As the authors point out, these findings compare extremely well with findings from many established medical, educational and behavioural interventions.

Weissberg et al's (1991) review on programmes for young people points to the following critical ingredients of the most effective programmes: 1) a focus on enhancing children's capacities, personal and social skills, attitudes and values, and 2) creating environmental settings and resources to support the development of young people's personal social and health behaviour. For children under the age of 5 years, high-quality family support and early childhood programmes have produced long-term benefits. The most widely quoted programme, the High/Scope Perry Preschool Program (Schweinhart & Weikart 1998) is a preschool educational programme which has produced multiple long-lasting positive effects across intellectual, social and mental health domains (see Ch. 5 for further details). Such findings indicate that, in addition to positive outcomes on academic achievement, these programmes have the potential to influence rates of delinquency, unwanted pregnancy, welfare and employment.

Adopting a Competence Enhancement Approach

Based on the models and frameworks reviewed in this paper, there is a compelling case for focusing on interventions that promote psychological strengths and competence. Programmes promoting positive mental health have a universal target group, they have been found to result in impressive long-lasting positive effects on multiple areas of functioning and also have the dual effect of reducing risk. Such programmes would, therefore, appear to hold the greatest promise as cost-effective interventions. The strength of evidence from systematic reviews and effectiveness studies would also support this orientation.

Mrazek and Haggerty (1994) clearly conclude from their review that there is currently little evidence that any specific mental disorder can be prevented. Tilford et al (1997), in their HEA review of mental health promotion programmes, also conclude that there is no strong evidence for the superiority of programmes directed at the prevention of specific disorders over broad skills-based interventions. The complex multifactorial aetiology of many mental health problems and disorders means that it is extremely difficult to identify risk and protective factors for specific mental health problems. Likewise, there are methodological difficulties in demonstrating that a negative outcome has not occurred, i.e. proving that interventions do actually prevent the onset of specific mental disorders (Durlak & Wells 1997, Mrazek & Haggerty 1994). Given the low base rate of diagnosed mental health problems and the episodic nature of some conditions, evaluation studies would require extremely large sample sizes and extensive follow-up periods in order to judge the effects of prevention and promotion programmes. With funding and other limitations, few current programmes meet these requirements as the majority of studies do not follow up beyond 12 months post intervention.

However, there is consensus that there are clusters of known risk factors and protective factors and there is considerable evidence that interventions can reduce identified risk factors and enhance known protective factors. Hosman and Jané-Llopis (1999) find ample evidence that mental health promotion programmes not only improve mental health and quality of life but also reduce the risk for mental disorder. For these conceptual and methodological reasons it is proposed that it may be more productive for programmes to focus on enhancing protective factors with the explicit goal of developing competence to promote well-being rather than preventing symptoms or the onset of disorders.

Moving from disorder prevention to a competence enhancement approach requires that current frameworks accommodate this shift in emphasis to locate the promotion of positive mental health within the broader spectrum of intervention activities. Mental health promotion reconceptualises mental health in positive rather than in negative terms and is concerned with the delivery of effective programmes designed to reduce health inequalities in an empowering, collaborative and participatory manner. While prevention programmes are primarily concerned with the reduction of the incidence and prevalence of mental disorders, mental health promotion also focuses on the process of enabling and achieving positive mental health and enhancing quality of life for individuals, communities and society in general. Mental health promotion endorses a competence enhancement perspective and seeks to address the broader determinants of mental health. In keeping with the fundamental principles of health promotion as articulated in the Ottawa Charter (WHO 1986) this calls for 'upstream' policy interventions across the non-health sectors in order to reduce structural barriers to mental health. This perspective underscores the importance of developing supportive environments for good mental health, e.g. in schools, workplaces and communities, reorienting existing services and advocating the development of

Box 1.4

Examples of positive mental health indicators

- improved mental well-being
- improved self-efficacy
- improved mental health literacy
- improved coping skills
- improved parenting skills and family functioning
- enhanced social support
- increased community participation and connectedness
- improved quality of life

healthy public policy designed to promote and protect positive mental health at a population level.

This shift in focus from negative to positive indicators of well-being (Box 1.4) calls for methodological refinement in establishing sound measures of protective factors and positive indicators of mental health outcomes. Zubrick and Kovess-Masfety (2005) provide a useful discussion of this issue and outline a socioecological framework for developing indicators of positive mental health that will contribute to improved monitoring and measurement of positive outcomes.

A focus on positive mental health also calls for more attention to the process and principles of programme delivery. Evaluation methods are needed that will focus on documenting the process as well as the outcomes, of enabling positive mental health and identify the intervening or mediating variables which act as key predictors of change (Barry 2002). This leads to a focus on evaluation methods aimed at capturing the dynamics of programmes in action and identifying the critical ingredients for successful programme development, planning and implementation. This requires that the core components of intervention strategies are clearly identified in order that they may inform the specification of proximal as well as distal programme objectives. The identification of such core intervention components calls for clear articulation of the underlying theories and constructs informing programme development. As Durlak and Wells (1997) point out, we need to challenge the idea of there being uniform primary prevention or mental health promotion programmes, as clearly programmes may draw from a range of different underlying theories, constructs and perspectives. Focusing on the level of developing distinct conceptual approaches and strategies for promoting positive mental health presents an opportunity for integration and establishing links across the spectrum of mental health interventions.

The Effectiveness of Mental Health Promotion

There have been important advances in establishing a sound evidence base for mental health promotion in recent years. There is consensus that there are clusters of known risk and protective factors for mental health (Mrazek & Haggerty 1994); there is a growing body of evidence that interventions exist which can modify these factors, and a number of model programmes evaluated in efficacy and effectiveness trials have been established and disseminated (Hosman & Jané-Llopis 2005, Jané-Llopis et al 2005). The IUHPE report for the European Commission (1999) clearly endorses that mental health promotion programmes work and that there are a number of evidence-based programmes to inform mental health promotion practice. The accumulating evidence base demonstrates the feasibility of implementing effective mental health promotion programmes across a range of diverse population groups and settings (Jané-Llopis & Barry 2005).

Programmes promoting positive mental health have been found to result in impressive long-lasting positive effects on multiple areas of functioning and have also been found to have the dual effect of reducing risks of mental disorders (Hosman & Jané-Llopis 1999). The strength of evidence from systematic reviews and effectiveness studies support the value of such programmes as cost-effective initiatives capable of impacting positively across multiple domains of functioning (Durlak & Wells 1997, Hosman & Jané-Llopis 1999, Jané-Llopis et al 2005, **mentality** 2003, Tilford et al 1997). Tilford et al (1997), based on their systematic review, concluded that 'Effective interventions have been identified which promote the mental health of the population at large and those known to be at risk of mental health problems'. In the IUHPE 1999 report, Hosman and Jané-Llopis (1999) attest to the impact of mental health promotion programmes on the reduction of a range of social problems such as delinquency, child abuse, school drop-out, lost days from work and social inequity. The available evidence supports the view that competence-enhancing programmes carried out in collaboration with families, schools and wider communities have the potential to impact on multiple positive outcomes across social and personal health domains (Jané-Llopis & Barry 2005). As discussed earlier, most interventions have been found to have the dual effect of reducing problems and increasing competencies.

An overview of effective mental health promotion programmes across different settings and stages of the lifespan is presented by Jané-Llopis et al (2005) and in other recent reviews (WHO 2004a, b). Jané-Llopis et al (2005) draw on different sources of evidence ranging from randomised controlled trials (RCTs) to case studies, and using the Ottawa Charter framework review the evidence across key settings (homes, schools, workplace, community and health services) in terms of effectiveness in health, social and economic impacts. This review, while acknowledging gaps in the evidence base, concludes that there is sufficient knowledge to move evidence into practice and provides recommendations for action in terms of addressing poverty, gender and mental health in a global society (Patel 2005), improving the quality of programme implementation (Barry et al 2005), integrating mental health into the health promotion and public health agenda (Herrman & Jané-Llopis 2005) and getting mental health promotion onto the government agenda (Moodie & Jenkins 2005). Marshall-Williams et al (2005), in the same volume, call for greater investment in mental health policies that are evidence based. They point to the fact that currently available programmes need to be brought to scale, disseminated, adopted and implemented across countries

Box 1.5

Characteristics of successful programmes

- a focused and targeted approach to programme planning, implementation and evaluation
- programme development based on underpinning theory, research principles of efficacy and needs assessment
- adopt a competence enhancement approach and an implementation process that are empowering, collaborative and participatory, carried out in partnerships with key stakeholders
- address a range of protective and risk factors
- employ a combination of intervention methods operating at different levels
- comprehensive approaches that intervene at a number of different time periods rather than once off
- include the provision of training and support mechanisms that will ensure high quality implementation and sustainability

and different cultural, social and economic contexts. While good progress is being made in building the evidence base for mental health promotion, a number of gaps in the evidence base may also be identified.

The Need for Evidence of the Effectiveness of 'Upstream' Policy Interventions

There is a need to generate evidence of the effectiveness of interventions operating at different levels, from the individual, community to macro level policies, in promoting positive mental health. However, much of the existing evidence has focused on individual-level interventions and, as highlighted by Petticrew et al (2005), there is a paucity of evidence on the effectiveness of upstream policy interventions such as improved housing, welfare, education and employment in improving mental health. There are many plausible policy interventions, which may be expected to directly or indirectly affect mental health, for which evidence appears to be absent. However, Petticrew et al (2005) caution that the 'absence of evidence' should not be mistaken for 'evidence of absence' and that plausible interventions such as improved housing can be reasonably expected to generate mental health gains. For example, a systematic review by Thomson et al (2001) found evidence of a consistent pattern of improvements in mental health linked to improved housing. Petticrew et al (2005) point to the fact that there is a clear potential for positive mental health to be promoted through non-health policies such as the building of new roads, new houses, area-based regeneration and the assessment of the 'spillover' effects of such policies will make an important contribution to the mental health evidence base. This requires the development of mental health impact assessment methods, which will monitor the mental health impacts, both positive and negative, of public policies. Petticrew et al (2005) point to the fact that we are still fishing for much of our evidence 'downstream' rather than 'upstream' where mental health is created. The need to generate better evidence of the benefits, harms and costs of 'upstream' interventions, such as non-health sector policies and programmes, remains a critical area for development.

Economic Evaluation

Economic data on the cost-effectiveness of mental health promotion interventions have an important contribution to make to the evidence for the promotion of mental health. Such data can usefully inform resource allocation decisions and lead to a better understanding of the long-term economic benefits of interventions for individuals and society and the related costs of inaction. These include economic benefits in terms of reduced hospital and treatment costs but also reduced indirect costs such as work disability and family burden. Examples of mental health promotion programmes which have demonstrated cost benefits include:

- the Prenatal and Infancy Home Visitation Programme (Olds 2002, Olds et al 1998), which reported that by the time children who participated in this early years intervention programme were 15 years old, the cost savings were four times the original programme investment in terms of reduced crime, welfare and health care costs and taxes paid by increased employment levels of the children's parents (Karoly et al 1998). Even the most expensive home-based programmes have been found to pay for themselves by the time the children are 4 years old (Olds 2002)
- the High/Scope Perry Preschool Program (Schweinhart & Weikart 1988, 1998) for 3–4 year-old children from disadvantaged backgrounds, which cost $1000 per child, but the cost-benefit produced was estimated to be over $7000–8000 per child (Barnett 1993) due to decreased schooling costs, reduced welfare, crime and justice system costs and increased taxes paid on higher earnings
- the JOBS programme for unemployed people (Price et al 1992, Vinokur et al 1991), which brought a three-fold return on investment after 2.5 years, and more than a 10-fold return after 5 years, due to increased employment and higher earning outcomes and reduced health service and welfare costs
- the Swedish educational programme to prevent depression and suicide introduced on the island of Gotland (Rutz et al 1992), which resulted in a significantly reduced suicide rate and produced considerable economic savings estimated as being a cost–benefit ratio of 1:30 in direct costs of care, but 1:350 in terms of productivity gains and mortality reductions.

Economic evaluation has yet to be applied to mental health promotion, and there exists very limited data on the cost-effectiveness of alternative mental health promotion strategies. There remain a number of methodological challenges in developing this further (Petticrew et al 2005) and a programme of evidence generation is currently underway at WHO (www.who.int/choice/en/). Of course, it is acknowledged that many of the related costs or benefits to society cannot be estimated in economic terms alone. However, the generation of reliable data on the short-term and long-term costs and benefits of interventions would usefully inform decision making on the best use of scarce resources and whether or not to implement interventions and which approaches to use. Mental health promotion interventions that can be implemented and sustained at a reasonable cost, whilst generating clear health and social gains in the population, represent a cost-effective use of resources and a strong case for policy investment (WHO 2002).

Evidence from Low-Income Countries

There is a particularly urgent need to expand the evidence base to be more relevant to the realities of those working and living in low-income countries. McQueen (2001) points to the fact that much of the relevant material that could broaden the discussion on evidence and its application in low-income countries is unpublished. Non-English language, unpublished programmes conducted outside of the European–American axis are under-represented in the current knowledge base. Voices from developing countries are absent as indeed are the voices of practitioners and programme users/recipients. This view is echoed in the WHO report which highlights that evidence is 'least available from areas that have the maximum need, i.e. developing countries and areas affected by conflicts' (2002:27). In many countries, implementing programmes usually entails working with minimal resources, little of which can be allocated to large research programmes. In the absence of dedicated funds from donors and governments to conduct research in middle- and low-income countries, the challenge is how to uncover and document innovative forms of practice. Traditional documentation may be lacking, yet nonetheless intervention programmes may be known through word of mouth and other traditional ways of spreading the word about good practice in the field. There has been much energy and resources devoted to establishing efficacy and effectiveness trials in high-income countries, and it is now timely to invest in dissemination research to examine how the existing evidence can be used effectively across diverse cultural settings. In particular, there is an urgent need to identify effective programmes that are transferable and sustainable in low-income country settings, particularly low-cost, replicable programmes based on empowerment principles that can be sustained in disadvantaged community settings (Barry & McQueen 2005).

Mental health promotion needs to be incorporated into the wider health development agenda in order that the broader determinants of poor mental health such as poverty, social exclusion, exploitation and discrimination can be successfully addressed. The innovative 'Voices of the poor' study, carried out under the auspices of the Poverty Reduction Group of the World Bank (Narayan & Petesch 2002), underscored the need to invest in poor people's assets and capabilities and to work in partnership with people living in poverty in order to develop strategies and solutions that can be locally owned and adapted. Patel (2005) points to the clear association between indicators of poverty and mental health and advocates that programmes aimed at empowering women and the poor, and policies which ensure gender equality and equity in economic development, are likely to play the greatest role in promoting mental health. Patel et al (2005), reviewing the impact of social and economic development policies and programmes on mental health, focus on the importance of programmes in three main areas: advocacy, empowerment and social support. Examples of such programmes include the impact of equitable economic development, micro-credit schemes, literacy promotion, promotion of gender equality, violence and crime reduction programmes in advancing mental health gains. The development of community banks in developing countries such as that implemented by the Bangladesh Rural Advancement Committee, has been shown to lead to improved health in terms of better nutrition, improved child survival, higher educational achievement, lower rates of domestic violence and improved well-being and psychological health (Chowdhury & Bhuiya 2001). The implementation of school-based programmes for young people would also appear to be a key area for development in low-income countries. Community development approaches, which include health sector reform, the participation of local community leaders and empowerment of the marginalised, are being implemented by non-governmental organisations in low-income countries as a way of promoting health among the poor (Patel 2005) and have been identified as a key strategy for mental health promotion (Arole et al 2005). These development programmes, some of the best examples of which come from low-income countries, provide a useful model within which to incorporate the promotion of mental health.

Adopting an Evidence-Based Approach to Mental Health Promotion Practice

An important challenge is strengthening the evidence base in order to inform best practice and policy globally. While researchers are more likely to be concerned with the quality of the evidence, its methodological rigour and contribution to the knowledge base, the different stakeholders in the area may bring different perspectives to bear on the types of evidence needed. As described by Nutbeam (1999a) each of the stakeholders will view the evidence from different perspectives:

- policymakers are likely to be concerned with the need to justify the allocation of resources and demonstrate added value
- practitioners need to be able to have confidence in the likely success of implementing interventions
- the potential users or populations who are to benefit need to see that both the programme and the process of implementation are participatory and relevant to their needs.

While acknowledging that there remain important gaps in the evidence base, a major task is to promote the application of existing evidence into good practice, particularly in disadvantaged and low-income countries and settings. The challenge is, therefore, two-fold: translating research evidence into effective practice on the ground, and translating effective practice into research so that currently undocumented evidence may make its way into the published literature and serve to build on and expand the existing evidence base. This calls for critical consideration of how best to assemble and apply evidence which is congruent with the principles of mental health promotion practice and which is inclusive of the realities of programme implementation across diverse cultural and economic settings (Barry & McQueen 2005).

A useful guide on translating mental health promotion evidence into practice, produced by the Scottish Development Centre for Mental Health (2004), defines evidence-based practice as a structured and systematic approach to using research-based knowledge of effectiveness to inform practice. The evidence-based practice of health promotion is a relatively recent phenomenon, therefore strengthening the evidence base in order to inform best practice and policy is an important challenge. However, there is considerable debate as to how this is best approached. Barry (2002) outlines some of the key issues, challenges and opportunities in strengthening the mental health promotion evidence base.

There has been much debate concerning the practical and ideological challenges of adopting an evidence-based approach in the field of health promotion. This has included discussion of what constitutes legitimate 'evidence' in health promotion evaluation and how best to respond to the challenge of assembling evidence in ways which are relevant to the complexities of contemporary health promotion (McQueen 2001, Nutbeam 1999b, Tones 1997). As health promotion is an interdisciplinary area of practice, the challenge has been identified as using evaluation methods and approaches which are congruent with the principles of health promotion practice (Labonté & Robertson 1996), which cross methodological boundaries and seek to evaluate initiatives in terms of their process as well as their outcomes (WHO EURO 1998). McQueen and Anderson (2001) discuss the complexity of the evidence debate in health promotion and call for the establishment of rules of evidence that take into account the diversity, multidisciplinary and contextualised nature of health promotion practice. Different methodological approaches are required to encompass the different elements of process, impact and outcome evaluation. While outcome-focused studies may lend themselves to more quantitative approaches, process-focused research requires more qualitative and naturalistic methods. Standards of rigour and quality can equally be applied to evidence derived from different methodological perspectives. The quality of the different types of evidence should be judged on criteria derived from their respective paradigms and ultimately on their appropriateness to the research questions being addressed.

In keeping with these developments, there has been a call for an expansion of the current range of evaluation methodologies and analytical frameworks applied in mental health promotion and a widening of the evidence base to be more inclusive of the realities of practical applications from a more global perspective (Barry 2002). A continuum of approaches is required ranging from RCTs to more qualitative process-oriented methods. Action research and participatory research methods are also highlighted as having important roles to play in developing more collaborative forms of research inquiry. The adoption of a more pluralistic range of evaluation methods signals a more inclusive approach to setting standards of evidence and evaluation research in mental health promotion. As mental health promotion draws on a diverse range of disciplines, different theoretical and methodological perspectives may be brought to bear in establishing a sound evidence base. As McQueen (2001) suggests, we need to identify the rules of different disciplines and where they fit into the process of building the evidence base in order to capitalise on the multidisciplinary nature of the field. This broad approach is the one endorsed and taken up by the IUHPE (1999) Global Programme on Health Promotion Effectiveness (GPHPE). This initiative aims to raise the standards of health-promoting policy making and practice worldwide by:

* reviewing and building evidence of effectiveness in terms of health, social, economic and political impact
* translating evidence to policy makers, teachers, practitioners, researchers
* stimulating debate on the nature of evidence of effectiveness.

Evaluation approaches are required that permit a better understanding of the actualities of programme activities and lead to a better informed assessment of programme processes and outcomes. The generation of practice-based evidence and theory is an important challenge in this area and will require researchers and practitioners to work in partnership in documenting and analysing the implementation of mental health promotion programmes. Through the development of more collaborative and participatory evaluation methods, there will be an opportunity to include the knowledge base of programme implementers and participants into the evaluation process, thereby incorporating the 'wisdom literature' into the evidence base. There is a need for analytic frameworks that integrate process and outcome data in a meaningful way so that clear statements can be made about how and why programme changes have come about. Contrasting and complementary perspectives and methods are needed to fill out the larger picture and to tap previously undocumented areas of knowledge and practice (Barry & McQueen 2005).

Translating Evidence into Practice

The key challenge in establishing the mental health promotion evidence base is how this evidence can be used to create change and bring about improved mental health for individuals, families and communities in most need. The evidence base should serve the needs of practitioners and policy makers concerned with the practicality of implementing successful programmes that are relevant to the needs of the populations they serve. This calls for the active dissemination of validated programmes and guidelines on best practices based on efficacy, effectiveness and dissemination studies. There is a need for investment in capacity building, the provision of technical support, designing dissemination strategies, publishing guidelines for effective implementation of low-cost sustainable programmes and providing training in programme planning and evaluation. The ultimate test is how the evidence base can be effectively used to inform practice and policy that will reduce inequalities and bring about improved mental health, especially where it is needed most.

While good progress is being made in building the research base of mental health promotion, there is a need to extend the focus to the quality of the intervention programmes and their wider practice and policy implications. As advocated by Mittelmark (2003), it is time to draw clear messages from the existing evidence base and establish guidelines based on best available evidence in order to inform best practice and policy on the ground. It is important that we seek to apply what we do know in order to inform decision making and bring about lasting change in the broader policy context. While continuing to build on systematic reviews of specific topic areas, it is important to identify cross cutting themes and generic processes that underpin the successful implementation of mental health promotion programmes (Speller et al 1997). There is a need for practice and policy guidelines based on the existing evidence to inform practitioners and decision makers concerning effective programme planning, delivery and evaluation and the critical factors that are needed to ensure the implementation of successful programmes. This information is beginning to emerge and there are some useful practitioner-oriented publications, e.g. Price et al (1988), the 'Blueprints' series by Elliott (1997), 'Making it happen' (DoH 2001), and 'Making it effective' (Mentality 2003), all concerned with providing practical guidance on programme implementation, strategy development and using the evidence base.

The development of user-friendly information systems and databases is required in order to make the evidence base accessible to practitioners and policy makers. A number of international and national organisations have developed databases on evidence-based promotion and prevention programmes. Examples include:

- the Cochrane Health Promotion Public Health and Field (www.cochrane.org and www.vichealth.vic.gov.au/cochrane)
- the Evidence for Policy and Practice Information Centre (EPPI-Centre) (http://eppi.ioe.ac.uk)
- the Centers for Disease Control and Prevention Guide to Community Preventive Services (www.thecommunityguide.org)
- the NHS Centre for Reviews and Dissemination (www.york.ac.uk/inst/crd/wph.htm)
- the US National Registry of Effective Prevention Programs, Substance Abuse and Mental Health Services Administration (SAMHSA) (www.samhsa.gov)
- the Social and Emotional Learning Library (The Collaborative for Academic, Social and Emotional Learning (CASEL) (www.casel.org/index)
- the Implementing Mental Health Promotion Action (IMHPA) database in Europe (www.imhpa.net).

However, databases are more of a passive than an active form of dissemination and there have been a number of initiatives to explore more active ways of disseminating and translating the evidence base into practice.

Publications specifically targeting policy makers and practitioners, such as the IUHPE 1999 report for the European Commission and research summaries produced by organisations such as VicHealth Mental Health and Well-being Unit (www.vichealth.vic.gov.au/MHWU), briefing papers by the UK-based Sainsbury Centre for Mental Health (www.scmh.org.uk) and Mentality (www.mentality.org.uk), have an important part to play in influencing national policy and encouraging good practice. Targeted evidence briefings, which consist of summaries and syntheses of existing systematic reviews on a range of topics, have been produced on mental health by the former Health Development Agency in

England (now incorporated into the National Institute for Health and Clinical Excellence) and on mental health promotion by Mentality and the Sainsbury Centre for Mental Health in England: Briefing 24 Mental Health Promotion. These documents are designed as a resource that can be used by a variety of audiences. However, as noted by Kelly et al (2004), for the evidence to be applicable in the field, a further step is required to make the evidence accessible, contextualised, usable and implemented by practitioners.

There is a need for dissemination research which will examine the documentation, replication and adaptation of effective programmes across diverse settings and countries. More active strategies are required for disseminating the evidence base and providing technical assistance and capacity-building resources for mental health promotion, especially in middle- and low-income countries. As Backer (2000) points out, dissemination entails not only distributing information about successful programmes and practices, but also the provision of technical assistance and capacity-building resources to enable practitioners to actually implement the programmes and engage successfully with the complex processes involved. This involves not only funding a particular programme but also identifying the overall ability and resources of the organisation or group needed to implement and sustain the programme in complex and challenging local contexts. Capacity building also entails increasing the organisation's ability to share new programmes and practices with others, including documenting innovative practice at the local level. Learning will then be a two way process in terms of innovation, adaptation and dissemination of promising programmes and creative practice.

Building the Infrastructure for Mental Health Promotion

The generation and provision of evidence of course is not enough in itself and there is a need for the development of the necessary infrastructures to support implementation and cross-sectoral collaboration. It is now accepted that many of the main determinants of mental health and mental health inequalities lie outside the health sector and that intersectoral collaboration is needed to effectively address them. There is a need for both the political will on the part of policy makers and skilful practice by practitioners to ensure that the evidence translates into policy and practice which will produce affirmative action on the ground. This requires a focus on both the policy and practice of creating positive mental health.

The Policy Context

The promotion and maintenance of mental health at a population level calls for a comprehensive approach, including effective policies and strategies at international, national, regional and community levels. A supportive and favourable policy context is critical to ensure that initiatives to promote mental health are sustained (Scanlon 2002). This includes dedicated resource allocation, investment in the necessary infrastructure such as research, training, policy and practice development and providing strategic leadership in driving forward the mental health promotion agenda. Factors such as poverty, housing, employment, education, safe neighbourhoods, cohesive and socially just societies are all recognised as influencing people's mental health potential. Creating a mentally healthy society entails addressing these broader socioenvironmental and political influences and working across diverse sectors in order to address the upstream determinants of mental health (Barry 2005). The political context of this work needs to be recognised as the development and implementation of policy, practice and research are mediated through political processes. This is evident in terms of the prioritisation of areas for action and the provision of dedicated funding and resources. There needs to be political will and commitment to ensure that the necessary resources are put in place to enable effective policies and plans to be put into action.

Saxena and Saraceno (2004) identify a clear need for advocacy as mental health is often an implicit rather than explicit part of health policy and remains hidden and not of high priority. In 2002 the World Health Assembly (WHA) adopted a resolution urging the WHO, as the lead international agency with responsibility for health, to facilitate the effective development of policies and programmes to strengthen and protect mental heath (WHA 2002). The resolution called for 'coalition building with civil society and key actions in order to enhance global awareness-raising and advocacy campaigns on mental health' (WHO 2002). Political commitment needs to be mobilised so that mental health is given greater priority in terms of policy development, including policies which promote mentally healthy living, working and social environments. Among the key agents are politicians, policy makers, educators, opinion leaders and members of civil society. There is a need to raise awareness of the determinants of mental health at public and policy making levels. Public participation is critical to this process, as policy development needs to be based on greater public awareness of, and engagement with, the importance of good mental health to overall health and social well-being. In other words, the visibility and value of mental health need to be enhanced (Jenkins et al 2001).

In addition, the public health potential of mental health promotion needs to be recognised in order to promote greater awareness of what mental health promotion can contribute to wider health and social gain (Bywaters 2005, Friedli 2001). As demonstrated by the systematic reviews in the area, effective mental health promotion strategies have the potential to contribute to a range of improved health and social outcomes in terms of educational achievement, employment, reduced crime and delinquency, improved sexual health, better family and social relationships and reduced inequalities. As Moodie and Jenkins (2005) point out, there is a persuasive case for governments to invest in mental health promotion as an effective strategy for creating health and social gain. The mental health declaration for Europe (WHO 2005b) advocates making mental health an inseparable part of public health and thus recognises the need for action across a range of areas and consideration of the impact of all policies on mental health.

Jenkins et al (2001) discuss the importance of mental health promotion and mental health monitoring in overall policy and point to the importance of national components, support infrastructure and service components. Among the national components of mental health policy that need to be considered are:

- legislation
- the national strategy to promote mental health
- policy links with other government departments (housing, employment, education, etc.)
- mechanisms for implementation and accountability
- the funding streams.

Support infrastructure includes the mental health information strategy, the research and development strategy and the human resource strategy. The service components include mental health promotion in schools, workplace, primary, secondary and tertiary prevention, good practice guidelines and health service links with justice, employment services, schools, non-governmental organisations and the community sector. There is a need for investment in building the necessary infrastructure and providing strategic leadership and capacity building for the workforce (Box 1.6).

The publication 'Mental health promotion and mental disorder prevention. A policy for Europe' (Jané-Llopis & Anderson 2005) provides a policy framework and a case for action in mental health promotion across the mental health,

Box 1.6

Developing the infrastructure for promoting mental health

- establish a policy framework that provides a mandate for action
- develop a strategic action plan which identifies priorities, key goals and objectives for action
- coordinate an intersectoral and partnership approach to policy implementation at governmental, regional and local levels
- invest in research to guide evidence-based mental health promotion policy and practice
- invest in human, technical, financial and organisational resources to achieve priority actions and outcomes
- support capacity building and training of the mental health promotion workforce to ensure effective practice and programme delivery
- identify models of best practice and support the adoption and adaptation of high quality, effective and sustainable programmes, particularly those meeting the needs of disadvantaged groups
- engage the participation of the wider community
- put in place a system of monitoring policy implementation and impact
- systematically evaluate programme process, impact, outcome and cost

public health and public policy sectors. A number of countries have also developed policies at a national level to provide a strategic framework for action on mental health promotion, e.g. Australia, Canada, New Zealand, England and Scotland. See, for example, New Zealand's 'Te Tāhuhu – improving mental health 2005–2015: the second New Zealand mental health and addiction plan' (Ministry of Health 2005), the Australian 'National mental health plan 2003–2008' (Australian Health Ministers 2003) and the Scottish Executive's 'National programme for improving mental health and well-being' (2003).

Intersectoral Approaches

The integration of mental health promotion across a range of health and social policies is an important element of infrastructure development. Mental health promotion is relevant across the entire spectrum of mental health and social services and effective strategies require engagement with a broad range of service and community sectors, such as the primary care, mental health, public health, community, prison, family and social welfare services and agencies. However, it is also clear that the promotion of population level mental health depends on much more than health policies alone. The socioenvironmental nature of the determinants of mental health demands that a cross sectoral approach is required involving the building of partnerships and collaboration across a range of agencies, organisations and community groups within and beyond the health sector. Collaboration across government departments and different sectors is key to effectively influencing the determinants of mental health. Rowling and Taylor (2005) describe the most significant components of an intersectoral approach as being:

- the adoption of a unifying language with which to work across sectors
- a partnership approach to allocation and sharing of resources
- a strengthening of capacity across the individual, organisational and community dimensions.

In keeping with the basic principles of health promotion, a multi-sectoral, integrated approach is needed that will ensure that mental health promotion is embedded firmly in policy across a range of sectors such as education, employment, housing, environment and equality/social inclusion. These efforts need to be coordinated across the various sectors and the impact of all public and social policies on population level mental health needs to be assessed. Mental health impact assessment, as a methodology for proofing the impact of public policies on mental health, is an important area for development and implementation.

Developing Effective Practice

In order to translate from research and policy into effective practice, the skills of effective implementation are required. This entails developing creative solutions to local problems and the implementation of innovative and effective programmes. The art of programme implementation is frequently not reported in published papers (Durlak 1998, Mihalic et al 2002) but is contained in what has been referred to as the 'wisdom literature' (Domitrovich & Greenberg 2000). This refers to the practical experience of programme delivery and the ground-work that needs to take place by practitioners in order to ensure effective implementation. These implementation skills include creatively working with local resources, engaging participation, mobilising support and successfully navigating the process of collaboration and partnership building with different stakeholders. Developing sustainable initiatives requires imagination, skill, high level motivation and the ability to foster a positive ethos and climate of collaboration. The generic processes underpinning effective implementation are discussed by Barry et al (2005) and recommendations for improving the quality of programme implementation are made. Adopting an evidence-based programme does not in itself guarantee success. Practice skills and creativity are required for quality planning and effective programme delivery. These factors will be discussed in more detail in Chapter 2.

Developing the Workforce

The development and sustainability of mental health promotion is dependent on having a skilled and informed workforce drawn from across different sectors such as health, education, employment, community and non-governmental organisations. Mental health promotion requires skills to work with populations and communities as well as individuals. Partnership working and the implementation of multiple strategies calls for high level expertise in order to engage and facilitate the participation of diverse sectors. Continuing education and training is required to disseminate knowledge related to mental health promotion and effective intervention programmes, to provide professional training and education of health professionals and the general public and to enhance the quality of practice (Commonwealth Department of Health and Aged Care 2000).

The development of skills, to support the implementation of policy initiatives on the ground and to ensure the development of best practice, is key to the future growth and development of mental health promotion as a multidisciplinary area of practice. Workforce education and training range from awareness raising about the promotion of mental health, to skills development needed to support and implement specific initiatives, through to dedicated mental health promotion specialists who facilitate and support the development of policy and practice across a range of settings. Much of the knowledge and skills required is inextricably linked to health promotion generally and as such can be provided through continuous professional education programmes and postgraduate training (Mittelmark 2004). In Australia, for example, both Ausienet and the Australian Federal Government identified the need to enhance the capacity of the workforce in the application of effective mental health promotion strategies. See, for example, the development of professional development courses, tools and resources by the Victorian Health Foundation (www.vichealth.vic.gov.au). Mentality in the UK (www.mentality.org.uk) has also produced a number of useful guides and resources to enhance the capacity of the workforce to engage in effective mental health promotion practice.

Investing in Research

In addition to practice skills, research skills are required to develop and evaluate programmes, to monitor mental health status and patterns at a population level and to improve our understanding of the determinants of mental health. Effective policies and strategies need to be based on sound epidemiological data and effective intervention approaches. While national health surveys of physical health status and its determinants are routinely collected in many countries, the situation with regard to mental health is quite different. There are quite limited data on mental health status at a population level or the pattern of differences among different population groups. To determine this information requires the assessment of mental health status and its determinants at a population level.

Investment in research and evaluation is critical to supporting the implementation of evidence-based policy and practice in mental health promotion. There is a need for different types of research including:

- monitoring and surveillance systems for assessing mental health status and its determinants at a population level
- efficacy studies which provide information on intervention outcomes under controlled research conditions
- effectiveness studies which evaluate programme impacts and outcomes in more uncontrolled 'real world' conditions
- dissemination research which documents programme replication and adaptation across diverse groups, settings and cultures.

A culture of research and evaluation needs to be cultivated in both the policy and practice fields. The undertaking of systematic evaluation studies plays an essential role in advancing knowledge on best practice in local settings. It is also critical to the effective dissemination of programmes and the effective translation of research evidence into best practice. It is important to ensure that mental health promotion programmes are operating effectively and efficiently and there is, therefore, a need to systematically evaluate both the process and outcome of mental health promotion activities. While there is often a clear awareness of the importance of evaluation and evidence-based practice, there is equally a need for awareness of the necessity to invest in the expertise and resources to undertake this work. Evaluation research has a critical role to play in demonstrating the success and added value of mental health promotion, and it is vital to justifying funding for sustaining initiatives in the longer term. The generation of evidence-based practice is an important challenge in mental health promotion and requires that researchers, policy makers and practitioners work in partnership in documenting and evaluating the implementation of programmes on the ground. The Scottish Development Centre for Mental Health has produced a series of four evaluation guides to encourage and improve standards in the evaluation of mental health improvement initiatives (Scottish Development Centre for Mental Health 2004). These guides, which form part of the NHS Health Scotland's programme of support for the National Programme for Improving Mental Health and Well-being (www.wellontheweb.net), are intended as resources for people working in mental health across all sectors and settings. Readers are also referred to a useful guide for practitioners on planning, monitoring and evaluating mental health promotion produced by VicHealth (2005) (www.vichealth.vic.gov.au).

Facilitating Partnerships and Collaboration

Mental health promotion cannot be undertaken by any one sector or any single organisation on its own. Effective policy and practice requires that the different sectors and organisations work together, including international organisations, national governments, non-governmental organisations, prospective donors and professional associations (WHO 2002). Active engagement with these different sectors is needed to promote greater understanding of the concept of positive mental health and its importance for overall health and quality of life. To increase the visibility of mental health promotion at a societal level, a public awareness strategy is needed in order to 'remove the shadows' of the stigma surrounding mental ill-health and to promote greater public and professional understanding of the importance of promoting positive mental health in its own right as a resource for everyday life and societal well-being.

In view of the insufficient resources for research and development of effective policies and programmes in the mental health promotion area, it makes sense to pool knowledge, expertise and resources. Based on the aims articulated by the IUHPE Global Programme on Health Promotion Effectiveness, in moving forward there is a need to:

- promote mental health promotion among decision and policy makers at all levels of governance
- communicate to a wider, more general public audience what mental health promotion is about, why it is important and the health, social and economic benefits that it can bring
- advocate for more support in developing policies, research, structures and capacity
- promote best practice in a variety of environments and with a range of key players.

Moving Forward: Strengthening the Links between Research, Policy and Practice

To advance mental health promotion, there is a need to combine the art, science and politics (i.e. practice, research and policy) of promoting mental health for effective action (Barry 2005). The research base needs to be strengthened in order to provide a strong foundation for effective policy and practice. Dissemination research and further systematic studies of programme implementation, adoption and adaptation are needed so that practice-based theory may be generated, which will guide the building of capacity for effective programme delivery. Political commitment needs to be mobilised so that mental health is given greater priority in terms of policy development, including policies which promote mentally healthy

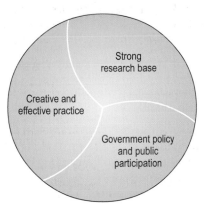

Figure 1.4 • The art, science and politics of promoting mental health (adapted from Barry 2005 with permission of the Journal of Public Mental Health)

living, working and social environments. There is a need to raise awareness of the determinants of mental health at public and policy making levels. Public participation is critical to this process, as policy needs to be accompanied by greater public awareness of, and engagement with, the importance of good mental health to overall health and social well-being. We, therefore, need to ensure that the art, science and politics of mental health promotion, as outlined in Figure 1.4, work in tandem so that practice, research and policy will support the development of a society which creates, promotes and maintains the mental health of its citizens.

References

Albee G W 1982 Preventing psychopathology and promoting human potential. American Psychologist 37:1043–1057

Albee G W, Joffe J M, Dusenbury L A (eds) 1988 Prevention, powerlessness, and politics: readings on social change. Sage, London

Antonovsky A 1996 The salutogenic model as a theory to guide health promotion. Health Promotion International 11:1118

Arole R, Fuller B, Deutschman P 2005 Community development as a strategy for mental health promotion: lessons from rural India. In: Herrman H, Saxena S, Moodie R (eds) Promoting mental health: concepts, emerging evidence, practice. A report of the World Health Organization, Department of Mental Health and Substance Abuse in collaboration with the Victorian Health Promotion Foundation and University of Melbourne, WHO, Geneva:243–251

Arsenault-Lapierre G, Kim C, Turecki G 2004 Psychiatric diagnoses in 3275 suicides: a meta-analysis. BMC Psychiatry 4(1):37

Australian Health Ministers 2003 National mental health plan 2003–2008. Australian Government, Canberra. Online. Available: http://www.mentalhealth.gov.au April 2006

Backer T E 2000 The failure of success: challenges of disseminating effective substance abuse prevention programs. Journal of Community Psychology 28(3):363–373

Barnett W S 1993 Benefit–cost analysis of preschool education: findings from a 25 year follow-up. American Journal of Orthopsychiatry 63(4):500–508

Barry M M 2001 Promoting positive mental health: theoretical frameworks for practice. International Journal of Mental Health Promotion 3(1):25–43

Barry M M 2002 Challenges and opportunities in strengthening the evidence base for mental health promotion. Promotion and Education 9(2):44–48

Barry M M 2005 Creating a mentally healthy society: lessons from a cross border rural mental health project in Ireland. Journal of Public Mental Health 4(1):30–34

Barry M M, McQueen D V 2005 The nature of evidence and its use in mental health promotion. In: Herrman H, Saxena S, Moodie R (eds) Promoting mental health: concepts, emerging evidence, practice. A report of the World Health Organization, Department of Mental Health and Substance Abuse in collaboration with the Victorian Health Promotion Foundation and University of Melbourne,WHO, Geneva:108–118

Barry M M, Domitrovich C, Lara M A 2005 The implementation of mental health promotion programmes. Promotion and Education Suppl2:30–35

Bronfenbrenner U 1979 The ecology of human development: experiments by nature and design. Harvard University Press, Cambridge, Massachusetts

Building Australia's capacity to promote mental health 1997 Review of the infrastructure for promoting mental health in Australia. Prepared for the AHMAC Mental Health Working Group by the Australian Centre for Health Promotion at the University of Sydney

Bywaters J 2005 Carpe diem: seize the day. Journal of Public Mental Health 4(1):7–9

Caplan G 1964 Principles of preventive psychiatry. Basic Books, New York

Caplan R, Holland R 1990 Rethinking health education theory. Health Education Journal 49:10–12

Caplan R D, Vinokur A D, Price R H et al 1989 Job seeking, reemployment, and mental health: a randomized field experiment in coping with job loss. Journal of Applied Psychology 74(5):759–769

Chowdhury A, Bhuiya A 2001 Do poverty alleviation programs reduce inequalities in health? The Bangladesh experience. In: Leon D, Walt G (eds) Poverty, inequality and health. Oxford University Press, Oxford:312–332

Commonwealth Department of Health and Aged Care 2000 Promotion, prevention and early intervention for mental health – a monograph. Mental Health and Special Programs Branch, Commonwealth Department of Health and Aged Care, Canberra

Cowen E L 1991 In pursuit of wellness. American Psychologist 46(4):404–408

DoH (Department of Health) 2001 Making it happen: a guide to developing mental health promotion. The Stationery Office, London

Domitrovich C E, Greenberg M T 2000 The study of implementation: current findings from effective programs that prevent mental disorders in school-aged children. Journal of Educational and Psychological Consultation 11(2):193–221

Drew N, Funk M, Pathare S et al 2005 Mental health and human rights. In: Herrman H, Saxena S, Moodie R (eds) Promoting mental health: concepts, emerging evidence, practice. A report of the World Health Organization, Department of Mental Health and Substance Abuse in collaboration with the Victorian Health Promotion Foundation and University of Melbourne,WHO, Geneva:81–88

Durlak J A 1998 Why program implementation is important. Journal of Prevention and Intervention in the Community 17(2):5–18

Durlak J A, Wells A M 1997 Primary prevention mental health programs for children and adolescents: a meta-analytic review. American Journal of Community Psychology 25(2):115–152

Elliott D S 1997 Blueprints for violence prevention. Center for the Study of Prevention of Violence, Institute of Behavioral Science, University of Colorado, Boulder, Colorado

European Commission 2005 Green Paper. Improving the mental health of the population. Towards a strategy on mental health for the European Union. European Communities, Brussels. Online. Available: http://europa. eu.int/comm/health/ph_determinants/ life_style/mental/green_paper/consulta- tion_en.htm June 2005

Friedli L 2001 Mental health promotion: per- spectives and practices. International Journal of Mental Health Promotion 3(1):20–24

Fryers T, Melzer D, Jenkins R 2003 Social inequalities and the common mental disorders: a systematic review of the evidence. Social Psychiatry and Psychiatric Epidemiology 38:229–237

HEA (Health Education Authority) 1997 Men- tal health promotion: a quality framework. Health Education Authority, London

Health Australia Project 1996 Building capacity to promote the mental health of Australians. Discussion paper. Health Australia

Herrman H, Jané-Llopis E 2005 Mental health promotion in public health. Promotion and Education Suppl2:42–47

Herrman H, Saxena S, Moodie R (eds) 2005 Promoting mental health: concepts, emerging evidence, practice. A report of the World Health Organization, Department of Mental Health and Substance Abuse in collaboration with the Victorian Health Promotion Foundation and University of Melbourne,WHO, Geneva

Hoffman K, Jackson S 2003 A review of the evidence for the effectiveness and costs of interventions: preventing the burden of non-communicable diseases: How can health systems respond? Unpublished: Prepared for the World Bank Latin America and the Carribean Regional Office. Online. Available: http://www.utoronto.ca/chp/ReportsandPresentations.htm November 2005

Hosman C M H 2000 Prevention and health promotion on the international scene: the need for a more effective and comprehensive approach. Addictive Behaviors 25(6):943–954

Hosman C, Jané-Llopis E 1999 Political challenges 2: mental health. In: The evidence of health promotion effectiveness: shaping public health in a new Europe. A Report for the European Commission. International Union for Health Promotion and Education, Paris, Chapter 3:29–41

Hosman C, Jané-Llopis E 2005 The evidence of effective interventions for mental health promotion. In: Herrman H, Saxena S, Moodie R (eds) Promoting mental health: concepts, emerging evidence, practice. A report of the World Health Organization, Department of Mental Health and Substance Abuse in collaboration with the Victorian Health Promotion Foundation and University of Melbourne,WHO, Geneva:169–184

Hosman C, Jané-Llopis E, Saxena S (eds) 2006 Prevention of mental disorders: effective interventions and policy options. A report of the World Health Organization, Department of Mental Health and Substance Abuse in collaboration with the Prevention Research Centre of the Universities of Nijmegen and Maastricht, Oxford University Press, Oxford (in press)

IUHPE (International Union of Health Promotion and Education) Global programme on health promotion effectiveness. A multi-partner project coordinated by the International Union for Health Promotion and Education in collaboration with the WHO. Online. Available: http://www.iuhpe.org October 2005

IUHPE 1999 The evidence of health promotion effectiveness: shaping public health in a new Europe. A Report for the European Commission by the International Union for Health Promotion and Education, Paris

Jackson S, Perkins F, Khandor E et al 2005 Integrated health promotion strategies: a contribution to tackling current and future health challenges. Technical paper prepared for the 6th Global Conference on Health Promotion, Bangkok, Thailand, 7–11 August 2005. WHO, Geneva

Jahoda M 1958 Current concepts of positive mental health. Basic Books, New York

Jané-Llopis E, Anderson P 2005 Mental health promotion and mental disorder prevention. A policy for Europe. Radboud University, Nijmegen

Jané-Llopis E, Barry M M 2005 What makes mental health promotion effective? Promotion and Education Suppl2:47–55

Jané-Llopis E, Barry M M, Hosman C et al 2005 Mental health promotion works: a review. Promotion and Education Suppl2:9–25

Jenkins R, Lehtinen V, Lahtinen E 2001 Emerging perspectives on mental health. International Journal of Mental Health Promotion 3(1):8–12

Joubert N 2001 Promoting the best ourselves: mental health promotion in Canada. The International Journal of Mental Health Promotion 3(1):35–40

Karoly L A, Greenwood P W, Everingham S S et al 1998 Investing in our children: what we know and don't know about the costs and benefits of early childhood interventions. Rand Publications, California

Kazdin A E, Kagan J 1994 Models of dysfunction in developmental psychopathology. Clinical Psychology: Science and Practice 1:35–52

Kelly M P, Speller V, Meyrick J 2004 Getting evidence into practice in public health. Health Development Agency, London

Kickbusch I 2003 The contribution of the World Health Organization to a new public health and health promotion. American Journal of Public Health 93:383–388

Kovess-Masfety V, Murray M, Gureje O 2005 Evolution of our understanding of positive mental health. In: Herrman H, Saxena S, Moodie R (eds) Promoting mental health: concepts, emerging evidence, practice. A report of the World Health Organization, Department of Mental Health and Substance Abuse in collaboration with the Victorian Health Promotion Foundation and University of Melbourne,WHO, Geneva:35–44

Labonté R, Robertson A 1996 Delivering the goods, showing our stuff: the case for the constructivist paradigm for health promotion research and practice. Health Education Quarterly 23(4):431–447

Lahtinen E, Lehtinen V, Riikonen E et al (eds) 1999 Framework for promoting mental health in Europe. National Research and Development Centre for Welfare and Health, Ministry of Social Affairs and Health, Hamina, Finland

Lehtinen V, Riikonen E, Lahtinen E 1997 Promotion of mental health on the European agenda. National Research and Development Centre for Welfare and Health, Helsinki

Lehtinen V, Ozamiz A, Underwood L et al 2005 The intrinsic value of mental health. In: Herrman H, Saxena S, Moodie R (eds) Promoting mental health: concepts, emerging evidence, practice. A report of the World Health Organization, Department of Mental Health and Substance Abuse in collaboration with the Victorian Health Promotion Foundation and University of Melbourne,WHO, Geneva:46–57

Lewin K 1951 Field theory in social science. Harper, New York

MacDonald G, O'Hara K 1998 Ten elements of mental health, its promotion and demotion: implications for practice. Society of Health Promotion Specialists, Glasgow

McQueen D 2001 Strengthening the evidence base for health promotion. Health Promotion International 16(3):261–268

McQueen D V, Anderson L M 2001 What counts as evidence: issues and debates. In: Rootman I, Goodstadt M, Hyndman B et al (eds) Evaluation in health promotion: principles and perspectives. World Health Organization Regional Publications, European Series, Copenhagen, No.92

Marshall-Williams S, Saxena S, McQueen D V 2005 The momentum for mental health promotion. Promotion and Education Suppl2:6–9

Melzer D, Fryers T, Jenkins R (eds) 2004 Social inequalities and the distribution of the common mental disorders. Maudsley Monograph 44, Psychology Press, Hove and New York

Mentality 2003 Making it effective: a guide to evidence based mental health promotion. Briefing paper 1. Mentality, London

Mihalic S, Fagan A, Irwin K et al 2002 Blueprints for violence prevention replications: factors for implementation success. Center for the Study of Prevention of Violence, Institute of Behavioral Science, University of Colorado, Boulder, Colorado

Ministry of Health 2005 Te Tāhuhu – improving mental health 2005–2015: the second New Zealand mental health and addiction plan. Ministry of Health, Wellington. Online. Available: http://www.moh.govt.nz April 2006

Mittelmark M B 2003 Five strategies for workforce development for mental health promotion. Promotion and Education 10(1):20–22

Mittelmark M B 2004 How to influence policy. In: Moodie R, Hulme A (eds) Hands-on health promotion. IP Communications, Melbourne:29–23

Mittelmark M B, Puska P, O'Byrne D et al 2005 Health promotion: a sketch of the landscape. In: Herrman H, Saxena S, Moodie R (eds) Promoting mental health: concepts, emerging evidence, practice. A report of the World Health Organization, Department of Mental Health and Substance Abuse in collaboration with the Victorian Health Promotion Foundation and University of Melbourne, WHO, Geneva:18–33

Moodie R, Jenkins R 2005 I'm from the government and you want me to invest in mental health promotion. Well why should I? Promotion and Education Suppl2:37–41

Mrazek P J 1998 Prevention science in the 21st century. In: Killoran Ross M, Stark C (eds) Promoting mental health. Symposium of the Ayrshire International Mental Health Promotion Conference, Ayrshire:77–87

Mrazek P J, Haggerty R J (eds) 1994 Reducing risks for mental disorders: frontiers for preventive intervention research. National Academies Press, Washington DC

Murray C J, Lopez A D 1996 The global burden of disease. Harvard University Press, Cambridge, Massachusetts

Narayan D, Petesch P (eds) 2002 Voices of the poor: from many lands. Oxford University Press, World Bank, Oxford

Nelson G, Prilleltensky I, Peters R De V 1999 Prevention and mental health promotion in the community. In: Marshall W, Firestone P (eds) Abnormal psychology perspectives. Prentice Hall, Scarborough

Nutbeam D 1999a Health promotion effectiveness – the questions to be answered. In: The evidence of health promotion effectiveness: shaping public health in a new Europe. A Report for the European Commission. International Union for Health Promotion and Education, Paris, Chapter 1:1–11

Nutbeam D 1999b The challenge to provide 'evidence' in health promotion. Health Promotion International 14(2):99–101

Olds D L 2002 Prenatal and infancy home visiting by nurses: from randomised trials to community replication. Prevention Science 3(3):1153–1172

Olds D L, Hill P L, Mihalic S F et al 1998 Prenatal and infancy home visitation by nurses. In: Elliott D S (ed) Blueprints for violence prevention, book seven. Center for the Study and Prevention of Violence, University of Colorado, Boulder, Colorado

Orford J 1992 Community psychology: theory and practice. John Wiley, Chichester

Patel V 2005 Poverty, gender and mental health promotion in a global society. Promotion and Education Suppl2:26–29

Patel V, Swartz L, Cohen A 2005 The evidence for mental health promotion in developing countries. In: Herrman H, Saxena S, Moodie R (eds) Promoting mental health: concepts, emerging evidence, practice. A report of the World Health Organization, Department of Mental Health and Substance Abuse in collaboration with the Victorian Health Promotion Foundation and University of Melbourne, WHO, Geneva: 189–201

Petticrew M, Chisholm D, Thomson H et al 2005 Evidence: the way forward. In: Herrman H, Saxena S, Moodie R (eds) Promoting mental health: concepts, emerging evidence, practice. A report of the World Health Organization, Department of Mental Health and Substance Abuse in collaboration with the Victorian Health Promotion Foundation and University of Melbourne, WHO, Geneva 203–213

Pilgrim D, Rogers A 1993 A sociology of mental health and illness. OPU, Buckingham

Price R H 1998 Progress on promotion of mental health and prevention of mental disorders in the United States. In: Killoran Ross M, Stark C (eds) Promoting mental health. Symposium of the Ayrshire International Mental Health Promotion Conference:101–109

Price R H, Vinokur A D 1995 Supporting career transitions in a time of organizational downsizing: the Michigan JOBS program. In: London M (ed) Employees, careers and job creation: developing growth orientated human resources strategies and programs. Jossey-Bass, San Francisco:191–209

Price R H, Cowen E L, Lorion R P et al (eds) 1988 Fourteen ounces of prevention: a casebook for practitioners. American Psychological Association, Washington DC

Price R H, Van Ryn M, Vinokur A D 1992 Impact of a preventive job search intervention on the likelihood of depression among the unemployed. Journal of Health and Social Behaviour 33:158–167

Raeburn J 2001 Community approaches to mental health promotion. International Journal of Mental Health Promotion 3(1):13–19

Rappaport J 1984 Studies in empowerment: introduction to the issue. In: Rappaport J, Swift C, Hess R (eds) Studies in empowerment: steps toward understanding and action. Hawthorn Press, New York:1–7

Rappaport J 1985 The power of empowerment language. Social Policy 16:15–21

Rowling L, Taylor A 2005 Intersectoral approaches to promoting mental health. In: Herrman H, Saxena S, Moodie R (eds) Promoting mental health: concepts, emerging evidence, practice. A report of the World Health Organization, Department of Mental Health and Substance Abuse in collaboration with the Victorian Health Promotion Foundation and University of Melbourne, WHO, Geneva

Rutz W, von Knorring L, Walinder J 1992 Long term effects of an educational program for general practitioners given by the Swedish committee for the prevention and treatment of depression. Acta Psychiatrica Scandinavica 85:83–88

Saxena S, Garrison P J (eds) 2004 Mental health promotion: case studies from countries. A joint publication of the World Federation for Mental Health and World Health Organization. WHO, Geneva

Saxena S, Saraceno B 2004 International collaboration and the role of WHO and other UN agencies. In: Herrman H, Saxena S, Moodie R (eds) Promoting mental health: concepts, emerging evidence, practice. Summary report. A report of the World Health Organization, Department of Mental Health and Substance Abuse in collaboration with the Victorian Health Promotion Foundation and University of Melbourne,WHO, Geneva 57–58

Scanlon K 2002 A population health approach: building the infrastructure to promote mental health in young people. In: Rowling L, Martin G, Walker L (eds) Mental health promotion: concepts and practice, young people. McGraw Hill, Sydney:56–69

Schweinhart L J, Weikart D P 1988 The High/Scope Perry Preschool Program. In: Price

R H, Cowen E L, Lorion R P (eds) Fourteen ounces of prevention: a casebook for practitioners. American Psychological Association, Washington DC:53–65

Schweinhart L J, Weikart D P 1998 High/Scope Perry Preschool program effects at age twenty-seven. In: Crane J (ed) Social programs that work. Russell Sage Foundation, New York:148–162

Scottish Development Centre for Mental Health 2004 Mental health improvement evaluation guides. Online. Available: http://www.hebs.com/researchcentre/specialist/mhevidprog.cfm November 2005

Scottish Executive 2003 National programme for improving mental health and well-being. Action plan 2003–2006. Scottish Executive, Edinburgh. Online. Available: http://show.scot.nhs.uk/sehd/mentalwell-being April 2006

Secker J 1998 Current conceptualisations of mental health and mental health promotion. Health Education Research 13(1):57–66

Speller V, Learmonth A, Harrison D 1997 The search for evidence of effective health promotion. British Medical Journal 315:361–363

Thomson H, Petticrew M, Morrison D 2001 Housing interventions and health – a systematic review. British Medical Journal 323:187–190

Tilford S, Delaney F, Vogels M 1997 Effectiveness of mental health promotion interventions: a review. Health Education Authority, London

Tones K 1997 Beyond the randomized controlled trial: a case for "judicial review". Health Education Research 12(2):1–4

Tudor K 1996 Mental health promotion. Routledge, London

US Department of Health and Human Services 1999 Mental health: a report of the Surgeon General. US Department of Health and Human Services, Substance Abuse and Mental Health Services Administration, Centre for Mental Health Services, National Institutes of Health, National Institute of Mental Health, Rockville, Maryland

VicHealth 1999 Mental health promotion plan foundation document 1999–2002. The Victorian Health Promotion Foundation, Carlton South, Victoria

VicHealth 2005 Mental health and well-being research summary sheets, No.1. Burden of disease due to mental illness and mental health problems. The Victorian Health Promotion Foundation, Carlton South, Victoria

Vinokur A D, Schul Y 1997 Mastery and inoculation against setbacks as active ingredients in the JOBS intervention for the unemployed. Journal of Consulting and Clinical Psychology 65(5):867–877

Vinokur AD, van Ryn M, Gramlich E et al 1991 Long-term follow-up and benefit–cost analysis of the JOBS program: a preventive intervention for the unemployed. Journal of Applied Psychology 76(2):213–219

Wallerstein N 1992 Powerlessness, empowerment and health: implications for health promotion programs. American Journal of Health Promotion 6:197–205

Weare K 2000 Promoting mental, emotional and social health: a whole school approach. Routledge, London

Weissberg R P, Caplan M, Harwood L 1991 Promoting competent young people in competence-enhancing environments: a systems-based perspective on primary prevention. Journal of Consulting and Clinical Psychology 59(6):830–841

WHA (World Health Assembly) 2002 55th World Health Assembly, May 2002

WHO (World Health Organization) 1946 Preamble: World Health Organization Constitution. WHO, Geneva. Online. Available: http://w3.whosea.org/aboutsearo/pdf/const.pdf October 2005

WHO 1985 Summary report of the working group on concepts and principles of health promotion, Copenhagen, 9–13 July 1984. The Journal of the Institute of Health Education 23(1):5–9

WHO 1986 Ottawa Charter for health promotion. WHO, Geneva

WHO 2001a Mental health: strengthening mental health promotion. WHO Factsheet No. 220. Online. Available: http://www.who.int/mediacentre/factsheets/fs220/en/ October 2005

WHO 2001b Mental health: new understanding, new hope. The world health report. WHO, Geneva

WHO 2002 Prevention and promotion in mental health: evidence and research. Department of Mental Health and Substance Dependence, Geneva

WHO 2003 Investing in mental health. Department of Mental Health and Substance Dependence, Non-communicable Diseases and Mental Health, WHO, Geneva

WHO 2004a Promoting mental health: concepts, emerging evidence, practice. Summary
report. World Health Organization, Department of Mental Health and Substance Abuse
in collaboration with the Victorian Health
Promotion Foundation and the University of
Melbourne, WHO, Geneva. Online. Available:
http://www.who.int/mental_health/evi-
dence/en/promoting_mhh.pdf October 2005

WHO 2004b Prevention of mental disorders:
effective interventions and policy options. A
report of the World Health Organization,
Department of Mental Health and Substance
Abuse in collaboration with the Prevention
Research Centre of the Universities of Nijmegen
and Maastricht. WHO, Geneva. Online. Available: http://www.who.int/mental_health/
evidence/en/prevention_of_mental_disorders_
sr.pdf October 2005

WHO 2005a The Bangkok Charter for health
promotion in a globalized world. WHO, Geneva

WHO 2005b Mental health action plan for
Europe: facing the challenges, building
solutions. WHO, Geneva. Online. Available:
http://www.euro.who.int/document/mnh/
edoc07.pdf October 2005

WHO EURO 1998 Health promotion evaluation: recommendations to policymakers.
WHO, Copenhagen

Zubrick S, Kovess-Masfety V 2005 Indicators
of mental health. In: Herrman H, Saxena S,
Moodie R (eds) Promoting mental health:
concepts, emerging evidence, practice. A
report of the World Health Organization,
Department of Mental Health and Substance
Abuse in collaboration with the Victorian
Health Promotion Foundation and University
of Melbourne, WHO, Geneva:148–166

Implementing Mental Health Promotion Programmes: A Generic Template for Action

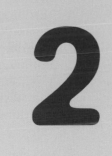

2

Introduction

Having overviewed the key concepts, principles and approaches to mental health promotion in Chapter 1, we now turn our attention to programme planning and implementation.

Before a programme can be put in place a great deal of groundwork in the form of programme planning needs to take place. This includes defining the target population, identifying their needs, strengths and capacities, designing a means of engaging their participation, selecting and adapting a suitable programme, working in partnership with key stakeholders and agencies in the community and building organisational linkages to make programme delivery possible. In this chapter we focus on the steps involved in programme planning and delivery. A generic template for action is outlined which can be used to guide programme planning and development across a range of programmes and settings. Before outlining the template for action, an overview is given of current research on programme implementation, why it is important and what we know from studies that have been carried out to date. This information will provide a useful base for informing the more practical steps involved in successfully putting programmes into practice.

Programme Implementation

Implementation refers to the actuality of putting a programme or intervention into practice. Durlak defines implementation as 'what a programme consists of in practice' (1995:5) and how much it is delivered according to how it was designed. As Bracht et al (1999) point out, implementation turns theory and ideas into practice and translates design into effectively operating programmes. Details on programme implementation are often not reported in the literature. In-depth descriptions and discussion of the implementation process in textbooks and journal articles have been limited in scope. Information on implementation is contained in what Domitrovich and Greenberg refer to as a 'wisdom literature generated from personal experiences and observations of programme implementation in context' (2000:209).

Zins et al (2000) identify the lack of attention to examining implementation as an increasing concern in the field. Implementation information is needed to know about what actually happens during programme delivery, what takes place on the ground, the quality of the programme as delivered and whether the target audience is reached. It allows for greater understanding of the internal dynamics and operations of the programme, how the pieces of the programme fit together, how the implementers and programme users interact and the obstacles they face and resolve in the process. Implementation data are also critical to interpreting positive or negative outcomes as they strengthen any conclusions that are made about the programme's role in producing change. Without measuring implementation quality, a programme may be incorrectly judged as ineffective when, in fact, negative outcomes are a result of poor quality implementation or shortcomings in the delivery process. This leads to the danger of a type III error, i.e. the programme is delivered so poorly as to invalidate outcome analyses. Information on implementation is also important in informing the replication and maintenance of programmes in other settings, thereby advancing knowledge on best practices. Careful delineation and monitoring of the implementation process provides a clear account of what was actually done, how well it was done and whether the outcomes were as a result of what was done. Programme monitoring and evaluation is sometimes feared or unwanted by practitioners and programme implementers. The purpose of this activity is not to evaluate the achievements of individuals in a competitive or critical manner but rather to assess the overall process of implementation in a constructive and collaborative way. The advantages of this information for the practitioner are multi-fold. Monitoring and documenting the process of programme implementation enables the practitioner and programme evaluators to highlight programme strengths and weaknesses, determine why certain things happened, enhance the validity of outcome evaluation and provide feedback for continuous quality improvement in programme delivery.

Overview of Implementation Research

It is clear from the research results available that to adequately assess implementation, information is needed about the specific programme components, how they are delivered and the characteristics of the context or settings in which the programme is conducted (Dane & Schneider 1998, Pentz et al 1990). In addition to the content and structure of the intervention, information is needed on what Chen (1998) refers to as the characteristics of 'the implementation system'. This includes the process and structure of the implementation and training system, the characteristics of programme implementers and participants and the nature of their relationship, characteristics of the setting in which the programme is being implemented (organisational climate, level of support, etc.) and a host of other system-level variables (Weissberg 1990). Chen (1998) points out that although an intervention is the major change agent in a programme, the 'implementation system' is likely to make an important contribution to programme outcomes as it provides the means and the context for the intervention. Therefore, as well as having a clear programme theory and establishing the essential programme components that contribute to outcomes, it is necessary to understand the conditions required for successful implementation and the factors that may affect and moderate their effects. A well-designed programme, based on a strong theory or conceptual model is, therefore, necessary but not sufficient to produce behaviour changes in target groups (Botvin et al 1990a, b, Connell et al 1985).

The 'how' of programme implementation is difficult to find out about. Evaluation studies and reports have largely focused on assessing outcomes while failing to examine the details of implementation. Implementation research is critical to understanding how and under what conditions programmes may be effective. Implementation has been relatively neglected in outcome research with the majority of studies conducted without any source of implementation information. Durlak (1997) reports that less than 5% of over 1200 published prevention studies provide data on programme implementation. Likewise, Durlak and Wells (1998), in a meta-analysis of indicated prevention programmes, found that 68.5% of the programmes were described too broadly to be replicated and very few included measurement of programme fidelity. Gresham et al (1993), in a review of school-based intervention studies published between 1980–1990, found that only 35% provided an operational definition of their intervention through a detailed description or reference to a manual. Only 14.9% of studies systematically measured and reported levels of programme fidelity. However, for those studies that have monitored implementation, it is clear that the variability in the quality of implementation is related to programme outcomes (Botvin et al 1995, Connell et al 1985). The research that has examined this issue reports two clear findings; first that implementation is variable across change agents and is sometimes seriously compromised, and second that the level of implementation influences outcomes.

Implementation is Variable

Durlak (1998) reviewed a number of representative field studies on the level of implementation attained in different prevention programmes and reported that:

- between 23–81% of programme activities may be omitted (Smith et al 1993, Wall et al 1995)
- only a minority of change agents may implement the programme with a high degree of integrity or fidelity (Bush et al 1989, Taggart et al 1990).

Two overall conclusions were drawn from this review: 1) we do not know what level of implementation is necessary for maximum programme impact and what levels are feasible under different circumstances, and 2) as a general rule researchers and implementers should not expect that the quantity or quality of implementation will be 100%.

Implementation Affects Outcomes

Dane and Schneider (1998) examined prevention trials in which dimensions of programme implementation (integrity or dosage measures) were analysed in relation to outcomes. The results confirm the importance of integrity information, particularly measures of programme adherence and exposure for outcomes. A number of studies have also reported that variation in the level of implementation may be directly related to the strength of outcomes:

- for some programmes, positive effects occur only when a certain level of implementation is attained (Pentz et al 1990, Taggart et al 1990)
- for other programmes, better or higher levels of implementation are associated with stronger or more positive outcomes (Botvin et al's 1995 drug prevention programme), e.g. Connell et al's (1985) health education programmes had to be implemented for at least 20 hours and also include parents, as the programme model specified, in order to produce a significant positive effect
- studies found that poorly implemented programmes were not successful (Botvin et al 1989, Taggart et al 1990).

This brief overview of the research clearly indicates the importance of programme implementation; the level of implementation influences outcomes and poor implementation can jeopardise programme impact. Programme implementation needs to be monitored extensively as variability in the quality of implementation is related to programme outcomes (Botvin et al 1990a, b, Botvin et al 1995, Connell et al 1985, Taggart et al 1990). Research indicates that there is considerable variability in the extent to which attention has been paid to the measurement of implementation. As a result there is often a dearth of information in the published literature to guide practitioners in making decisions regarding the practical aspects of programme adoption and replication. Some exceptions

Box 2.1

Useful sources of information on programme implementation

Price R H, Cowen E L, Lorion R P, Ramos-McKay J 1988 Fourteen ounces of prevention: a casebook for practitioners. American Psychological Association, Washington DC. In this text, 14 model programmes are described. Each author describes how the programme actually works, discusses the research evidence for programme effectiveness, highlights the programme's limitations as well as its positive aspects and offers practical suggestions for replicating the programme. The book is aimed at practitioners who may be interested in replicating these programmes in their local settings.

Elliott D (ed) Blueprints for violence prevention series, published by the Center for the Study and Prevention of Violence, University of Colorado in Boulder. Each Blueprint describes an exemplary programme in the area, outlining the theoretical rationale for the intervention, the core components for the programmes as implemented, the evaluation designs and findings, and the practical experiences the programme staff encountered while implementing the programme at multiple sites. The Blueprints are designed to be very practical descriptions of effective programmes which allow individuals or agencies to determine the cost estimate of each intervention, provide an assessment of the organisational capacity required to ensure the successful start-up and operation over time and give some indication of the potential barriers and obstacles which might be encountered when attempting to implement each type of intervention. A particularly useful publication based on this series is Mihalic S, Fagan A, Irwin K, Ballard D, Elliott D 2002 Blueprints for violence prevention replications: factors for implementation success.

There is also a series of research papers that explores and studies aspects of programme implementation. See, for example, the special issue by guest editors Zins et al in the *Journal of Educational and Psychological Consultation* 2000, Volume 11(2), titled 'Measurement of quality of implementation of prevention programs'.

to this may be found in the publications listed in Box 2.1 to which the reader is directed for further details.

The research cited in Box 2.1 demonstrates that successful implementation is not guaranteed by the decision to adopt a best practice programme. To ensure the quality of the implementation system, the following points have been highlighted by Domitrovich and Greenberg (2000):

- assess the clarity of the programme's theory and how it directly relates to how staff should be trained and supported
- if training is required the quality of the training should be assessed, including the skills needed to become proficient in the programme
- when implementation begins determine whether or not the essential components are actually being delivered
- information on the quality of the delivery of the programme should be gathered

- use of participant feedback, such as satisfaction surveys, to assess the reaction of both participants and implementers to the programme and their views on its merits and benefits.

Durlak (1998) also provides the following suggestions for improving implementation:

- specify the essential ingredients of an intervention
- collaborate with change agents in field settings to tailor the programme to the target setting
- obtain a clear commitment to administer the agreed-upon intervention
- train change agents to conduct the programme effectively
- provide on-going supervision and consultation once the programme has begun
- be ready for unexpected problems
- do pilot work
- designate staff with responsibilities for implementation.

To implement effectively and then maintain quality programmes, both researchers and practitioners will need to play an important role in the measurement and support of the implementation process. The remainder of this chapter addresses these issues and provides a step-by-step guide to programme planning and implementation.

Generic Template for Action

In this section a generic template or framework for the implementation process is outlined. This includes the stages involved in the process of programme planning and delivery, including developing mechanisms for consultation and collaboration, identifying the target population, assessing the local context, selecting possible intervention strategies and building a base of support and interagency links for project implementation, maintenance and evaluation. These different steps may be divided up into different phases as follows.

Phase 1: Programme Initiation and Initial Planning Stages

- needs assessment and consultation
- assess the local context
- select intervention programmes and activities
- mobilise support and develop partnerships
- management of the project.

Phase 2: Develop Delivery Plan

- formulate project goals, objectives and activities
- develop a sequential work plan that facilitates the systematic implementation of the programme

- specify programme components
- identify and recruit intended programme recipients
- assign resources, including the necessary staffing, skills and training that are needed to implement the plan of the programme
- develop and pilot programme materials
- build networks for ongoing sustainability of the programme.

Phase 3: Deliver Intervention

- implement programme components
- monitor quality of programme implementation
- feedback and communication
- ongoing consultation and collaboration
- manage resources.

Phase 4: Programme Maintenance and Consolidation

- integrate intervention activities
- assess programme effectiveness in terms of process, impact and outcomes
- feedback findings to ensure continuous quality improvement
- put in place strategies to sustain the programme over time.

Before detailing each of these steps in turn, it may be useful at this point to briefly outline some key principles of practice that should underpin the implementation of mental health promotion programmes. Many of these concepts have already been described in Chapter 1. Here we remind the reader of their relevance and importance in underlying the delivery of programmes in practice.

Applying Generic Principles of Practice

Adopting a Socioecological Perspective

Adopting a socioecological perspective to programme implementation means recognising the importance of the broader context of programme delivery, such as the socioenvironmental influences on individual behaviour and attitudes. An ecological perspective highlights the interdependencies among social systems operating at different levels, e.g. parent–child dyad, the family system as a whole, the interrelations among these systems and larger socioeconomic influences operating at the level of the community and wider society (Bronfenbrenner 1979). This perspective shifts the focus of mental health promotion programmes beyond an individualistic focus to also consider the influence of broader social, economic and political forces. The implications of this model are wide-ranging including, for example, an awareness that the behaviours and attitudes of different social and cultural groups need to be understood in terms of the multiple interacting influences on their everyday circumstances. This means paying due attention to the wider structural influences on behaviour, such as the role of poverty and discrimination, and how these are mediated through local community norms and values. As pointed out by Olds (1988), programmes need to be able to influence in significant ways the enduring environment in which the individual, family, group or community is functioning. For example, parents are influenced by culturally defined norms of appropriate behaviour during pregnancy and early childhood rearing. Most of these norms are shared by members of the society. Programmes seeking to influence parents' skills and practices must start from where parents are at and take account of these shared community values and beliefs in the development and design of any new programme. The ecological model underscores the importance of supportive environments and highlights the role of schools, workplaces and communities as providing key contexts or settings for promoting positive mental health.

Embracing an Empowerment Philosophy

Adopting an empowerment philosophy requires that programmes be delivered in an empowering and participatory manner, building on the strengths and skills of the programme participants. The style or manner of delivery may be just as important as what is delivered. Empowering programmes seek to engage the active participation of programme recipients and implementers in order to build on existing capacities and strengths and to enhance their sense of control over their lives. An empowerment approach to mental health promotion requires that attention be focused away from an exclusive concern with individual factors to consider the interface between the individual and the wider community and social forces. This approach underscores the importance of interventions addressing systems of socialisation, social support and control and tackling the wider context of poverty, disadvantage, social injustice and discrimination. Embracing an empowerment philosophy signifies an emphasis on 'process', seeking to engage the active participation of programme users in gaining understanding, knowledge and skills in controlling the determinants of their lives as encountered in their everyday circumstances. In terms of programme delivery, this requires that practitioners and programme implementers change their role from one of 'experts' delivering programmes in a didactic fashion to that of facilitators adopting an interactive and participative approach. As outlined by Rappaport, adopting an empowerment agenda means being 'committed to identifying, facilitating, or creating contexts in which heretofore silent and isolated people, those who are "outsiders" in various settings, organizations and communities, gain understanding, voice and influence over decisions that affect their lives' (1990:52).

Engaging in Consultation and Collaboration

Collaborative working is at the core of mental health promotion practice. Programmes need to be delivered in an empowering manner with clear strategies for partnership working and participation at all stages. Implementing effective programmes requires good collaboration with key stakeholders in the community, schools, or workplace settings. Consultation needs to begin at the earliest stage of programme development. The consultative process fosters early involvement by stakeholders, promotes greater ownership of the programme and facilitates capacity building (Everhart & Wandersman 2000). Consultation is key to understanding how mental health issues are understood and dealt with in the local setting and how the resources and capacities of the local school or community can be mobilised to implement the intervention with quality. The need to understand local beliefs and values regarding both why problems arise and how they may be alleviated is critically important, especially in the area of mental health which may be shrouded with prejudices, fear and stigma. The nature of these beliefs and attitudes has been shown to vary by place, culture, age, gender and socioeconomic status. For example, teachers in a school may be uncomfortable about implementing a mental health promotion programme due to fears that the introduction of the programme may stigmatise the school and its students as having problems in this area. Understanding and addressing these concerns from the outset is critically important in securing teachers' cooperation and support, so vital in ensuring successful programme implementation. Consultation, therefore, plays a critical role in establishing readiness for involvement in the programme and this process takes time and should be allowed for in the programme plan. Early consultation and collaborative working is also critical to ensure the meaningful input and participation of key stakeholders and works to increase their sense of programme involvement and ownership. This process produces a better ecological fit for the programme, actively engages participation and generally increases the chances of successful implementation and future sustainability.

Phase 1: Programme Initiation and Initial Planning Stages

Successful implementation of a mental health promotion programme is dependent on good planning. Planning entails a number of interrelated activities involving clear analysis of the need for the programme, identifying key target groups/ programme recipients, resources needed, understanding of social structures and values in the local context, interagency and organisational involvement to build collaborative partnerships and facilitating broad level participation. There are a number of systematic guidelines and models available for the practitioner to use in planning health promotion programmes (see, for example, Green & Kreuter 1999), which may also be employed in relation to mental health promotion programmes. Only the major steps will be highlighted here by way of illustration (Box 2.2).

Box 2.2

Phase 1: Programme initiation and initial planning stages

- needs assessment and consultation
- assess the local context
- select intervention programmes and activities
- mobilise support and develop partnerships
- management of the project

Before proceeding on the detailed steps outlined in Box 2.2, it may be useful to engage in a collaborative planning session with key stakeholders in order to formulate a broad picture of the intervention. Initial planning stages need to be characterised by consultation and collaboration with all key groups who will be involved in the project's development. In planning an intervention it is, therefore, important to address these issues early on in order to understand the perspectives and attitudes in the local context and to mobilise local involvement. Reiss (1981) refers to this process as understanding 'community frames' and it is a critical step before proceeding to design an intervention. Price and Smith (1985) advise using an interactive workshop format for this early stage planning session. Based on this format, Box 2.3 outlines a number of steps to guide this process. Interactive programme planning with key stakeholders and agencies may include programme funders, implementers, members of the target group/potential programme recipients and programme evaluators. A planning workshop is a useful way of engaging key persons in the programme and mobilising their participation and interest. At this stage, it may be useful to also consider setting up an advisory group or core-planning group to guide the planning process. The inclusion of programme evaluators at this point in the process is also useful in order to help with initial clarification of programme aims and objectives and to document and monitor the planning process from the outset.

At the beginning of the project, initial clarification of the overall plan of the project is needed. It is important to be clear about what the project can and cannot do when informing the community about its existence. In collaboration with key stakeholders, it is useful to agree on preliminary goals and objectives, which can be fine-tuned at a later stage (Box 2.4). Early clarification will help to ensure smooth running of the implementation and development phase. These initial ideas, once formulated, then need to be anchored in the realities of the local context, both in terms of the organisational context of the delivery agency and in the community or setting context of the target population. This requires a clear understanding of both the culture and structure of the organisations involved and the infrastructure, capacities and possible barriers in the local setting.

Box 2.3

Steps in initial programme planning

- clarify the identified need for the programme
- identify a population subgroup or setting
- identify key project stakeholders
- have a broad model for intervention in mind
- engage in interactive planning with key stakeholders
- have some preliminary ideas about the positive mental health outcomes that need to be promoted
- consider intervention approaches in the context of the local setting
- develop a plan for implementation

Box 2.4

Worksheet for programme planning
(based on interactive workshop format developed by
Price & Smith 1985)

- agree on the characteristics of the target population
- identify key strengths, resources and major stresses affecting the target population
- what positive mental health outcomes (attitudes, behaviours) within the target population should be promoted with a mental health promotion intervention?
- what skills does the target population need to develop?
- identify the agencies or the groups in the community that must be involved in planning for this target population. Which persons need to be involved?
- what steps will be taken to secure the interest and cooperation of the community groups or agencies?
- establish several tentative objectives for the intervention project
- identify intervention strategies to achieve these objectives
- how will the programme be evaluated to identify needed administrative changes while the project is underway?
- how will the programme be evaluated to determine the extent to which intervention objectives have been/are being met for the target population/group?
- what level of resources (information, money, support, space, expertise) will be needed? What sources for these resources should be approached?

Substantiating the Need for a Programme

The need for the programme may be highlighted from a number of sources. These include:

- emerging local concerns, such as a call for school-based programmes in order to counter rising rates of adolescent mental health problems
- topics identified by policy makers or health service decision makers as areas for strategic action, e.g. a need to promote parenting skills among first time low-income teenage mothers
- practitioners' interest in implementing 'best practice' programmes in order to fill a gap in existing service provision, e.g. implementation of a successful workplace mental health promotion programme.

In all cases the initial planning for the programme requires that there is a clear understanding of why the programme is needed and what the programme can realistically hope to achieve within a given timeframe. This is referred to as having a clear rationale for the programme development. It is useful from the outset to consult previous research and theory in the area when deciding on how best to address an identified problem or need. Take the example of tackling the issue of increasing youth suicides, which may give rise to calls for suicide prevention programmes in schools. Consultation of the research in this area, however, shows that suicide prevention programmes have not been found to be effective and there is some evidence that they may actually increase the risk for vulnerable young people, particularly boys (Lister-Sharp et al 1999). Reviews of research in this area have called for generic competence-building interventions that promote mental health rather than narrow suicide-specific prevention programmes (Garland & Zigler 1993). There is a growing body of evidence that high-quality comprehensive programmes that focus on young people and their socialising environments produce long-lasting positive effects on mental, social and behavioural development (Durlak & Wells 1997, Hosman & Jané-Llopis 1999, Tilford et al 1997, Weissberg et al 1991). This evidence clearly points the practitioner in the direction of more broad-based, competence-enhancing programmes, which when carried out in collaboration with families, schools and wider communities have the potential to impact on multiple positive outcomes across social and personal domains.

Undertaking a Needs Assessment

In planning for a new programme the first objective is to carry out a comprehensive needs assessment. This entails:

1. assessing the unique characteristics (strengths, problems, obstacles, facilitating factors) of the community, school or workplace setting in which the programme will be implemented
2. clearly identifying the target population (age, gender, socioeconomic status, geographic area, level of risk)
3. choosing a programme that has a good fit with the targeted population or community; selecting a programme that does not fit with the local context, even if carried out with fidelity, can lead to unsuccessful outcomes (Mihalic 2001).

Identifying the Target Population Identifying the target population involves deciding who the programme will be designed for and delivered to. Needless to say the available resources need to be considered when making decisions about the scope and reach of the programme. Mrazek and Haggerty's prevention framework (1994) identifies three main categories of prevention programmes according to the population groups that are targeted. These include:

1. universal programmes – targeting all members of the general population on the basis that everybody has mental health needs, e.g. a mental health awareness programme
2. selected programmes targeting groups known to be at higher risk of developing mental health problems, e.g. high-quality pre-school programmes for young children from low-income disadvantaged backgrounds
3. indicated programmes targeting high-risk individuals or groups already displaying symptoms, e.g. early diagnosis and intervention for primary care patients showing early signs of depression.

Programmes may, therefore, range from a universal audience, i.e. open to everybody within a defined community, school or work site, or it may entail selecting only those most likely to benefit from the programme or those most in need. Criteria such as identified need or more general vulnerability factors may be used in making this selection. Consulting the literature is also useful as it frequently points to groups where a programme has been known to have most success. For example, in relation to maternal and child health programmes, being a teenage mother, unmarried and poor increases the likelihood of poor health and developmental outcomes on the part of the child and arrested personal development on the part of the mother (Olds 1988). The programme may, therefore, be targeted at low-income unmarried women having their first child, on the grounds that they are most in need of such an intervention, would be more receptive to offers of help and that the skills developed would be carried over to subsequent children, thereby increasing the long-term impact of the programme. However, in targeting the programme in this way, the practitioner needs to take into account the risk of stigmatising the programme as being for poor parents at risk for child abuse and neglect. This may have the effect of turning people away from the programme and hence not reaching those who are most in need. A balance needs to be struck and in this case it may be wiser to leave the programme open to include all first time parents, regardless of their risk status. In this respect it is useful to note that a mix of high- and low-risk participant groups has been found to have a beneficial effect in depression prevention programmes for the unemployed (Vinokur et al 1995).

Assessing the Local Context

Here we consider the process of assessing and identifying needs, barriers, opportunities and resources involved in initiating a mental health promotion programme. Needs assessment is a first step in shaping the design of the project and in adapting implementation plans to the unique characteristics of the local setting or community. It is important that the assessment identifies strengths as well as problems including local perceptions and attitudes, current resources, readiness, capacity for mental health promotion and infrastructure for successful programme implementation. The process of undertaking a needs assessment provides a unique opportunity for local involvement in the project. As Rissel and Bracht point out, 'In genuinely empowering and participatory health projects, analysis is not done on the community but with the community' (1999:59). Involvement in the needs assessment provides an opportunity for local people and organisations to develop an awareness of the project and to build commitment to local action. The cooperation of local people is needed to undertake a comprehensive local needs assessment, as this involves gleaning information on local power structures, views and perceptions. Participatory research methods and structured planning models may be used to actively engage members of the local community or setting in this process (see Ch. 3 for further discussion).

In undertaking a focused needs assessment of the identified population for the purposes of planning, consulting existing data sources may be useful in providing readily available information and also identifying gaps in knowledge. However, the planning information needed for a specific project will more often than not require the collection of original data from the local site. This includes specialised studies such as systematic surveys, key informant interviews, focus groups with target groups, agency staff, local organisations/groups and influential people in the local setting. A focused needs assessment seeks to gather information from people most likely to be interested in or affected by a new programme. In addition to its planning function, the process of needs assessment may be designed to identify potential collaborating organisations, groups and individuals which can actively participate in the building of a sustainable intervention.

There is a wide range of strategies that may be used for needs assessment. Among the methods most commonly employed are the following:

Utilising existing sources of data
- demographic, social, educational, employment and economic profiles related to the mental health profile or needs of people in the area
- local mental health status data or studies concerning behavioural, social and environmental risks and protective factors
- health service data including patterns of service use from which inferences may be made about future needs, such as identifying high demand groups or groups with significantly low uptake
- previous surveys of relevance to the topic that have been carried out in the area.

Collecting new data
- resource surveys entailing a broad level analysis of general characteristics of the setting or community including its role, structure and history, current level of provision, local organisational infrastructures and capacities, potential barriers and receptivity to change
- local surveys on perceptions of mental health needs, awareness, attitudes, stigma, knowledge of support services, specific areas of concern
- key informant interviews with knowledgeable community members and agency staff regarding their perceptions of local issues, strengths, obstacles and areas of concern
- focus groups with key members of the target population to garner their views and understandings of particular issues of importance locally and how they might best be dealt with locally
- community meetings and open fora for inviting discussions with a wide range of participants on their perceptions of local issues, concerns, strategies for tackling these issues and the potential for change.

Successful implementation depends on accurate analysis and understanding of the local context and conditions for the programme including wider community, social and political factors. Once collected, the needs assessment data should be converted into programme operations in order to inform the next stage of planning. This may be done by compiling a summary report which synthesises the data, in order to prioritise areas for action. This information can then be disseminated in an appropriate manner to key stakeholders who will play an active role in the design of the programme. For example, the findings from a community survey can be fed back to the local residents via a project newsletter which outlines the key findings and the issues raised in a format that is easy to understand. In setting priorities, it may also be useful to invite local key players to review in a collaborative manner the information gathered in order to arrive at a consensus concerning priority areas and action strategies. This consultative approach helps to ensure that programmes will be sensitive to the local culture and will also provide the basis for continuing local participation and collaboration.

Selection of Intervention Programmes and Activities

In selecting intervention strategies, it is useful at this stage to review the literature for examples of similar programmes which have been successfully evaluated. Practitioners and policy makers are developing greater awareness of the need to utilise empirically validated programmes and their best practices. Applying these programmes to the specific context of a school or community, there are numerous challenges in creating readiness, developing an effective model of training, garnering contextual support, monitoring implementation and evaluating outcomes. Alternative interventions can be considered in the light of available evaluation information and their appropriateness to the specific context of the project. Talking with others who have practical hands-on experience of implementing such programmes is useful, as this will provide valuable advice that is often absent from published studies and reports.

In selecting specific interventions it is useful to clarify the rationale behind the choices that are being made, whether adapting existing programmes or developing new ones, and to articulate assumptions about why a particular programme or intervention method should or should not work in the context of the project.

- Is there theoretical and empirical backing for the intervention approach?
- Has the programme been used in a similar environmental context?
- Are there manuals or clearly outlined programme guidelines for implementation available?
- Importantly, has the programme been shown to work and achieve its objectives?

61

The intervention needs to be clearly defined in order that all stakeholders and implementers are clear about the purpose of the initiative and that progress toward the desired goals and objectives of the project can be assessed.

In exploring the theories on which the programmes are based, the association among various mental health promoting and mental health compromising behaviours is one of the clearest facts to have emerged from the past decades of research (Botvin & Tortu 1988, Jessor 1982). A number of problem behaviours appear to be associated with the same underlying vulnerability factors. Likewise, clusters of protective factors have been identified as playing a critical role in promoting positive mental health outcomes. Intervention programmes should be developed which target the underlying determinants of several theoretically and empirically related problem behaviours. For example, the rationale or basis for the Life Skills Training programme (Botvin & Tortu 1988, Botvin et al 1990a, b) is derived from the knowledge that programmes increasing students' general personal and social competence positively affect factors that underlie many types of problem behaviours, including drug abuse. Further details on the Life Skills Training programme may be found in Chapter 5. The known clustering of risk and protective factors strongly supports comprehensive programme initiatives that seek to enhance protective factors such as self-esteem, self-efficacy, sense of personal control, social and communication skills, within the context of supportive socioenvironmental structures.

Mobilising Support and Developing Partnerships

When developing a new intervention, take time to consider whose approval and support is needed to get the project off the ground. It is extremely important to secure the interest and cooperation of key stakeholders early on in the planning process. Building a strong base of support requires time and effort and this should be budgeted for. Support may need to be garnered from a number of different levels, e.g. among decision makers, organisations and individuals who will be directly or indirectly involved in implementing and using the programme. In order to mobilise the necessary local support, it is important to assess the local political structure and to understand the power structure in the community or setting and its value system. Some of this information will already have been gathered in the needs assessment. For example, there is a need to identify the influential individuals or groups whose support is vital to the successful implementation of the programme and to build in a mechanism for user involvement in the planning process at the earliest stages of programme design. This will set the stage for continuing user participation in the process of implementation and ensures that the programme will be tailored for and acceptable to the local population. Programme designers should also seek to engage with the professionals already working with the target population about the new intervention or programme to be offered. The purpose of this is not to inform them about the project but to ask their assistance in developing a project that is congruent with the values and resources of that community. As Price and Smith (1985) point out, the presentation of the project in its early days is critical to its successful implementation. The project or programme needs to be tailored for the local audience and setting. It is important to invite, and hear the views of, local groups and agencies that are well positioned to know about what will and will not work in the local setting. Begin to identify agency staff and community members who are particularly interested in the project and those who are not. Identify 'project champions' who will support the project and provide needed support to see it through its various stages of development and maintenance.

Develop a plan for collaboration with the agencies and groups that might become involved. Consider what the project has to offer these groups, what they would like to see resulting from the project, whether it fits in with their existing work and how current levels of interagency links and cooperation may influence programme delivery. Questions to consider include:

- What goals and objectives would other professionals like to see for the project?

- How does the proposed programme fit in with their existing work?
- How do these professionals or groups interact with each other; are there interagency links and cooperation?
- Are there coordinating agencies or organisations that should be contacted?
- Are key stakeholders and agency staff clear about the aims and objectives of the project and characteristics of the target group who will participate in the project?

Failure to enlist the active involvement of all key players, including implementing staff and recipients, from the start can seriously jeopardise programme success. Once involved, keep partner groups informed at regular intervals as the study proceeds in order to ensure ongoing cooperation and programme partnership and sustainability.

Management of the Project

The planning stage also entails putting in place a mechanism for project management in order to oversee the smooth running of the programme and the management of resources. This involves choosing an organisational structure such as a steering group or advisory group who will play an active role in overseeing the implementation of the programme at the local level. The steering or advisory group should represent the key partners who have an investment in the project and careful attention should be given to how the members of the group are selected. This is particularly important in relation to community steering groups where representation in terms of race, gender, age, class, religious and ethnic affiliations need to be carefully considered. The function and purpose of the group should be clearly identified from the outset and the key roles and responsibilities of the group members should be agreed on in a collaborative fashion. It is worth putting some time into clarifying the functions of the group and also attending to the internal dynamics and working relationships of the members (see Ch. 3 for further discussion of these points).

In terms of managing resources, it is useful to draw up a plan of all the required resources for programme planning and implementation, including tangible and non-tangible resources. This includes securing appropriate funding for assessment, planning, start up and maintenance of the programme. A written budget with projected costing should be drawn up, together with an outline of required resources in terms of staffing, staff skills, training needs, any required accommodation, programme materials, transportation costs for programme recipients and any incidental costs such as crèche and meal costs. Failure to understand and secure all the resources necessary to implement a programme can result in poor implementation and possibly programme failure down the line. A comprehensive plan should aim at securing appropriate administrative and managerial support for the programme as it develops through its various stages of implementation.

In summary, these initial planning tasks all need to reflect a concern for detailed documentation and a commitment to working in an open, participatory and collaborative manner. Negotiation and consensus building early in the life of the project sets the tone for the working relationships and helps to minimise barriers and resistance. As Price and Smith (1985) highlight concerning early stages of planning 'The first phase is characterised by careful observation and documentation, systematic thinking, and an effective interactive style'.

Phase 2: Develop Delivery Plan

This next phase involves shifting from needs assessment and consultation to the formulation of project goals and objectives and developing a sequential work plan for programme delivery (Box 2.5). By this stage needs assessment data relevant to the population will have been collected, and some preliminary arrangements and organisational linkages with other agencies in the community will have been developed. Focus groups with the local population may also have been undertaken to help in prioritising the interventions to be delivered and determining the modes of delivery that will best suit the local audience. Alternative programme intervention strategies relevant to the target population and setting may also have been identified. A focus on programme goals and objectives provides an opportunity to use the information collected to clearly formulate the actual programme and to prioritise the menu of interventions to be delivered.

The Development of Project Goals and Objectives

The formulation of goals and objectives is an important conceptual phase in the planning of the programme and should be a collaborative exercise which brings people together and helps to focus more precisely on what the project aims to achieve. It is also an opportunity to develop a shared understanding of the key purpose of the project and to mobilise interested parties towards a common goal. Focusing on the goals and objectives provides a common ground for identifying

---

Box 2.5

Phase 2: Develop delivery plan

- formulate project goals, objectives and activities
- develop a sequential work plan that facilitates the systematic implementation of the programme
- specify programme components
- identify and recruit intended programme recipients
- assign resources including the necessary staffing, skills and training that are needed to implement the plan of the programme
- develop and pilot programme materials
- build networks for ongoing sustainability of the programme

criteria by which the project will be judged; it also focuses on what to assess or measure in evaluating the impact of project interventions.

Price and Smith (1985) propose a specific framework for developing intervention programme goals and objectives. They provide a quite detailed account of the process involved, and readers may find this source useful to consult, particularly with regard to specifying how operational statements of goals and objectives serve as criteria to be used in evaluation and accountability. In brief, a project goal is a general statement that specifies the condition or state of affairs that is desired as a result of the project. A project objective, on the other hand, is a specific statement of the outcomes that indicate progress towards the goal or the removal of barriers within a specific timeframe. A programme outcome may be stated as 'improved understanding of mental health'. However, the criteria that allow us to know whether the results are being achieved must be specified. This will be linked to the programme components delivered and may be stated as '70% of the classroom students will show improved attitudes and reduced stigma as measured on x questionnaires by the end of the programme'. The characteristics of well-formulated objectives have been identified as follows: Explicit, Specific, Measurable, Scheduled, Prioritised, Owned by those involved, Related to each other and Communicated.

Develop a Sequential Work Plan

Having developed an initial list of project goals and objectives and how they might be achieved, a detailed action plan for the intervention needs to be drawn up. The major elements of the plan for programme implementation need to be clearly defined and operationalised in order to guide the implementation process and generate a record of programme implementation. Once the intervention has been defined, the exact details of the intervention and what will need to be delivered by project staff should be clarified, i.e. what activities actually make up the intervention and the order in which they will be delivered. Careful documentation of planned programme activities is recommended early on in the life of the project. The exact details of what is being delivered, how often and under what circumstances calls for detailed monitoring and documentation throughout the process of implementation. Programme activities may be documented through independent observation, structured ratings and reports by project staff and implementers. These various sources will inform on how the intervention is actually being delivered on the ground and will detail what obstacles or critical sources of support were encountered and any unanticipated effects.

The delivery plan needs to detail who does what, with whom and when. Who is actually going to implement the programme? Depending on the programme, implementers may range from teachers delivering curricula in classroom settings, health visitors/nurses carrying out home visits, employment and training agency staff delivering a jobs search programme, mental health service staff delivering mental health awareness talks and workshops, to peer-led youth and community programmes. In all cases, the delivery plan needs to consider what staffing, including necessary qualifications/backgrounds, skills and training, are required to adequately deliver the programme. The delivery plan will also specify clearly the intended scope of the programme, including the number of participating agencies, and a recruitment strategy for engaging the expected number of programme recipients. These areas will now be discussed in more detail.

Written action plans or programme protocols have been shown to be a critical forerunner of successful change efforts (Fawcett et al 1997). They also maximise the use of available community resources in the plan and adapt to local constraints and values. Intervention cost estimates should also be included, along with the time frames. Developing a sequential plan or practical plan of work includes setting out both short-term and long-term goals and scheduling the process in a sequential fashion with incremental implementation steps. The programme goals, principles and key programme components must be identified and clearly communicated to all relevant players involved in the implementation. Failure to commit to the underlying philosophical principles and to implementation of the key programme components can seriously undermine programme success (Mihalic 2001).

Specify Programme Content

It is extremely useful from the outset to clarify and obtain agreement on the exact details of the intended programme, i.e. the specific activities to be delivered and the process by which they should be implemented. Programme managers and staff, in collaboration with evaluators, should identify and spell out the components that make up the intended programme. These include the strategies, activities, processes and technologies to be used. Programme evaluators can often help in this process, using tools such as evaluability assessment and application of programme theory. This involves identifying the key programme elements or activities, what Durlak refers to as 'the active ingredients of an innovation, that is, those elements believed to be responsible for a program's effects' (1998:7). A full description of programme components is needed to provide the foundation for assessing programme delivery (Scheirer 1994:45). Components are the strategies, activities, behaviours, media products and technologies needed to deliver the programme, along with the specification of the intended recipients and delivery situations. For example, the Nurse Home Visitation Programme by Olds (1988) identified three major activities carried out by the nurses during their home visits to enable parents to create a healthy environment for their child's development:

1. parent education about influence on fetal and infant development
2. the involvement of family members and friends in the pregnancy, birth, early care of the child and support for the mother
3. the linkage of family members with other formal health and human services.

The manual for the Life Skills Training programme (Botvin 1983) lists five major programme components, each of which consists of two to six classroom lessons designed to be taught in sequence:

1. knowledge and information
2. decision-making component

3. self-directed behaviour change
4. coping with anxiety
5. social skills.

Many programmes develop a structured manual for delivery which clearly specifies the core elements of the programme, their objectives, amount of time given to each component together with the sequence and the manner in which they should be delivered. For example, programme materials for school-based curriculum programmes are frequently included in a structured teacher's manual containing detailed lesson plans, describing both the content and activities to be included in each session. Student guides, including classroom exercises, homework and space to keep notes, audiotape relaxation tapes, etc., may also be included. The JOBS depression prevention programme also includes a detailed implementation and training manual for teaching people successful job search strategies (Curran et al 1999). The instruction manual specifies all the programme components for training and programme delivery including the workshop protocols and handouts for participants. In the absence of an already created manual, it is useful to develop a detailed written programme protocol specifying as far as possible the component elements and the intended sequence in which the activities are to be delivered.

Identify and Recruit Intended Programme Recipients

Specification of the intended recipients may include criteria such as background characteristics appropriate for the programme, e.g. age, gender, socioeconomic group or income level, ethnicity, health status. In some cases eligibility requirements for the programme may need to be specified, e.g. only those unemployed for 6 months or more, first time low-income mothers or students aged 14–16 years. These decisions can be made based on prior studies and evaluation findings concerning identified levels of need and/or optimal programme effectiveness.

Appropriate mechanisms for recruiting participants will also need to be identified. This may include recruitment through existing community organisations, e.g. women's groups, youth groups, rural organisations, schools, work sites, health services (hospitals, GPs, antenatal clinics, community health centres), via mass/local media ads and word of mouth. Once the recruiting mechanism is identified it may also be necessary to agree on a selection process, i.e. random selection, self-selection, first-come first-served, competitive application or screening by predetermined criteria, e.g. high-risk status, etc. The full details of the recruitment arrangements need to be planned in advance and the necessary cooperation secured from recruiting agencies.

Staffing and Training for Programme Delivery

The importance of quality training and staff development for successful implementation cannot be overemphasised. Good training is critical to good implementation.

Staff charged with programme implementation may feel uncomfortable with the new programme methods and materials and as a result may feel poorly equipped to use the new intervention techniques. High quality training ensures that implementers become more comfortable with their new roles by providing a situation in which they can learn and practise new techniques prior to actual implementation. Many programmes provide comprehensive training, including extensive training materials and a facilitator certification process.

Where training is required, conducting a formal training workshop is recommended. Structured training will provide a general understanding of the area and a thorough grounding in the programme approach. For example, Botvin and Tortu (1988) outline the elements of a teacher training workshop for the Life Skills Training (LST) programme as follows:

- provide an understanding of the issue of substance abuse and LST's theoretical rationale
- provide a full description of the programme and the curriculum materials needed to implement it successfully
- familiarise participants with programme contents and activities
- demonstrate the techniques needed to implement the programme
- provide participants with opportunities to practise the techniques in small group settings and receive feedback on their performance
- provide guidelines for scheduling and implementation
- generate a sense of enthusiasm and commitment among those who will be delivering the programme.

In general, training should aim to provide a conceptual framework for the programme, guidelines for implementation, skill demonstration and skill practice.

The selection of staff who will deliver the programme is a critical component of programme implementation. In selecting staff, it is useful to consider the essential and desirable staff characteristics that are required for successful programme delivery. These may range from appropriate qualifications and background to necessary skills or appropriate attributes, attitudes and level of interest. A useful distinction can be made between personal qualities such as self-confidence, sensitivity and liking working with people, to skills and experience such as group facilitation and teaching experience. The JOBS implementation manual, for example, advises distinguishing between attributes that can be improved through training (e.g. active listening skills) and those that should already be possessed by the person (e.g. empathy and reliability). The teacher selection for the LST training, described above, specifies such qualities as good student rapport, commitment to the programme and motivation to teach LST. Likewise, 'The Incredible Years: parent, teacher, and child training series' (Webster-Stratton et al 2001), which provides a programme to overcome conduct problems in children, specifies that the programmes can be delivered by trained professionals from a variety of backgrounds and disciplines including teachers, school counsellors and psychologists. Experience in working with children and parents, or in individual counselling, together with group leader experience is highlighted as being desirable. In this programme, successful facilitators have been characterised as those who have a background in social learning theory and child development principles, are warm, caring and collaborative in their interpersonal style and are able to provide effective leadership using the skills of persuading, coaching, humour, role play and practice. It is interesting to note that reports from the programme have found that the facilitators' effectiveness is determined not by their educational or professional background but by their degree of comfort with a collaborative process and their ability to promote intimacy and assume a friendship role with families.

In this respect, it is useful to highlight that a collaborative model of training has the added value of increasing engagement in the intervention, building good quality relationships with programme users and creates a climate of support and trust. Research suggests that the collaborative process has the multiple advantages of reducing attrition rates, increasing motivation and commitment, reducing resistance, increasing situational generalisation and giving participants a joint stake in the outcome of the intervention (Webster-Stratton et al 2001). In short, collaborative training empowers participants by strengthening their knowledge, self-confidence, skill base and their autonomy, instead of creating dependence and a sense of inadequacy. Following initial training, many programmes recommend providing ongoing support, supervision and additional training as necessary.

Develop and Pilot Programme Materials

The materials needed for delivery may include a wide range, from the use of instructional manuals, leaflets and take-home instructional packs to audio tapes, videos, use of drama and interactive workshops. It is important to ensure that any material used should be culturally meaningful, in terms of presentation, content and sensitivity to the local situation. The delivery plan should include provision for the piloting of an initial trial of the intervention materials in the hands of local staff. Using formative evaluation techniques, the pilot should be carefully evaluated. It is important to include feedback from both programme implementers and programme recipients at this stage. The findings from the formative evaluation may then be used to make any necessary changes and to fine tune the programme before being implemented more widely. Cost data from the pilot may also be useful in informing projected programme expenditure through the lifetime of the project.

Build Networks for Ongoing Sustainability

When applying a new programme to the specific context of a school, workplace or community, there are numerous challenges in establishing readiness, developing an effective model of training, garnering contextual support, monitoring implementation and evaluating outcomes. Implementation of new programmes will often require the active participation of health and support agencies in the community. To elicit the cooperation of these multi-sectoral agencies it is important to identify and communicate with individuals or groups with a vested interest in programme delivery and who are in a position to make decisions about adopting a new programme. These may range from mental health service staff, voluntary agencies, community groups, schools, parents, teachers, employers, managers to local health departments. Botvin and Tortu describe the planning phase of implementing a new curriculum as a process 'fraught with psychological, socio-logical, political, and economic concerns' (1988:105–106). Support for imple-menting a new school-based programme will be needed from several levels, from district level down to school board members, principals, classroom teachers and parents. Parent support is critical and it is, therefore, important to ensure that parents are fully informed and supportive of any new programme that is being introduced. Regardless of the setting, the programme details, including its back-ground rationale together with results of previous evaluations, should be clearly described to all interested parties. The concerns of the key stakeholders should be heard and resolved in the process of refining the programme and all parties kept informed of progress at regular intervals as the programme proceeds. As the programme is implemented, good communication ensures ongoing coopera-tion and lays the groundwork for strengthening programme partnerships and sustainability.

Phase 3: Deliver Intervention

This next stage involves implementation of the programme together with careful monitoring and support of the implementation process (Box 2.6). It is important that the programme be delivered as planned with clear agreed-upon objectives for each intervention component. Shortening or omitting particular programme com-ponents is not recommended as this may dilute the effectiveness of the interven-tion. If any last minute changes are made, these should be carefully documented in order to monitor their effects. Likewise, particular obstacles or unexpected bar-riers to implementation that are encountered should be documented and notified as the programme proceeds. As far as possible, the already developed programme protocol should be followed in the recommended order and format. This is referred to as maintaining programme integrity and methods of ensuring this will now be outlined.

Box 2.6

Phase 3: Deliver intervention

- implement programme components
- monitor quality of programme implementation
- feedback and communication
- ongoing consultation and collaboration
- manage resources

Monitoring Implementation and Programme Integrity

As outlined earlier in this chapter, current research indicates that implementation is often variable and imperfect in field settings and that the level of implementation influences outcomes. A weakness in many programmes is the absence of detailed information on the quality and quantity of programme implementation. Durlak (1995, 1998) suggests that a starting point for measuring implementation is for a programme to specify its programme components, or active ingredients. These should be observable and include all materials and activities used in the intervention (Scheirer 1994). It is unclear whether factors such as the quality of trainers, quality of training, feedback from implementers or other system level variables (e.g. organisational support) may indeed also constitute active programme ingredients. Chen (1998) argues that although an intervention is the major change agent in a programme, the implementation system is likely to make an important contribution to programme outcomes. The implementation system provides the means and a context for the intervention and is affected by a number of factors such as characteristics of the implementers, the nature of the implementing organisation and the quality of the linkages between the organisation and the broader community. The level and extent of these aspects of the implementation system should be carefully documented. Once the programme's active ingredients are established, an objective assessment system is needed to monitor the quantity and quality of the programme.

Assessing implementation is a complicated process, as the gaps between plans and delivery may be either positive or negative (Scheirer 1994). It is likely that successful implementation requires more than just faithfully replicating programme components. Programmes are adjusted to meet the needs and capacities of local communities, or to allow consumers to gain ownership of programmes. It is critical to consider the debate between fidelity and adaptation. Programmes may need to be adapted to meet the perceived ecological needs of the context in which the programme is being delivered. This type of local adaptation should be documented and requires to be systematically researched.

The concept of implementation integrity, also referred to as fidelity or adherence, is a determination of how well the programme is being implemented in comparison with the original programme design. Four primary components of programme fidelity have been identified by Dane and Schneider (1998):

1. adherence – whether the programme is being delivered as it was designed or written, i.e. with all the core components being delivered to the appropriate population, staff trained appropriately, using the right protocols, techniques, and materials and in the locations and contexts prescribed
2. exposure – may include the number of sessions implemented, length of each session or the frequency with which programme techniques were implemented
3. quality of programme delivery – manner in which a teacher, volunteer, or staff member delivers a programme (e.g. skill in using the techniques or methods prescribed by the programme, enthusiasm, preparedness, attitude)

4. participant responsiveness – extent to which participants are engaged by and involved in the activities and content of the programme.

Although the concept is not new, research studies on the measurement of programme integrity are relatively recent phenomena. Domitrovich and Greenberg (2000), in a review of implementation in 34 exemplary school-based prevention programmes, report the following findings:

*   59% included some rating of fidelity and adherence in their implementation data, i.e. tracking the programme's essential components with ratings made by independent observers or implementers
*   33% of the studies reported dosage or the amount of the intervention administered to participants
*   12% assessed participant responsiveness such as degree of participant satisfaction or involvement
*   6% assessed programme differentiation which involves verifying the content of experimental conditions
*   only 32% utilised implementation information as a source of data for outcome analyses. Therefore, in the majority of cases the implementation data were not related to programme outcomes.

It is worth noting that the dimension of 'quality of programme delivery' was not included in this review. There is considerable variability in the extent to which attention has been paid to the measurement of implementation. As a result, there is a dearth of information in the published literature to guide practitioners in decisions regarding programme adoption and replication. In contrast to the absence of formal measurement there is, however, a wealth of information based on practitioner experience that does not enter the literature. Domitrovich and Greenberg (2000) refer to this as the 'wisdom literature', namely the body of knowledge that is based on practical experience of programme delivery on the ground. There is a need for greater attention to documenting and accessing this body of knowledge in order to become better informed about the circumstances and practices that enhance programme implementation. Process evaluation techniques, based on careful project description, documentation and monitoring, may be used to assess both the quantity and quality of programme delivery and implementation (Dehar et al 1993).

Monitoring Implementation and Process Evaluation

Mihalic et al (2002) outline the primary purpose of process evaluation as being to improve our understanding of how a programme achieves what it does. It is used to interpret programme outcomes and to inform others wishing to learn from the experiences of the programme (Dehar et al 1993). If programme implementation is not monitored and assessed, an outcome evaluation may be assessing a programme which differs greatly from that originally designed and planned. This seriously limits the strength of conclusions that can be drawn from outcome results. Process evaluation is critical to the validity of programme evaluations. This includes:

* making confident connections between programmes and outcomes (internal validity)
* replicating interventions in other settings (external validity)
* determining how or why a programme works (construct validity)
* variability in implementation – introduces error variance that reduces the power of statistical analyses (statistical conclusion validity).

Implementation or process data are critical for interpreting both positive and negative outcomes; positive findings cannot be attributed to the programme unless you know that the programme was actually conducted. Negative results can arise when a programme is poorly implemented and thus never put to a fair test. Programme evaluations that fail to consider implementation lead to a type III error, i.e. potentially useful programmes will be prematurely and unfairly rejected not because the programme per se does not work but because it has not been properly implemented (Dobson & Cook 1980). As Durlak (1998) points out, unless we assess implementation we do not really know what we are evaluating and run the risk of making a type III error.

Process evaluation may also be viewed as a feedback mechanism that provides data on the range and extent of programme delivery and whether key objectives are being achieved. This information helps to identify areas where the programme may be working well or where objectives are not being met. This information may lead to modifications in order to improve and fine tune aspects of the programme and its delivery, thereby ensuring continuous quality improvement as the programme progresses.

The collection of systematic data on programme implementation also plays an important role in advancing knowledge on best practices for replication in 'real world' settings. Comprehensive documentation of programme delivery provides data on the practical realities of implementation, including programme modification or drift/adaptation for the local setting. This information provides the basis for developing a useful practical guide for others contemplating implementation of a similar programme.

For all of the above, we need to know how well the proposed programme was actually conducted. Both the quantity and quality of implementation need to be assessed; how much of the programme was administered and how well was each part conducted? Process evaluation involves assessing the active ingredients or components of the programme. In addition to the content and structure of the intervention, information is needed on the process and structure of the wider implementation system. This entails gaining an insight into the internal dynamics and operations of the programme; how the various parts of the programme fit together, how the users interact with each other and with the trainers or implementers. Information is also needed on organisational processes, any obstacles encountered and how they were resolved, together with any unexpected benefits. In essence, programme monitoring seeks to understand the strengths and weaknesses of the programme as implemented in the local setting.

Data for process evaluation are primarily gathered from programme records (i.e. forms and activity logs kept by project staff), focus groups, direct observation by the evaluator and information gathered from programme staff and participants through written questionnaires, telephone or in-person interviews. Monitoring implementation is important at each stage, from initial pilot studies through to large-scale implementation.

The following are among the key questions to be asked:

- Are members of the target population being reached successfully?
- What is the profile of actual participants?
- Are the interventions being delivered as intended – frequency, intensity, quality of implementation, feedback from observations, interviews with participants and trainers/programme providers?
- Is the project progressing towards key objectives – are key objectives being addressed and is there preliminary evidence that the objectives are being met?
- Are members of the target group and local agencies/professionals being successfully engaged in the project – interviews with key players and recipients on their perceptions of the project?
- Is there evidence of interagency cooperation?
- What is the added value of the project?

Feedback and Communication

Feedback from the results of the process evaluation may be used to inform key players, managers and programme sponsors of programme performance. Reviewing programme activities and using results from process evaluation could be undertaken in an interactive workshop format. Ongoing planning and review sessions with key stakeholders may be put in place to take stock of what has been achieved, identify strengths and weaknesses, and alter, where needed, the course of action. Evaluators and key stakeholders have an important contribution to make in these sessions and it is important that findings are presented in a format targeted for specific audiences and that there is a willingness and openness to consider both problems and achievements. Putting in place a transparent and frequent feedback system is critical to ensuring good quality communication and cooperation as the project develops.

Ongoing Consultation and Collaboration

Ongoing consultation and collaboration are needed as the programme moves through the different stages of planning and implementation. For example, the training process may not end with the formal training workshop, as it may be necessary to offer continuing support, guidance and consultation as the programme is being implemented. Regular site visits are also helpful in maintaining contact with implementation and provide an opportunity to get feedback, review satisfaction levels and learn first hand of any concerns and difficulties. Ongoing consultation plays an important role in consolidating collaboration and enhancing the sense of efficacy of staff in relation to the programme, and also decreases the likelihood of loss of interest or that the programme will be abandoned due to lack of support services.

Manage Resources

Ongoing management of staff and financial resources is needed as the programme unfolds. Once materials and training have been purchased, the ongoing costs of implementation of each intervention activity including instructors' fees, facilities and equipment should be estimated and actual expenditure carefully monitored. A budget for programme delivery should be developed and potential sources of support, both in kind and financial, should be identified. Budgeting for sustainability should also be taken into account at this point, i.e. what further investments in terms of training, staff and other resources are needed to ensure the ongoing maintenance of the programme in the long term. Due to the likely turnover of project volunteers, paid staff and even steering group members, it may be necessary to recruit and involve new people in the project on an ongoing basis. New sources of energy, commitment and support may be needed as the programme progresses.

Phase 4: Programme Maintenance and Consolidation

By this stage project staff will be experienced with the programme. Implementation problems may have been encountered and resolved, and the programme is being successfully embedded into the local organisational context or setting (Box 2.7).

Integrate Intervention Activities

Programme integration may be planned for early in the life of the programme, or it may take place later, as programme staff and the local organisation gain confidence and become more comfortable with the programme. Putting in place

---

Box 2.7

Phase 4: Programme maintenance and consolidation

- integrate intervention activities
- assess programme effectiveness in terms of process, impact and outcomes
- feed back findings to ensure continuous quality improvement
- put in place strategies to sustain the programme over time

ongoing training opportunities and capacity building for project group members should be considered at this stage. Capacity building will assist with the continuing quality improvement of programme delivery and consolidates the programme by building on achievements to date.

A positive project climate, with good communication and relationships between key players, is a critical factor in promoting and maintaining programmes in the longer term. Fostering good quality relationships is central to building the programme on a foundation of respect, an appreciation of different strengths and an acknowledgement of the contribution of different members. As Bracht et al (1999) point out, good group process is developed and nurtured through an attitude of openness and trust. This applies at all levels, from the steering or advisory group through to project trainers, implementation staff, evaluation personnel and programme recipients. A positive project climate, which fosters an ethos of participation, collaboration and empowerment, provides the right environment in which enthusiasm, creativity and good quality work can be promoted and maintained.

Assess and Feed back Findings on Programme Effectiveness

A formal system of evaluation needs to be put in place in order to systematically assess programme inputs, process, impact and outcomes. The ongoing monitoring of programme activities makes possible the periodic review of project achievements and progress towards desired goals and objectives. A variety of quantitative and qualitative indicators of success can be evaluated (Zubrick & Kovess-Masfety 2005). These include information on awareness, participation, knowledge, attitudes and behaviour change together with programme reach, participant engagement, partnership building, interagency and cross-sectoral cooperation. These indicators provide evidence of programme performance; they can be used to demonstrate programme accountability and provide feedback to programme managers, sponsors and key stakeholder groups. Results from the various types of process and outcome data will be helpful in assessing the programme's successes and challenges. Further details on the different types of evaluation methods employed in specific programmes and case studies are outlined in later chapters. However, it suffices to highlight at this point the importance of providing feedback of evaluation findings together with opportunities for key stakeholders to systematically review programme results in order to take stock of programme achievements and identify areas for modification. This allows for decisions concerning the programme's future to be made based on empirical data as well as more anecdotal evidence.

Moving from Implementation to Sustainability

As a programme progresses to more widespread implementation, another critical step involves identifying what factors increase the potential for sustainability of effective interventions. There is a need to consider the organisational structures and policies that are necessary to support long-term maintenance and sustainability of quality programmes. To effectively maintain quality programmes, practitioners in collaboration with programme evaluators will need to identify key programme elements needed for a high probability of success such as organisational capacity, quality training, funding, stability, commitment and resources. Some programmes may need new sponsors; other programmes may need to be significantly changed. Developing a strategy or plan for continued collaboration and partnerships is critical to the continued sustainability of the programme. Such a plan should include key players such as agencies motivated by the programme, programme participants, project staff and programme sponsors. Disseminating information on project activities and evaluation results increases the project's visibility, acceptance and level of interest among potential support sources. Maintaining high visibility and ensuring that key decision makers learn about the project or programme may also be critical in determining whether resources will be made available for the project's continuance. An opportunity to witness the programme in action and to speak with programme implementers and recipients may also be useful in convincing decision makers about the value and worth of the programme. A combination of good quality relationships, a high standard of implementation and rigorous evaluation together with widespread programme acceptance and support provides the basis for effective and long lasting mental health promotion practice.

Conclusions and Recommendations

In this chapter we have outlined the various stages and steps involved in programme planning and implementation. It is important to note that these stages begin as early as when a progamme is being considered and planned (pre-adoption), through to programme implementation (delivery) and programme consolidation and maintenance (sustainability). Barry et al (2005) provide a useful overview of the strategies that can be used to improve the overall implementation and delivery of mental health promotion programmes. Recommendations, based on the work of Barry et al (2005), for practitioners and programme developers to support effective implementation across the various stages are reproduced in Box 2.8. As a programme moves to more widespread implementation and replication, practitioners in collaboration with programme evaluators will need to identify key programme elements needed for a high probability of success and identify factors that increase the potential for sustainability of effective programmes. This entails clearly identifying core elements of the programme content together with the implementation system and organisational structures needed to support the long-term maintenance and sustainability of the programme. Based on Barry et al (2005), the recommendations for policymakers and researchers in supporting and evaluating the quality of programme implementation are outlined in Box 2.9.

Box 2.8

Recommendations for practitioners in improving programme implementation

(adapted from Barry et al 2005 and reprinted by permission of the IUHPE journal *Promotion and Education*)

Programme initiation and planning phase

- assess the characteristics and resources available in the local community
- identify the problems and associated risk and protective factors for that community
- verify that the programme model is appropriate for implementation in the target community
- involve key stakeholders in the decision-making process including implementing staff, management and potential programme recipients
- ensure buy-in of all parties by providing documentation that supports the need for the programme (e.g. the evidence base for the programme and the match between the approach adopted and the needs in the community)
- identify the key components of the intervention based on underlying programme theory
- identify and communicate programme objectives, principles and the mechanisms that will be used to achieve them to all relevant players at the planning stage
- provide decision makers and stakeholders with the necessary information to secure adequate resources to implement the programme
- lay the foundation for successful cooperation and collaboration by clearly defining the roles of all parties involved and establish a system for discussing and resolving problems
- plan for the long-term sustainability of the programme

Delivery phase

- assess readiness to implement the programme
- make modifications or adaptations in delivering the programme, balancing programme fidelity with the needs of the local site
- draw on the 'wisdom knowledge' of those with experience of the programme
- develop a structured manual or detailed programme description to facilitate programme implementation
- train programme staff to conduct the programme effectively
- provide ongoing support and supervision once the programme has begun
- partner with an evaluator to develop an implementation monitoring system that includes assessment of the programme (i.e. programme fidelity, exposure, quality of delivery, participant responsiveness and programme differentiation), support system, and key system factors

Box 2.8 Continued

Programme maintenance and sustainability phase

- develop a plan for the sustainability of the programme based on existing funding, long-term priorities and resources
- use implementation information and process evaluation data to fine tune and improve programme delivery
- provide regular updates and evaluation information to key stakeholders
- document the provision of feedback and any subsequent changes that are made to the programme

Box 2.9

Recommendations for policymakers and researchers in improving programme implementation

(adapted from Barry et al 2005 and reprinted by permission of the IUHPE journal *Promotion and Education*)

Policymakers

- the decision to adopt a best practice programme does not guarantee success without attention to good quality implementation
- provide adequate resources for programme development and replication including the necessary staff skills, training, supervision and organisational support needed to implement the programme to a high level of quality
- invest in process evaluation in order to facilitate and enhance knowledge and best practice in programme implementation

Researchers

- systematically monitor and assess programme implementation as a core part of programme evaluation
- collect qualitative data on the barriers, obstacles and facilitating factors encountered in the course of programme delivery
- gather information from multiple sources including programme recipients, implementers and researcher observation, in order to to reduce bias in assessing the quality of implementation
- identify key mediating variables that are theorised to be responsible for the programme outcomes
- relate variability in implementation to short-term and long-term programme outcomes
- work in partnership with practitioners, employing collaborative evaluation methods, in order to feed back implementation findings and to ensure continuous improvement of programme quality

References

Barry M M, Domitrovich C, Lara M A 2005 The implementation of mental health promotion programmes. Promotion and Education Suppl2:30–35

Botvin G J 1983 Life skills training: teachers manual. Smithfield Press, New York

Botvin G J, Tortu S 1988 Preventing adolescent substance abuse through life skills training. In: Price R H, Cowen E L, Lorion R P et al (eds) Fourteen ounces of prevention: a casebook for practitioners. American Psychological Association, Washington DC:98–110

Botvin G J, Dusenbury L, Baker E et al 1989 A skills training approach to smoking prevention among Hispanic youth. Journal of Behavioral Medicine 12:279–296

Botvin G J, Baker E, Dusenbury L et al 1990a Preventing adolescent drug abuse through a multi-modal cognitive-behavioral approach: results of a three-year study. Journal of Consulting and Clinical Psychology 58:437–446

Botvin G J, Bauer E, Filazzola A et al 1990b A cognitive-behavioral approach to substance abuse prevention: a one-year follow up. Addictive Behavior 15:47–63

Botvin G J, Baker E, Dusenbury L et al 1995 Long-term follow-up results of a randomized drug abuse prevention trial in a white middle-class population. Journal of the American Medical Association 273:1106–1112

Bracht N, Kingsbury L, Rissel C 1999 A five-stage community organization model for health promotion: empowerment and partnership strategies. In: Bracht N (ed) Health promotion at the community level 2: new advances. Sage, California:83–117

Bronfenbrenner U 1979 The ecology of human development: experiments by nature and design. Harvard University Press, Cambridge, Massachusetts

Bush P J, Zuckerman A E, Taggart V S et al 1989 Cardiovascular risk factor prevention in black school children: the "Know Your Body" evaluation project. Health Education Quarterly 16:215–227

Chen H 1998 Theory-driven evaluations. Advances in Educational Productivity 7:15–34

Connell D B, Turner R R, Mason E F 1985 Summary findings of the school health education evaluation: health promotion effectiveness, implementation and costs. Journal of School Health 55:316–321

Curran J, Wishart P, Gingrich J 1999 JOBS: a manual for teaching people successful job search strategies. Michigan Prevention Research Center, Institute for Social Research, University of Michigan

Dane A V, Schneider B H 1998 Program integrity in primary and early secondary prevention: are implementation effects out of control? Clinical Psychology Review 18(1):23–45

Dehar M A, Caswell S, Duignan P 1993 Formative and process evaluation of health promotion and disease prevention programs. Evaluation Review 17:204–220

Dobson D, Cook T J 1980 Avoiding type III error in program evaluation: results from a field experiment. Evaluation and Program Planning 3:269–276

Domitrovich C E, Greenberg M T 2000 The study of implementation: current findings from effective programs that prevent mental disorders in school-aged children. Journal of Educational and Psychological Consultation 11(2):193–221

Durlak J A 1995 School-based prevention programs for children and adolescents. Sage, California

Durlak J A 1997 Successful prevention programs for children and adolescents. Plenum Press, New York

Durlak J A 1998 Why program implementation is important. Journal of Prevention and Intervention in the Community 17(2):5–18

Durlak J A, Wells A M 1997 Primary prevention mental health programs for children and adolescents: a meta-analytic review. American Journal of Community Psychology 25(2):115–152

Durlak J A, Wells A M 1998 Evaluation of indicated preventive intervention (secondary prevention) mental health programs for children and adolescents. American Journal of Community Psychology 26:775–802

Elliott D (ed) 1997 Blueprints for violence prevention (Vols 1–11). Center for the Study and Prevention of Violence, Institute of

Behavioral Science, University of Colorado, Boulder, Colorado

Everhart K, Wandersman A 2000 Applying comprehensive quality programming and empowerment evaluation to reduce implementation barriers. Journal of Educational and Psychological Consultation 11(2):177–191

Fawcett S B, Lewis R K, Paine-Andrews A et al 1997 Evaluating community coalitions for the prevention of substance abuse: the case of Project Freedom. Health Education and Behavior 24:812–828

Garland A F, Zigler E 1993 Adolescent suicide prevention. Current research and social policy implications. American Psychologist 48(2):169–182

Green L W, Kreuter M W 1999 Health promotion planning: an educational and ecological approach, 3rd edn. Mayfield, Mountain View, California

Gresham F M, Cohen S, Rosenblum S et al 1993 Treatment integrity of school-based behavioural intervention studies: 1980–1990. School Psychology Review 22(2):254–272

Hosman C, Jané-Llopis E 1999 Political challenges 2: Mental health. In: The evidence of health promotion effectiveness: shaping public health in a new Europe, Chapter 3: 29–41. A Report for the European Commission. International Union for Health Promotion and Education, Paris

Jessor R 1982 Critical issues in research on adolescent health promotion. In: Coates T, Petersen A, Perry C (eds) Promoting adolescent health: a dialog on research and practice. Academic Press, New York:447–465

Lister-Sharp D, Chapman S, Stewart-Brown S et al 1999 Health promoting schools and health promotion in schools: two systematic reviews. Health Technology Assessment, London

Mihalic S 2001 The importance of implementation fidelity. Online. Available: http://www.colorado.edu/cspv/blueprints/newsletter/pdf/BPNewsVol2Issue1.pdf October 2005

Mihalic S, Fagan A, Irwin K et al 2002 Blueprints for violence prevention replications: factors for implementation success. Institute of Behavioral Science, University of Colorado, Boulder

Mrazek P, Haggerty R (eds) 1994 Reducing risk for mental disorders. National Academy Press, Washington DC

Olds D L 1988 The prenatal/early infancy project. In: Price R H, Cowen E L, Lorion R P et al (eds) Fourteen ounces of prevention: a casebook for practitioners. American Psychological Association, Washington DC

Pentz M A, Trebow E A, Hansen W B et al 1990 Effects of program implementation on adolescent drug use behavior: the Midwestern Prevention Project (MPP). Evaluation Review 14(3):264–289

Price R, Smith S 1985 A guide to evaluating prevention programs in mental health. US Government Printing Office, Washington DC

Price R H, Cowen E L, Lorion R P et al (eds) 1988 Fourteen ounces of prevention: a casebook for practitioners. American Psychological Association, Washington DC

Rappaport J 1990 Research methods and the empowerment social agenda. In: Tolan P, Keyes C, Chertok F et al (eds) Researching community psychology: integrating theories and methodologies. American Psychological Association, Washington DC:51–63

Reiss D 1981 The family's construction of reality. Harvard University Press, Cambridge, Massachusetts

Rissel C, Bracht N 1999 Assessing community needs, resources and readiness: building on strengths. In: Bracht N (ed) Health promotion at the community level 2: new advances. Sage, California:59–71

Scheirer M A 1994 Designing and using process evaluation. In: Wholey J S, Hatry H P, Newcomer K E (eds) Handbook of practical program evaluation. Jossey-Bass, San Francisco:40–68

Smith D W, McCormick L K, Steckler A B et al 1993 Teachers use of health curricula: implementation of Growing Healthy, Project SMART and the Teenage Health Teaching modules. Journal of School Health 63:349–354

Taggart V S, Bush P J, Zuckerman A E et al 1990 A process evaluation of the District of Columbia "Know Your Body" project. Journal of School Health 60:60–66

Tilford S, Delaney F, Vogels M 1997 Effectiveness of mental health promotion interventions: a review. Health Education Authority, London

Vinokur A D, Price R H, Schul Y 1995 Impact of the JOBS intervention on unemployed workers varying in risk for depression. American Journal of Community Psychology 232(1):39–74

Wall M A, Severson H H, Andrews J A et al 1995 Pediatric office-based smoking intervention: impact on maternal smoking and relapse. Pediatrics 96:622–628

Webster-Stratton C, Mihalic S, Fagan A et al 2001 Blueprints for violence prevention. Book eleven: The Incredible Years: parent, teacher and child training series. Center for the Study and Prevention of Violence, Institute of Behavioral Science, University of Colorado, Boulder, Colorado

Weissberg R P 1990 Fidelity and adaptation: combining the best of two perspectives. In: Tolan P, Keys C, Chertok F et al (eds) Researching community psychology: issues of theories and methods. American Psychological Association, Washington DC:186–190

Weissberg R P, Caplan M, Harwood R L 1991 Promoting competent young people in competence-enhancing environments: a systems-based perspective on primary prevention. Journal of Consulting and Clinical Psychology 59:830–841

Zins J E, Elias M J, Greenberg M T et al 2000 Promoting quality implementation in prevention programs. Journal of Educational and Psychological Consultation 11(2):173–174

Zubrick S, Kovess-Masfety V 2005 Indicators of mental health. In: Herrman H, Saxena S, Moodie R (eds) Promoting mental health: concepts, emerging evidence, practice. A report of the World Health Organization, Department of Mental Health and Substance Abuse in collaboration with the Victorian Health Promotion Foundation and University of Melbourne, WHO, Geneva:148–166

Community Mental Health Promotion

3

Introduction

Working at the community level presents possibly one of the most challenging and exciting settings for mental health promotion practice. Community settings are complex and dynamic, composed of many sub-settings such as schools, workplaces and neighbourhoods, with population groups ranging from childhood through to old age. As such the community setting offers important opportunities to work with diverse groups across a range of different settings and sectors. A community approach to mental health promotion views mental health as a positive resource for individuals and communities embedded within the cultural, social and economic contexts of everyday life. This approach is based on a socioecological perspective of mental health, which conceptualises mental health as the interaction between the person, social settings and systems, including the structure of social support and power (Orford 1992). This approach, therefore, underscores the importance of social interventions addressing systems of socialisation, social support and control operating at multiple levels.

Community working is essentially characterised by collaborative practice, based on the facilitation of active community participation and the enhancement of community empowerment. These are fundamental guiding principles of a community model of practice. This style of practice is often characterised as a 'bottom-up' approach and is derived from community development or community organisation models of health promotion. These approaches are well documented in the health promotion literature and there are many excellent examples of their application which the reader may wish to consult (see, for example, Bracht et al 1999). The area of community mental health promotion is probably less well documented in the literature. However, many of the fundamental principles of community health promotion programme planning and delivery apply equally well to community mental health promotion. In this chapter we explore the application of these principles in practice and examine the main factors which influence their successful implementation. Practical examples from tried and tested model programmes, as well as new programmes in development, are used to illustrate the translation of these concepts into reality. This chapter addresses a range of different implementation strategies that may be applied with diverse groups across different settings within the community context. These include implementing comprehensive multi-level programmes, community partnerships, empowerment and peer support strategies. Case studies illustrating the practical implementation of programmes employing these different strategies are used to guide the reader in applying the research and theory to practice. Prior to outlining these different implementation strategies, the rationale and underlying principles of working at the community level in mental health promotion practice are discussed. Many of these principles, for example those relating to good practice in developing collaborative partnerships, will equally apply when working in other settings such as the home, schools, workplaces and health services, as discussed in subsequent chapters.

Rationale for Community Mental Health Promotion

Community mental health promotion provides a unique opportunity to put into practice the principles of community participation and empowerment as outlined in the Ottawa Charter (WHO 1986). Both of these concepts occupy a special importance in mental health promotion practice. Strengthening community action is one of the five key action areas identified in the Ottawa Charter (WHO 1986):

> Health promotion works through concrete and effective action in setting priorities, making decisions, planning strategies and implementing them to achieve better health. At the heart of this process is the empowerment of communities... their ownership and control of their own endeavours and destinies.

The community has been described as the new 'centre of gravity' for health promotion (Green & Kreuter 1991), signalling a shift from the more traditional individual or lifestyle approach to the community as the locus of practice

(Robertson & Minkler 1994). There is growing recognition that lasting, wide-spread change is more likely to occur if a broad range of stakeholders, including citizens, community groups, health professionals, statutory and voluntary agencies are involved in a process to bring about change within a supportive environmental context.

Participation

The principle of participation, central to community-based approaches to health, is based on the premise that change is more likely to occur when the people it affects are involved in the change process. Participation by local people is posited as having the greatest and most sustainable impact in solving local problems and in setting local norms. As articulated by Thompson and Kinne, 'Change is more likely to be successful and permanent when the people it affects are involved in initiating and promoting it' (1999:30). The process of community participation and engagement is recognised as promoting a sense of ownership of the programme, which in turn leads to increased 'capacity' or competence and promotes programme maintenance (Bracht & Kingsbury 1990, Flynn 1995, Robertson & Minkler 1994). Shediac-Razallah and Bone argue that at the core of all these related concepts is the idea of 'the process of enabling individuals and communities, in partnership with health professionals, to participate in defining their health problems and shaping solutions to those problems' (1998:95).

Socioecological Perspective

At a theoretical level, community health promotion practice draws on a socio-ecological model of health which points to the importance of the larger socio-environmental context within which individuals, group systems and social settings are embedded. The social ecology perspective recognises that the potential to change individual behaviour is best considered within the social and cultural context in which it occurs (Goodman 2000). Interventions that are informed by this perspective are directed mainly at social factors such as community norms, structures and services. Stokols et al describe ecologically informed programmes as addressing '... interdependencies between socioeconomic, cultural, political, environmental, organizational, psychological, and biological determinants of health and illness' (1996:247). A key concept underpinning the socioecological perspective is that of interdependence; the fact that behaviour is influenced by multiple interacting systems. As outlined in Chapter 1, Bronfenbrenner's (1979) model of nested systems (micro, meso, exo and macro systems), operating at individual, family, community and broader societal levels, interact with and mutually influence each other. The community may be seen as the interface between these multiple interacting systems, i.e. the individual, group, organisational, environmental and policy systems. As such, community programmes have the capacity to address these multiple interacting levels thereby increasing the synergistic or interactive effect of the intervention. Based on this theoretical perspective, which draws on Lewin's (1951) person-in-context principle, mental health is conceptualised as the interaction, over time, between the person and social settings and systems including the influence of broader social, economic and political forces. This perspective, which has been most clearly elaborated

85

within community psychology (see, for example, Orford 1992), underscores the importance of mediating structures such as schools, workplaces and community settings as providing key contexts for social interventions operating from the micro to the macro levels.

Social Inclusion and Mental Health

Belonging to a social network of communication and supportive relationships is protective of good health and positive well-being (Wilkinson & Marmot 2003). There is a large body of evidence which shows that more socially isolated people have poorer health and increased mortality (Berkman & Glass 2000, House et al 1988) and that more socially cohesive societies are healthier and have lower mortality rates (Kawachi & Kennedy 1997). A socially inclusive society may be defined as one where 'all people feel valued, their differences are respected, and their basic needs are met so that they can live in dignity' (VicHealth 2005). Durkeim (1897) was one of the first to propose that a lack of cohesion in society or 'anomie' contributes to negative mental health and is a leading factor influencing rates of suicide. Variations in suicidal behaviour and anti-social behaviour have been traced to the presence or absence of social cohesion (OECD 2001). Davey Smith et al 2001 report that suicide is strongly associated with social fragmentation characterised by neighbourhoods with high levels of private renting, mobility, unmarried persons and persons living alone. A culture of cooperation and tolerance between individuals, institutions and diverse groups in society; a sense of belonging to family, one's school, workplace and community, and a good network of social relationships have all been identified as protective factors for positive health and social outcomes (Moodie & Jenkins 2005). It is now widely recognised that social exclusion damages mental and physical health and contributes significantly to inequalities (Mentality 2003). Communities can feel marginalised, fearful, excluded and disempowered in their ability to influence decisions and to participate fully in the social, economic, political and cultural systems that affect their lives. Perceptions of racial discrimination have been identified as a significant factor in the poor health of black and ethnic minority communities, over and above the contribution of socioeconomic factors (Nazroo 1998, Nazroo & Karlsen 2001).

The concept of social capital has emerged as important in describing the features of social relationships within a social group or community. Putnam defines social capital as 'the connections among individuals – social networks and the norms of reciprocity and trustworthiness that arise from them' (2000:19). Social capital is not conceived as an individual resource but is seen as an ecological characteristic, which emerges from the interactions and shared norms that are inherent in the structure of social relationships and that are external to the individual (Henderson & Whiteford 2003). Research on social capital and inequality points to the importance of community cohesion, such as levels of trust, reciprocity and participation in civic organisations, as important influences on health status (Mentality 2003). Putnam (2001) indicates that economic inequality and civic inequality are less in areas with higher values of social capital. Similarly, Putnam (2001) reports that in areas with low levels of social capital and high levels of perceived inequality, self-reported well-being and levels of happiness are lower. Wilkinson (1996) also emphasises the importance of psychosocial pathways in examining the relationship between income inequality, social capital and health. Whiteford et al (2005) provide an interesting overview of the relationship between social capital, health and mental health and the potential of mental health promotion to enhance social capital.

Community initiatives aimed at building social capital, seeking to strengthen community networks and increasing participation by excluded groups have an important contribution to make in mental health promotion. Urban regeneration projects, which address the psychosocial aspects of deprivation, may have a significant mental health impact. A large prospective controlled trial by Thomson et al (2003) has shown that housing improvements can reduce anxiety, depression and self-reported mental health problems. Likewise, access to open spaces and the quality of the built environment have a beneficial impact on mental health (Dalgard & Tambs 1997).

The mental health benefits of participation in community arts, drama, sports and culture have also been recognised both for the general population and for people with a mental disorder who may experience higher levels of social exclusion due to prejudice and stigma. Moodie and Jenkins (2005) and Mentality (2003) report on a number of initiatives, such as Arts on Prescription in the UK, the Women's Circus in Melbourne for survivors of physical and sexual abuse and VicHealth's Sport and Active recreation programme (VicHealth 2004a), all of which promote self-esteem, identity, strengthen communities and social inclusion. In a review of 60 community-based arts projects, Matarasso (1997) found that the benefits of participation included increased confidence, community empowerment, self-determination, improved local image and greater social cohesion.

Intersectoral Working and Partnerships

As our understanding of the nature of mental health and its determinants broadens, so also does our appreciation of the need to address the factors outside of the health area that influence mental health. A community perspective recognises that many public and private sectors and players can have a critical influence on mental health at the community level. Sectors outside of the health area are recognised as having an important role to play, for example, educational institutions such as schools, the media, local government and planning authorities, economic and commercial organisations, employment and transport sectors, faith groups, voluntary organisations, social, cultural, sports and civic groups. Partnership working and intersectoral collaboration are now very much at the core of modern health promotion practice where community members, health professionals, governmental and non-governmental agencies work together in achieving agreed goals and objectives in promoting health and well-being. Collaborative community partnerships based on existing strengths and resources are, therefore, recognised as a key strategy for community mental health promotion (Box 3.1). Community programmes that are based on community resources and collaborative structures are also more likely to be relevant, meaningful and ethnically and culturally more appropriate for that community and are also more likely to be owned by that community. An ecologically valid programme fits the community context because its design is driven by community needs and its implementation process complements existing community strengths and resources (Foster-Fishman et al 2001).

Box 3.1

Arguments for a community-based approach

- community-based programmes have the capacity to address multiple interacting levels of the person, situation and environment, thereby increasing the synergistic effect of intervention programmes
- community-wide interventions have the potential to reach a wider range of population groups across a range of setting and sectors
- cross-sectoral community approaches provide an opportunity to engage with multiple stakeholders through collaborative partnerships in addressing the broader social determinants of mental health
- community programmes reinforce social norms, and promote structures and environments that are supportive of positive mental health across multiple segments of the community
- community programmes which target the whole community are more likely to avoid the stigma and negative labelling associated with programmes targeted at specific groups, such as those who are disadvantaged or regarded as being at higher risk of mental health problems
- the process of participation, which is central to community practice, is recognised as promoting a sense of ownership of the programme and enhancing overall community competence and capacity
- programmes that are planned and designed through community partnerships and collaboration are more likely to be ecologically valid, i.e. relevant, meaningful and culturally appropriate for the community in which the programme is implemented
- collaborative community programmes, through the empowerment of community members, contribute to the development of local expertise which increases the possibility of sustaining local initiatives after initial funding

Conceptual Approaches

A community perspective to promoting positive mental health calls for appropriate models and implementation strategies to ensure that the desired process of implementation and programme outcomes are achieved. In broad terms, two main conceptual approaches to community working can be identified: programmes which adopt a community-based or community organisation approach and programmes which embrace a community development approach. Programmes adopting a community-based approach are those where the main purpose of the community setting is to consult with and reach as wide a range as possible of community members. Community organisation approaches have been defined as those involving and mobilising major agencies, institutions and groups in a community to work together to coordinate services and create programmes for the united purpose of improving the health of a community (Robinson & Elliott 2000). These universal programmes are frequently prevention oriented, addressing single issues such as violence reduction or substance abuse. Examples of these approaches are the large-scale community programmes such as the Communities that Care initiative (Hawkins et al 2002) and the Midwestern Prevention Project (Pentz et al 1997), as described in this chapter. Community development approaches, on the other hand, are often described as 'bottom-up' approaches or grassroots initiatives where community members actively participate in identifying their own needs and organise themselves in planning and devising strategies for meeting shared needs. An example of this approach is illustrated in this chapter by a case study from South Africa on developing partnerships with women and children from disadvantaged communities. The principles of active participation and empowerment are central to this collective process. As a health promotion practice, community development has been defined as 'the process of organising and/or supporting community groups in identifying their health issues, planning and acting upon their strategies for a social action/change, and gaining increased self-reliance and decision-making power as a result of their activities' (Labonté 1993:237).

The community development approach, in which local communities identify and address local concerns, appears to hold much promise for community mental health promotion programmes, especially when working in low-income settings and countries. A community health development continuum is a useful way of conceptualising the process of translating community participation and empowerment principles into programmes on the ground. Community development may be portrayed as involving a series of stages each with varying degrees of potential for maximising community empowerment (Jackson et al 1989, Labonté 1989). These stages cover personal development, mutual support, issue identification in community organisations, participation in organisations and coalitions and collective political and social action. These stages represent a continuum from personal to collective levels of empowerment. Both the psychological and community empowerment process is embraced with the potential for empowerment being maximised as one moves from the individual to the collective action end of the continuum. Individual level empowerment may entail personal development and capacity building such as skills training or improved self-efficacy. This level of empowerment may be necessary for a person to function within and participate in a group process or, indeed, in society. Likewise, social involvement may lead to increased personal development. Active participation in community groups or partnerships is recognised as offering important opportunities for both personal and community empowerment (Florin & Wandersman 1990). Participation in the group collective process is a way of increasing awareness of the influence of wider social structures on health issues and also of acquiring skills and capacities required to strengthen local community capacities. Ideally, community participation should lead to increased empowerment among community members and increased capacity and control as a result of the process. Programmes operating at these different levels of the continuum are discussed in this chapter to highlight the application of empowerment principles in mental health promotion practice.

There are clearly ideological differences between the community organisation and community development approaches with consequent implications for planning and implementation processes such as consultation mechanisms, community participation and ownership. However, as Tones and Tilford (2001) point out, both types of programme acknowledge the importance of supportive environments and community involvement in bringing about sustainable change.

The reader is directed to Bracht et al (1999) for a useful overview of the origins of these different models and the general theories and principles underpinning community and system level change (Thompson & Kinne 1999). While models may vary in the degree and extent of community participation, control and ownership, a key feature of community approaches is that community members are actively involved in community change. Adopting a community approach calls for a change in the style of practice and the role of the professional in implementing such programmes within the community setting. Professional skills and competencies are required in facilitating effective community structures and collaborative mechanisms for the implementation of community programmes. Minkler (1994) outlined ten 'commitments' to community health education practice, which apply equally well to community mental health promotion. These commitments, listed in Box 3.2, efficiently sum up the perspectives and attitudes required when embarking on community practice and provide a good starting point in orienting the practitioner to some of the key challenges of working in the community setting.

Box 3.2

Minkler's ten commitments for community health education
(based on Minkler M 1994 Health Education Research: Theory and Practice 9(4):527–534, with permission of Oxford University Press)

1. Start where the people are at
A commitment to starting where the people are emphasises the importance of health agencies and organisations listening to the community's assessment of its strengths and needs, following the community agenda rather than their own in order to benefit both communities and the organisations that serve them.

2. Recognise and build on community strengths
Identifying, fostering and working through natural helping networks in a community, respecting local customs and beliefs and involving community members in the design of 'culturally competent' programmes are among the ways to demonstrate a commitment to the principle of identifying and building on community strengths and assets.

3. Honor thy community – but do not make it holy
Respecting and working in partnership with communities and recognising them as part of the critical context in which the individual is embedded. Develop and use an 'epidemiology of strengths' rather than relying on the traditional 'epidemiology of pathologies' (Greiger 1993). However, this does not mean romanticising communities and argues instead for following a social justice principle of practice and avoiding exclusionary agendas which may arise in some communities.

Box 3.2 Continued

4. Fostering high level community participation

The principles of participation reflect a belief in the need for high level community involvement at every stage of the work. This means tackling the realities of power, control and ownership including the structural distinctions between communities and professionals.

5. Laughter is good medicine – and good health education

Given the nature of the issues confronted such as substance abuse, violence, suicide, etc., it is important to recognise and appreciate the healing benefits of laughter. Incorporating humour into the work, whether with communities or professional colleagues, is encouraged.

6. Health education is educational – but it is also political

Highlights the role of political analysis and activism and also the importance of reframing health problems and their solution in terms of political, economic and social contexts (Minkler 1994).

7. Thou shalt not tolerate the bad 'isms'

Reminder that health education and promotion is about inclusion, not exclusion, and attitudes and practice predicated on racism, sexism, ageism, homophobia and other forms of exclusion must be fought at all levels of professional involvement.

8. 'Think globally, act locally'

Highlights the importance of helping to meet local needs without losing sight of the larger global picture and advocating the need for macro level social change efforts.

9. Foster individual and community empowerment

Refers to working with communities in creating environments in which individuals and communities can take the power they need to transform their lives (Miller 1985).

10. Work for social justice

Using skills in organising and advocacy to work for public health and social justice on a broader level; 'blending science and politics with a social justice orientation to… make the system work better for those with the least resources' (Wallack et al 1993).

The Process of Implementing Community Mental Health Promotion Programmes

Given the breadth and complexity of the area, the process of implementing community mental health promotion programmes requires special attention. The impact of community programmes may depend as much on how the programme is implemented, i.e. methods and style of delivery, as on what is implemented, i.e. programme content. Working at the community level calls for skills in collaboration, partnership working and political savvy concerning local power structures. Programmes need to be tailored to the local setting and have the flexibility to evolve organically in response to local needs, interests, capacities, emerging opportunities and challenges. For all these reasons the implementation of community-based programmes calls for clearly defined goals and objectives and a structured plan to guide collaborative programme planning and delivery. These factors have already been discussed in Chapter 2. Community programmes are committed to the principles of collaborative working, facilitating meaningful participation and enhancing community empowerment.

Implementing Collaborative Community Programmes

A core feature of all community working is collaborative practice or intersectoral collaboration as referred to in the Ottawa Charter (WHO 1986). This model of collaborative working builds on existing community organisations and structures to address community issues. The process of collaborative working involves building links among a diverse range of organisations, groups and agencies across a range of sectors that have a stake in the issues being addressed (see, for example, the World Health Organization (WHO) Healthy Cities initiative by the WHO Regional Office for Europe 1997).

The collaborative style of working leads to the development of interorganisational and intersectoral collaborative structures, varyingly titled as community coalitions, community partnerships and strategic alliances between health agencies and different sectors. Hauf and Bond (2002) use the term 'community-based collaboration' to refer specifically to collaborative efforts that are anchored in partnerships among individuals and groups within the community, bringing together local stakeholders who affect and are affected by the issue being addressed.

> Good collaboration both facilitates desired programme outcomes and supports the functioning and development of the people, organization and agencies committed to promoting mental health in their communities. (Hauf & Bond 2002:52)

Hauf and Bond (2002) highlight that the sharing of resources, power and authority differentiates collaboration from other less dynamic forms of intergroup cooperation. Hauf and Bond point out that the strength of community-based collaboration is that many different stakeholders contribute to and facilitate a programme by working together to achieve its goals: 'Successful community-based collaborations include stakeholders who contribute the understanding, skills and contacts necessary for working effectively with and within the local political environment' (2002:48). Therefore, effective community-based collaborations need to include community representatives, local leaders, activists, policy makers, local organisations and agencies as well as local mental health and health professionals. Adequate start-up time is needed for a new programme to develop linkages in the community, building trust, establishing common goals and agreeing a common vision thereby laying the foundation for effective programme implementation and sustainability. The breadth and diversity of membership is one of the key strengths of collaborative working and needless to say is also one of the key challenges in making them work effectively. Adopting effective collaborative practice is not without its difficulties and this fact has been well recognised. Hauf and Bond (2002) discuss recommendations for some of the more common challenges encountered in this style of working (Box 3.3).

Box 3.3

Recommendations for overcoming challenges to community-based collaboration in prevention and mental health promotion

(based on Hauf & Bond 2002, with permission of The Clifford Beers Foundation)

- create a team approach
- involve all stakeholders in planning the programme design
- negotiate clear roles, responsibilities and contributions for each stakeholder
- develop joint goals and mutual priorities
- share responsibilities for achieving explicitly stated and agreed goals
- agree upon procedures for handling grievances
- work to develop buy-in and commitment from each stakeholder
- establish strong leadership and effective coordination among stakeholders
- provide (and support involvement in) training and professional development activities that collaborators can participate in together throughout all phases of the project
- help stakeholders to become familiar with each others' skills and expertise
- explore differences, assumptions, biases and confusion related to differences in professional culture
- work to develop skills and relationships that support collaborative partnerships
- maintain frequent communication among collaborators
- negotiate areas of tension and fear among stakeholders
- identify and negotiate on-going contributions of resources for meeting unanticipated needs

The processes of collaborative working and maintaining collaborative partnerships call for a wide range of skills and also provide an important context for the sharing and developing of those skills among key players in programme planning and delivery. Different forms of structures and partnerships have been identified in the literature for organising collaborative working. These include community coalitions, advisory boards, community boards, task forces, steering committees, informal networks and consortia, among others. The reader is directed to Bracht et al (1999), Butterfoss et al (1993) and related papers in a special issue on community coalitions in the journal *Health Education Research* 1993, volume 8(3), for a more detailed discussion of these various structures and their defining characteristics. In general terms, the coalition or alliance of several community groups and health organisations has now become a popular vehicle for implementing community health promotion programmes. 'Coalitions, partnerships and other collaborative efforts bring together representatives of community institutions in order to combine resources and foster relations needed to address threats to the community' (Chavis 2001:311). Coalitions have built community health and resilience by promoting economic development, intergroup relations, civic participation and other community strengths. Himmelman (2001) delineates four levels of partnerships; networking, coordinating, cooperating and collaborating. Himmelman identifies partners as collaborating when they demonstrate their willingness to enhance each other's capacity for mutual benefit and a common purpose by sharing risks, responsibilities, resources and rewards.

Wolff (2001) provides an attractively simple definition of a community coalition as being a group that involves multiple sectors of the community and comes together to address community needs and solve community problems. Wolff uses the following criteria to characterise a community coalition:

- composed of community members
- focuses mainly on local issues
- addresses community needs, building on community assets
- helps resolve community problems through collaboration
- is community wide and has representatives from multiple sectors
- works on multiples issues
- is citizen-influenced if not necessarily citizen-driven
- is a long-term, not an ad hoc, coalition.

In Wolff's practitioner's guide to successful coalitions (2001) he also identifies the characteristics of the most effective community coalitions as follows:

- adopt a holistic and comprehensive approach to addressing community priorities
- are flexible and responsive to community needs
- build a sense of community by creating a forum where the community can gather to solve local problems
- build and enhance resident engagement in community life by providing a structure through which people can engage with others in addressing local concerns
- provide an opportunity for civic engagement thereby building social capital
- provide a vehicle for community empowerment through opportunities for citizen participation and making an impact at the local level
- allow diversity to be valued and celebrated as different community groups and sectors identify common ground and share common goals
- incubators for innovative solutions for challenging problems with relevance to larger national issues.

Many of the key elements which make community coalitions successful tend to be recorded in the 'wisdom literature' and are passed on among community practitioners. However, there now exists a growing literature, which the community mental health practitioner needs to be aware of, which identifies best practice in building collaborative mechanisms and effective community coalitions (Fawcett et al 1995, Foster-Fishman et al 2001, Gillies 1998, Goodman et al 1996, 1998, Kreuter et al 2000, Weiss et al 2002, Wolff 2001). VicHealth

(2004b) have developed 'the partnerships analysis tool' to assist organisations in developing a clear understanding of the purposes of collaborations, to reflect on the nature of the partnerships that they have established and develop ways to strengthen new and existing partnerships. The literature highlights a number of key factors and skills which are identified as being critical to the effectiveness of community partnerships and coalitions. These critical implementation features, which make the difference between the success and failure of community collaborative partnerships, will now be examined and a number of model programmes and case studies illustrating their application in practice will then be outlined.

Building Effective Collaborative Partnerships

The key features that have been highlighted as being critical to building effective collaborative partnerships will now be outlined.

Choosing an Organisational Structure

As indicated earlier in this chapter, there are many different forms of organisational structures involving people from more than one sector working together in order to achieve a common goal. These include healthy alliances, community partnerships, coalitions, community boards, task forces and grassroots structures. Drawing clear distinctions between various terms can often be difficult as they are often used interchangeably. Community boards and task forces tend to bring together key leaders from different segments of the community to work together toward achieving project goals and initiating programme change. The involvement of high profile persons in the community is used to garner local support and resources. Grassroots structures on the other hand are more akin to community development approaches and are characterised by Wittig as 'a local form of collective action by community members employing various techniques, primarily as strategies for addressing the root causes of social problems' (1996:4). One of the features of grassroots organisations is that the initiators and leaders are not professionals whose job it is to run a programme but rather the process is owned and driven by local members acting collectively to pursue shared goals. The choice of structure will depend on the degree of commitment to an underlying philosophy of community working, the issue being addressed and, to a certain extent, the context of a particular community setting. However, it is worth noting that they may vary considerably in the degree of community and citizen participation, influence and ownership that they engender and as a consequence may differ substantially in the types of planning, consultation and implementation processes employed.

Developing a Shared Mission and Clear Objectives

Critical to the early success of community partnerships is the development of a clear vision and mission of purpose and agreement on what the partnership is to achieve. The project goals and objectives need to be clear to all participants; they need to be concrete, attainable and measurable. A visioning process may be used in helping to shape the shared goals and objectives at the early stages of project development. The active engagement of community citizens in setting goals and determining priority objectives is an important step in setting the groundwork for building community ownership. A collaborative process for fine tuning objectives in conjunction with project evaluators has already been outlined in Chapter 2. The setting of goals and objectives may need to be revisited at regular intervals in the course of the project and reshaped in response to changing community and project developments.

Creating Clear Structures

There is no single set structure that has emerged from the literature as the most effective for running community partnerships. Whatever structure is selected needs to reflect the usual organisational capacities in terms of clear roles and responsibilities, clear decision-making processes, adequate staffing and resources necessary to run the organisation and achieve its objectives. The decision-making structure in community partnerships may be particularly complex due to the range and diversity of interests and members involved. In this case, clarifying roles and responsibilities for group members is identified as a critical process. Explicitly identifying, writing down and agreeing the key roles and responsibilities of group members is an important exercise that should be undertaken. Bracht et al (1999) refer to this as 'responsibility charting' and provide a sample form which may be used to list the specific tasks or responsibilities assigned to members.

Establishing Clear Communication

The importance of clear communication, both within the coalition and in communication to other parties externally, is crucial to effective functioning. Meetings need to be facilitated to enhance clear lines of communication and also to provide time for more informal networking and flow of information. Keeping detailed minutes and recording the details of planning and review sessions are all part of this process and serve as explicit reminders to members of what has been collectively agreed upon. Formal rules and procedures, clearly defined roles and expectations, written goals and objectives, and memoranda of understanding among participating organisations have all been associated with successful implementation (Butterfoss et al 1993, Kreuter et al 2000).

Engaging Active Membership

A unique characteristic of community partnerships is that they seek to engage with the whole community. Recruiting members from a broad section of the community is, therefore, essential to success. Deciding on how to engage with community members is a key challenge for community groups. The match of mission and membership is identified by Kreuter et al (2000) as being critical to a partnership's long-term survival. Partners or coalition members must have a strong enough sense of common purpose to set aside individual allegiances and conflicts. As the participating members are recognised as the partnership's greatest asset, issues of representation and trust need to be addressed from the outset. Projects need to consider how well partners represent the most and least powerful members of the community. Are members representative of the age, ethnic and cultural diversity and make up of the community? In discussing community representation, McKinney (1993) distinguishes between substantive and descriptive representation. In substantive representation, members are selected and accountable to different interests in a community, while in descriptive representation, members may simply mirror social or demographic profiles but have little accountability to groups. The building of partnerships is an ongoing task as new players and partners may need to be recruited as the project develops. Likewise, sustaining active membership in partnerships is also an ongoing challenge. Kaye (1997) summarises the reasons people participate as the six Rs: recognition, role, respect, reward, results and relationships. A supportive culture engenders a sense of ownership and a stake in the project and its activities and achievements. By recognising the six Rs identified above, partnerships and coalitions can create and foster an ethos where participation is facilitated and members gain a sense of ownership of the process.

Building Relationships

Relationships are at the heart of the community partnerships. The bringing together of diverse groups of people around a shared or common goal is what makes partnerships work. However, facilitating groups to work together collaboratively calls for skilled facilitation and management of group dynamics. Early stages of partnership formation are frequently marked by initial distrust among members and there is a need to focus on building relationships that foster real collaboration. This requires recognising the needs and strengths of group members and managing conflicts and tensions within the group. Fostering good quality relationships that are based on trust and mutual respect is vital to the smooth and efficient functioning of the coalition or group. 'Trying to "leapfrog" past the important phase of building trust with key stakeholders risks damaging or significantly delaying even the best intentioned efforts' (Potapchuk et al 1997:39). It is important that due attention is given to the dynamics of the group and that opportunities are created for enhancing the relationships between members. Both during and after meetings, build in a space for members to meet and chat, informally socialise and network. An induction process early in the life of the group together with facilitated workshops around the group process can play an important role in setting the stage for creative use of tensions and productive management of conflicts, which inevitably arise.

Developing Collaborative Leadership

Leadership skills such as group organisation, securing resources, motivating and facilitating group activities have long been identified as crucial in effective community working. However, an important point highlighted by Wolff (2001) is that the leadership of a community coalition is not usually located in a single charismatic person who launches and sustains the coalition. Rather successful coalitions and partnerships disperse their leadership and develop it among all participating members. Leaders who practise a democratic decision-making style and who demonstrate strong conflict resolution, communication and administrative skills are recognised as being particularly effective (Kumpfer et al 1993). This is known as collaborative or facilitative leadership and seeks to expand leadership among members by identifying leadership roles and delegating responsibility.

Building Core Competencies and Capacities

It is important that groups embarking on community partnerships identify and develop core competencies and capacities within the partnership structure. Foster-Fishman et al (2001), based on a review of the coalition and collaboration literature, identified core competencies and processes needed within collaborative bodies in order to facilitate their success. Collaborative capacity is defined as the necessary conditions for promoting effective collaboration and building sustainable change (Goodman et al 1998). Strategies for building these core capacities within community coalitions are outlined by Foster-Fishman et al (2001) and these are summarised in Box 3.4. The four capacity types are described as being highly interdependent with each other, as a shift on one level of capacity will affect the others. Ongoing training and development of these skills needs to be incorporated into the working programme of the group and is recognised as being critical to the ongoing sustainability and functioning of the working partnerships.

Box 3.4

Strategies for building core collaborative capacities
(based on Foster-Fishman et al 2001 Building collaborative capacity in community coalitions: a review and integrative framework. American Journal of Community Psychology 29(2):241–261, with kind permission of Springer Science and Business Media)

Building member capacity
- understand current member capacity in terms of core skills and knowledge sets
- value the diversity of member competencies; reinforce and maximise use of existing skills
- enhance current capacities; train in technical areas, disseminate knowledge and recruit new members with needed skills
- engage in incentives management; build on members' motivations, address members' dissatisfaction, reassess goals and vision
- foster positive intergroup understanding; share relevant expertise and experience, discuss differences in attitudes and traditions
- build diverse membership from a representative array of stakeholders
- support diversity and reduce barriers that may impede participation

Creating relational capacity
- build positive intergroup interactions, opportunities to socialise and celebrate successes
- create group norms about participation, member involvement, decision making and conflict resolution

Box 3.4 Continued

- develop superordinate shared goals, emphasise shared concerns and build consensus
- create inclusive decision-making processes by ensuring all members have a voice
- value member diversity by encouraging unique concerns and incorporating diverse goals
- build external relationships by seeking input from sectors and community residents not represented

Building organisational capacity

- proactively build leadership through developing and training the leadership skills of members
- develop task focus, e.g. time management, structure meetings
- formalise roles and processes by clearly defining members' roles and responsibilities, and making explicit agreements on policies and rules
- develop quality plans outlining strategies for action and monitor progress
- create committee infrastructure with respect to active sub-committees with specific responsibilities
- promote active communication among and between members and the community
- build financial resources through planning for, and actively seeking, needed resources
- develop skilled staff trained in needed skills
- develop an outcome orientation by developing explicit short- and long-term goals and tracking progress
- develop a monitoring system through reassessing objectives and strategies and evaluating progress

Building programmatic capacity

- seek community input through regular needs assessment and input in planning processes
- develop innovative programmes to meet needs avoiding duplication of effort

Fostering Action

The partnership's ability to effect change and to achieve outcomes that impact on the local community are vital to the partnership members, funders and the overall credibility of the project at the wider community level. Wolff (2001) identifies a number of ways in which community partnerships can foster action, such as developing written action plans, creating task forces or sub-committees that set clear goals, objectives and realistic work plans and outlining measurable indicators of success.

Management Skills

Management expertise to effectively manage the operations of the partnership is required. In addition to the communication, leadership and decision-making skills outlined above, these skills include securing and managing the necessary resources and funding to achieve the project's core objectives. An appropriate funding strategy needs to be in place, which clearly identifies the funds required and sources of funding to ensure continuity. Very often partnerships may be formed in response to available funding opportunities. In such cases it is vitally important that appropriate management of funds takes place and that a strategy for securing additional funding for the sustainability of project activities is put in place. In-kind resources from partner organisations are also recognised as a major source of support for community projects; these include specialist expertise, support, secretarial and other services which can make a huge contribution to the development and sustainability of project activities.

Planning Community Mental Health Promotion Programmes

Building on the theoretical base and rationale for comprehensive community programmes, such interventions cannot succeed unless they are adequately planned and implemented. The importance of good planning in implementing mental health promotion programmes has already been outlined in Chapter 2. These same steps are followed in working in the community setting. Adopting a planning model or framework for guiding programme planning at the community-wide level is strongly recommended. The five-stage community organisation model by Bracht et al (1999) provides an overarching and structured framework for programme planning and delivery. This model, outlined in Box 3.5, is based on the principles of partnership and empowerment. Employing a theoretical model such as this ensures that the development of the project is guided by a systematic framework and allows each stage of the process to be viewed within the context of an overarching structure. This model draws on earlier models of community organisation practice which have been successfully applied to community health promotion and public health strategies across the globe since the 1970s. The model proposes five stages, each of which has a number of key elements. Bracht et al (1999) point out that the stages are, in fact, overlapping and that citizen involvement is recommended at all stages. These stages correspond quite closely with the stages of the generic template for action already outlined in Chapter 2.

The Rural Mental Health Project in Ireland (Barry 2003, 2005) and the Maryborough Mental Health Promotion Project in Australia (VicHealth 2002) are examples of mental health promotion projects which employ community models. Both projects are based on community partnerships with project planning and implementation being undertaken in collaboration with a wide range of community members. These projects illustrate the process of engaging the participation of local communities in planning and implementing a range of initiatives designed to improve mental health at the community level.

The Rural Mental Health Project in Ireland (Barry 2003) applied Bracht's five-stage model in planning and implementing a community-based project concerned with promoting positive mental heath in rural communities. The adoption of this structured planning model, based on community participation principles,

---

Box 3.5

Model of community organisation
(Bracht et al 1999, with permission)

1. Community analysis and assessment
   - define the community
   - collect data
   - assess community capacity, barriers and readiness for change
   - synthesise data and set priorities
2. Design and initiation
   - establish a core planning group and select a local organiser or coordinator
   - choose an organisational structure
   - identify and recruit organisation members
   - define organisation's missions and goals
   - clarify roles and responsibilities of citizen members, staff and volunteers
   - provide training and recognition
3. Implementation
   - determine priority intervention activities
   - develop a sequential work plan
   - generate broad citizen participation
   - plan media interventions
   - obtain resource support
   - provide a system for intervention monitoring and feedback
4. Programme maintenance and consolidation
   - integrate intervention activities into community networks
   - establish a positive organisational climate
   - establish an ongoing recruitment plan
   - acknowledge the work of volunteers
5. Dissemination and reassessment
   - update the community analysis
   - assess the effectiveness of intervention programmes
   - summarise results and chart future directions

---

was identified as being critical to the successful implementation of a complex, multifaceted, community-based mental health promotion project (Barry 2005).

A more comprehensive system which aims to provide communities with a framework or operating system to assist them in focused planning is the 'Communities That Care' (CTC) initiative (Hawkins et al 2002). The CTC system is described by Hawkins (1999) as a research-based system that helps to guide and empower communities in engaging in planning through objectively assessing their own profiles of risk and protection, and choosing and implementing effective strategies to address their unique strengths and needs. The system has been applied in organising the promotion of positive social development for young people and the prevention of problems such as youth crime and substance abuse. It is a comprehensive community-wide strategy that mobilises and trains communities in reducing risk factors and increasing protective factors for adolescent problem behaviours. This programme has been introduced in over 500 communities in the USA and is also being replicated in the UK, the Netherlands and Australia.

The CTC system consists of five phases:

1. the readiness phase – defining the community, identifying and gaining the support of key stakeholders, assessing current capacities and barriers
2. involving the community – educating key community stakeholders about the intervention and engaging them in the CTC planning process; choosing an organisational structure to oversee planning and implementation activities; citizen recruitment to form a community board
3. training in compiling a baseline community profile – a community board develops a databased profile of the community's strengths and challenges including risk and protective factors; inventory of existing community resources; the data are used to prioritise areas for action
4. training to develop a comprehensive youth development plan for the community – specification of clear measurable outcomes; the selection of tested policies, actions and programmes; an action plan for implementing new programmes and an evaluation plan to measure progress
5. implementation and evaluation of the plan – identification of resources to support the plan; clarifying roles; developing good communication and monitoring of progress toward desired outcomes.

The CTC system has been applied across a range of diverse communities in relation to both youth crime and substance abuse (Harachi et al 1996, Harachi Manger et al 1992). Hawkins (1999) reports evaluation studies which found that, with adequate training, communities can effectively use the CTC in assessing their own profiles of risk and protection, and in implementing effective strategies to address their needs. Hawkins cites a report by the Office of Juvenile Justice and Delinquency Prevention (OJJDP) prepared in 1997 which found that communities trained in the CTC system improved interagency collaboration, reduced duplication of services, coordinated allocation of resources, strategically targeted prevention activities to priority areas, increased use of research-based approaches and increased professional and community involvement. The OJJDP (1997) report also points to desired reductions in risk factors and crime in communities using CTC. To date, the CTC system has been tested in the USA comparing 40 communities in seven states as part of a 5-year study. Among the positive outcomes reported include improvements in youth cognitive skills, parental skills, family and community relations and decreases in school problems, weapon charges, burglary, drug offences and assault charges. The CTC framework provides an effective system of training and technical assistance in involving communities in planning and implementing their own programmes.

Community Implementation Strategies

In this section we will examine intervention strategies and methods for translating the key principles of community-based programmes into action. In particular, we will focus on the following:

* implementing comprehensive multi-component community programmes
* implementing collaborative community partnerships
* facilitating empowerment through developing capacities and mutual support.

Implementing Comprehensive Community Programmes

The implementation of comprehensive community programmes calls for the use of appropriate implementation models and strategies in order to guide the sequencing of programme delivery and to ensure that desired programme outcomes are achieved. These complex community interventions are typically composed of multiple programme components targeting different population groups and settings. Programme components may be planned to occur across different levels of the social ecology: individual, interpersonal, organisational, community and macro-policy. Programmes at each level may in turn be composed of multiple programme elements. Interventions may be linked across levels with each programme element logically connected to supportive activities at the next level, i.e. individual skills building linked to supportive community organisation activities. This type of multi-component programme requires an implementation and evaluation model which will plot the sequence of events that are needed for effective outcomes at each level. Based on social ecology principles, Goodman (2000) recommends four key strategies for implementation of complex community programmes. These are:

1. developing logic models as a strategy for mapping out complex community-based interventions as recommended by Kumpfer et al (1993) and Scheirer (1996). Kumpfer defines logic models as '... a fancy term for what is merely a succinct, logical series of statements that link the problems your program is attempting to address, how it will address them, and what the expected result is' (1993:7–8). Logic models provide a framework for collecting data as events occur, permitting the accurate monitoring and recording of the programme as it unfolds. This type of qualitative data forms the basis of a detailed process analysis of programme implementation

2. using the logic model as a strategic blueprint for assuring the fidelity of implementation as planned

3. staging the implementation of the multiple programme interventions or elements (as represented in the logic model) sequentially across the different social ecological levels, i.e. individual, organisation, community, policy levels. Each intervention may require its own staging so that it fully matures

4. employing strategies that foster the development of community capacities to implement multifaceted programme interventions and to manage complex programme exchanges.

A good example of such an ecologically oriented multi-component programme is the Midwestern Prevention Project (Pentz et al 1990, 1997).

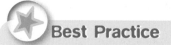

Best Practice

The Midwestern Prevention Project

(Pentz et al 1997)

The Midwestern Prevention Project (MMP) is a comprehensive multi-component community-based programme which targets adolescents' use of 'gateway' drugs such as tobacco, alcohol and marijuana. This model programme, which runs over a 3–5 year period, involves schools, parents and community organisations. The project integrates demand and supply reduction strategies by combining programmes aimed at teaching youth drug resistance skills with local school and community policy change aimed at institutionalising intervention programming and limiting youth and community access to drugs. It also uses mass media to communicate messages regarding non-drug use, and seeks to bring about changes in health policies and community practices to reduce youth access to targeted substances. Although initiated in a school setting, it extends beyond this into the family and community contexts. Each ecological domain – the school, home, community and policy – is targeted in a specific timeline beginning with the school intervention in the first year and ending with the health policy changes. The policy changes are implemented by parents together with school and community leaders as part of the parent and community organisation programmes. The MPP has been shown to be equally effective with both high-risk and low-risk samples. A very detailed account of the implementation of the programme may be found in Pentz et al (1997), which the reader is advised to consult. Here we will summarise the main points and highlight key implementation issues demonstrated in this programme.

Programme Content

The intervention consists of five programme components: school programme, parent programme, community organisation, health policy change and mass media coverage and programming.

1) The school programme focuses on increasing student skills to resist and counteract pressures to use drugs and to change the social climate of the school to accept a drug-free norm. The school curriculum consists of 10–13 resistance skills training classes, six or seven homework assignments which require parental and family involvement, five booster sessions in the second

year, together with follow up counselling and support. Active social learning techniques including modelling, role play and discussion, with student peer leaders assisting teachers in programme implementation are used in the school programme.

2) The parental programme focuses on family support of non-drug use through the provision of skills training in parent–child communication and a review of school drug policy. The programme is delivered by a trained core group comprising the school principal, four to six parents and two student leaders from each school.

3) The community component involves community leaders in planning and implementing drug abuse prevention and referral services within the community.

4) The health policy change component is implemented by a sub-committee of the community organisation and local government leaders. This component focuses on changing local ordinances such as restricting cigarette smoking in public places, increasing alcohol pricing, limiting availability, and including prevention and support provision in drug policies aimed at deterrence. Community leaders are trained in promoting policy change.

5) The mass media campaign uses TV, radio and print broadcasts which are delivered throughout the project and convey messages that support the student and parent skills training components of the programme.

Evaluation

The programme was first evaluated in Kansas City (Johnson et al 1990, Pentz et al 1989) and replicated 3 years later in Indianapolis/Marion County. Employing a quasi-experimental design, evaluation of the MPP has demonstrated impressive results including net reductions of up to 40% in adolescent daily smoking and marijuana use and similar, athough smaller, reductions in alcohol use, which have been maintained through high school graduation (Pentz et al 1997). Significant reductions in heavy marijuana use and some hard drug use (e.g. LSD and amphetamines) have been shown for participating youth through to 23 years of age. The programme has also demonstrated significant reductions in parent alcohol and marijuana use, and increased positive parent–child communication about drug use. Communities participating in MPP have also reported that the programme facilitated development of prevention programmes, activities and services among community leaders. Pentz et al (1997) report that costs per student/family unit average $28 per year for the school and parent programme.

Programme Implementation Focus

The following key features of the planning and implementation of this multifaceted programme are highlighted for attention.

Organisational structure: The MPP employed a highly structured coordinating mechanism to facilitate programme planning and implementation across the different programme modalities. The community organisation structure consisted of:

- a steering committee of community leaders
- a community task force or council that monitors overall project direction
- a number of subcommittees with responsibility for implementation of specific tasks and programme objectives such as education, media, etc.

Community mobilisation: High profile community leaders were engaged initially as programme 'champions' and through the use of snowball-sampling techniques, these community leaders in turn nominated and recruited other community members into the coalition. Pentz et al (1997) stress that the programme is tailored to specific community interests, needs, norms and solutions and highlight the importance of this in working with multi-ethnic communities. Induction or orientation sessions were conducted with key stakeholders in the community in order to introduce the programme concepts and mobilise participation. Strong school principal and parental support was also secured for the school and parent programmes. Initial introduction of the programme in the schools was used as a means of engaging parents and gaining visibility for the programme at the wider community level.

Use of a logic model to guide planning and implementation stages: A detailed process model was used to guide the practical steps that needed to be taken in planning, implementing and evaluating the different programme elements. These steps included:

- identifying the target population and community leaders
- conducting introductory workshops
- establishing a coordinating structure
- training programme implementers.

Each of these steps was followed in relation to each of the programme components across the different modalities of schools, parents, community, etc. Pentz et al (1997) report that the process involved continual programme planning even after community acceptance and support of each programme component.

Sequencing programme components: MPP involved structured sequencing of the programme components across the 5 years of programme implementation. Year 1 involved the school programme, year 2 the parents, year 3 the community organisation element, policy change across years 4 and 5 and the media running throughout the 5 years. This sequencing of programme components ensured that resources were spread across the various years of the programme and that there was an element of novelty in terms of programming in each year.

Building on existing resources: Programme delivery involved employing existing resources where possible with programmes being delivered by personnel who were already in place and paid for in other positions, e.g. teachers delivered the school programme and the local media delivered the mass media component. Community services were made available through establishing interagency links and facilitating referrals and collaboration across agencies.

Training provision: Programme implementation involved the provision of training for community leaders, school staff, teachers and parents in delivering the programme elements. The teacher training included use of a training-of-trainers model, thereby putting in place a largely self-sustaining training mechanism that could be used in subsequent years.

Integrity of programme implementation: Programme implementation and training was standardised through the use of training manuals, protocols and planning manuals to maximise the integrity of programme delivery. In addition there was continuous quality control of programme implementation including use of teacher-completed and independent observer-completed forms. Booster and refresher training in programme delivery were also provided.

Use of evaluation findings to inform the programme: Extensive process and programme implementation data were collected, including data on programme duration, exposure and difficulties experienced, in order to determine if the programme had been implemented as planned. These process data and interim evaluations were reported back to coalition members and key stakeholders as the programme developed. Feedback of the evaluation findings was used to fine tune the programme on an annual basis.

Key Recommendations for Replication

Based on the experience of programme implementation in communities in Kansas and Indianapolis, Pentz et al (1997) make the following recommendations to others interested in developing a community-based programme:

- involve business and community leaders who are well respected early in the process of coalition formation
- include educational administrators in all phases of the coalition and include a school programme as the reference point for the community coalition
- use programme evaluation results as feedback to the community to promote community awareness and support of the coalition
- centralised communications may be necessary to maintain a primary focus of the community coalition on the programme
- maintenance of the coalition may depend on early planning for securing outside funds as a stated objective
- programme institutionalisation may depend on the coalition's willingness to re-review and respond to community needs on a regular basis.

The evaluation results attest to the value of comprehensive, community-based programmes such as MPP, which have a dual focus on universal mental health promotion for youth and 'strategic' prevention for high-risk youth. It is interesting to note that Pentz et al (1997) advise that future interventions should be designed to focus on risk and protective factors known to impact on more than one outcome. This recommendation is in recognition of the fact that there is a clustering of risk and protective factors for many problem behaviours such as delinquency, drug use, school failure, teen pregnancy and unsafe sex. This line of thinking is very much in keeping with mental health promotion programmes suggesting that the overall framework of this successful community model could be used in designing programmes which target the promotion of generic life skills in the broader community setting. The MPP is a clear example of a highly structured and well coordinated community-based programme which illustrates the importance of a systematic planning and implementation process in successfully implementing multifaceted programmes. While the mobilisation of community leaders is highlighted as being key to the success of the programme, less emphasis is given to the importance of the active engagement of less powerful community members in the community organisation process. In the next section we go on to consider implementation strategies for working with disadvantaged individuals and communities.

Implementing Community Empowerment Programmes

Community-based practice provides an opportunity to work with marginalised and disenfranchised groups in their local surroundings. The engagement of disadvantaged groups is a particular challenge in community health programmes. Adopting a community approach in addressing inequalities in health has been recognised by community initiatives such as the Health Action Zones in the UK (Barnes et al 2005) and the Healthy Communities Movement in the USA (Norris 2001). Mental health promotion may be incorporated as part of these wider community initiatives and included as an integral component of a community strategy for tackling health inequalities. As Israel et al (1994) point out, a clear rationale for a community empowerment approach is provided by epidemiological, sociological and psychological evidence of the relationship between control and health, and the association between powerlessness and mental and physical health status. There is also an accumulating body of evidence that poverty, or economic powerlessness, is linked to high rates of social dysfunction, poor mental health and increased morbidity and mortality (Narayan & Petesch 2002, Patel et al 2005).

Empowerment may be defined as a social action process through which individuals, communities and organisations gain mastery over their lives in the context of changing their social and political environment to improve equity and quality of life (Rappaport 1985, Wallerstein 1992). Community empowerment may be differentiated from empowerment at the individual level, since as a multilevel concept it operates at the different system levels of the group, organisational and wider community levels. Labonté (1990) links these levels of empowerment through the idea of a continuum. This continuum ranges from personal and small group empowerment to community organisation, coalition building and political action. Israel et al (1994) point out that empowerment at the individual level is linked with the organisational and community levels through the development of personal control and competence to act, social support, and the development of interpersonal, social and political skills. An empowered community is where individuals and organisations apply their skills and resources in collective efforts to meet their respective needs. Through participation, individuals and organisations within an empowered community provide enhanced support for each other, address conflicts within the community and gain increased influence and control over the quality of life in their community. An empowered community has the ability to influence decisions and make changes in the larger social system. Therefore, empowerment at the community level is connected with empowerment at the individual and organisational levels. A community empowerment approach recognises the cultural, historical, social, economic and political contexts within which the individual exists. A model of empowerment that links all three levels provides the most effective means to collectively provide the support and control necessary to develop needed skills, resources and change.

Patel (2005) and Patel et al (2005) discuss how community empowerment programmes in low-income countries have a significant role to play in promoting mental health. As outlined in Chapter 1, these programmes include economic empowerment initiatives such as micro-credit schemes and community banks, literacy promotion, policies that promote gender equality and violence and crime reduction in marginalised communities. These community development programmes, based on the empowerment of the marginalised and the participation of local community leaders, provide a useful model for promoting mental health in low-income settings. Arole et al (2005) provide an interesting account of how a community development approach, without specific targeted mental health objectives, can impact very positively on mental health. They describe the effects of poverty and inequality on mental health in village settings in rural Maharashtra, India and provide examples of how building the social capital of communities through the Comprehensive Rural Health Programme has worked to achieve outcomes for mental health. This community development programme directly targets poverty, inequality and gender discrimination and has led indirectly, through empowerment and increased participation of women, to significant gains in mental well-being. A meta-analysis of 40 case studies from diverse cultures by Kar et al (1999) found that even the most disenfranchised and deprived women and mothers can and do lead successful social action movements that are self-empowering and significantly enhance the quality of life of their families and communities. They report that involvement in social action movements, ranging from a 'Community Kitchen Movement' in Peru to a 'Committee to Rescue our Health' in Puerto Rico and 'Women against Gun Violence' in the USA, regardless of their specific goals, methods used or outcomes, has strong empowering effects in terms of both the enhancement of the women's subjective well-being, self-esteem and self-efficacy and, as a result, their quality of life and social status in the community. Raeburn (2001) also argues that community development economic and ecological projects undertaken in low-income countries, e.g. building schools or saving the natural environment, have a direct and beneficial mental health promotion impact, whether that is their explicit aim or not. Employing examples of community projects from New Zealand, Raeburn (2001) outlines how the same principles of collective community effort can also be applied in relation to mental health promotion in high-income countries. Raeburn describes the process used as the PEOPLE approach, where PEOPLE stands for planning and evaluation of people-led endeavours. The principle underpinning this approach is that of 'people building their own strength and resilience through empowering processes that use resources, support and good organisation' (Raeburn 2001:18). Where professionals and community agencies are involved, their role is seen as being facilitatory rather than top down.

A case study on developing partnerships with women and children from disadvantaged communities in South Africa is presented as an example of a low-cost community programme with clear mental health benefits. The 'Community

Mothers Programme' (Johnson & Molloy 1995), outlined in Chapter 7, is also a good example of a programme with a focus on empowering women in disadvantaged communities. The enabling and empowering approach used is a critical feature of these programmes and makes the programmes well suited to delivery in disadvantaged community settings. In addition to the direct impacts of such programmes on, for example, the child's development and the mother's mental health, the programme developers also note that contact with the programme has empowering effects leading to further education, personal development and employment opportunities.

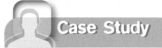

Case Study

Promoting Mental Health through Developing Partnerships with Women and Children from Disadvantaged Communities

Shona Sturgeon

Background: the Programme

This case study describes a replicable, low-cost programme that addresses promotion of mental health and prevention of mental illness among poor rural women and children. It was initiated and managed by a mental health non-profit organisation (NPO), Cape Mental Health Society (CMHS), in collaboration with a rural non-profit organisation, Diakonale Dienste, and funded and monitored by a provincial governmental department, the Department of Social Services. Ekin Kench of CMHS both pioneered and managed the project, and Professor Chris Molteno of the Department of Psychiatry, University of Cape Town acted as consultant.

Although an urban-based organisation, CMHS prioritised addressing the promotion of mental health in rural areas that, as in many developing countries, largely lack mental health programmes. CMHS was aware that in the western Cape there is a large number of poor, unemployed, unskilled, rural female-headed households. Their lack of economic resources and income-generation skills make them largely dependent on state grants. Many of these women display behaviour patterned on a classical cycle of poverty, unemployment and dependency. Children from these disadvantaged rural communities have poor access to community facilities and early childhood development opportunities and are, therefore, vulnerable to the development of mental health problems.

An opportunity to change these conditions was afforded when the state recognised that the poverty of these people would be exacerbated by the planned termination of the state grant in March 2001 and, therefore, made funding available for projects addressing poverty alleviation. CMHS accessed this funding to address the needs of mental health promotion and prevention in one rural community as a pilot project.

CMHS believes that communities can respond to their own needs for upliftment by being given choices and opportunities, which contribute to positive mental health. A sustainable solution would be to address both the needs of these women for income-generation skills and the needs of the children for day care. The CMHS has considerable experience in offering training to women from disadvantaged backgrounds in the care of children with special needs, and these training programmes could be adapted for this project, should the community indicate willingness to participate.

CMHS had a prior relationship with a NPO and the Department of Social Services in the rural community of Beaufort West, approximately 450 km from Cape Town. A needs assessment in the community revealed that 100 women were interested in participating in the programme. A partnership was thus formed between CMHS, the state on a local and provincial level, a local NPO and the community itself.

The goals and objectives of the programme, therefore, were to help 100 women in the Beaufort West community to:

* overcome patterns of dependency on public assistance
* establish cooperative services for pre-school children, after-care children and children with disabilities in order to generate a modest income
* acquire childcare skills.

A clear delivery plan was agreed on, and generally adhered to, by all the partners. The trainees (single mothers who had previously obtained a state grant) were identified, training materials were designed for the different levels of literacy of the trainees, quarterly training seminars of 4 days each, with a fifth day for site visits and evaluation were provided by staff from CMHS and the trainees were supervised and supported by the local NPO between sessions. When visiting to provide training, CMHS provided supervision to the local NPO.

The training programme included material on the mental health of children, mother and child interaction, language development, observation and evaluation of children, women and mental health, stress awareness and management, identification of disability and the development and management of cooperative childcare centres.

The cooperative model of the proposed centres enabled the women to share resources and gave them more bargaining power and mutual support. The project aimed at empowering the community and the women responded with initiatives such as making toys and equipment out of discarded household material and seven group leaders volunteered their homes as venues for day-care centres.

Ongoing evaluation was undertaken, a formal assessment was submitted to the state after a year and an assessment planning exercise 2 years into the programme was completed to direct forward planning. The outcomes of the project exceed the original expectations, particularly regarding the motivation of the women. Because of their life experiences and current situation, a high degree of apathy and even anger was anticipated. However, of the 78 women who signed up for the programme, only three withdrew after a year, and these have used the training provided to access jobs elsewhere. The training model was found to be appropriate, as there was rapid progress in the training seminars and the women grasped the concepts well.

The project has had both promotion and prevention results. The women demonstrated increased self-esteem, development of leadership abilities and increase in skills levels. There has also been promotion of mental health in the community generally through the education of the women. Seven informal day-care facilities were established initially in the poor community, providing stimulating day care to 153 poor children. These have since been collapsed into four more viable centres with approximately 45 women still in the programme working in shifts, resulting in a more practical arrangement. It is known that many of the other women have obtained employment elsewhere, using the skills developed on the programme, but this still needs to be researched properly.

The proactive preventive measures taught were valuable to the women's own mental health (e.g. depression, PTSD), and they were able to provide early assessment and prevention possibilities to the children under their care (e.g. early identification of fetal alcohol syndrome, behaviour problems).

However, the poverty impact of the project has been limited, as the centre fees have had to be low. This is being addressed in phase two of the project through proposals that the centres be subsidised by the Department of Social Services and that other income generation activities be initiated, such as the establishment of market gardens attached to the day centres which enable the day centres to be more sustainable.

Key Factors that Made the Programme Possible and Ensured its Successful Planning and Delivery

This programme would not have been possible without the combined resources of the partners. The leading organisation, CMHS, had the initiative, experience and expertise to see the opportunity for promotion of mental health afforded by state funding, to access the money, to form viable partnerships and to manage the process.

This funding was not earmarked by the state for 'mental health promotion' and, sadly, funding seldom is. Mental health professionals need to be alert to such opportunities, as was CMHS in this case. Prior relationships had been developed with the state, so a level of trust already existed which facilitated both access to funding and cordial relationships throughout the programme.

NPOs are often better placed than the state, certainly in developing countries, in partnering with communities and initiating empowering programmes. They are more accessible to communities and have more flexibility and, therefore, projects can be largely owned and driven by the communities. They also often have community members on their boards.

Mental health promotion requires a philosophy of equality, respect and empowerment of the target community, which needs to be reflected in all phases of the project and in all interactions with the community. The success of the project can largely be attributed to the fact that these principles were adhered to throughout. For example, adult learning principles needed to be followed in the training courses, which had to be developed in such a way that the community would not feel further disadvantaged.

Rural work is only possible if the community has access to a local organisation in which it has some confidence and from which it can receive ongoing support. Such NPOs often lack skills and capacity, but if assisted by an experienced NPO, can follow appropriate community development principles and provide the community with the local assistance needed.

Implementation Challenges

Two issues that arose during the programme have already been noted; the need for capacity building of the local NPO and the need for improved income generation of the community.

Limited structured financial systems and inadequate project reporting methods in the local NPO became apparent during the project. In retrospect, it would have been helpful to have identified these issues at the outset and either offered training in this area or structured the reporting differently. Training would also have been helpful for some of the NPO's counselling staff engaged in the project. The lesson was learned that it is essential to build capacity prior to implementation.

Regarding improved income generation for the community, it became clear that additional financial resources were required to supplement the income that the poor community could generate within itself. However, the process of starting within their own community was probably correct in that, having built confidence within their own community, the women were more prepared at this point to use their skills elsewhere. Additional creative income-generating ideas have also been generated to supplement the income of the day centres.

Programme Replication

The programme is replicable and CMHS is prepared to assist other NPOs to embark on similar projects. The main constraints would be securing seed money and duplicating the character of the training model which draws on childhood education, developmental disability and mental health practice.

The project is also sustainable in terms of low cost. There was no payment for attendance at the training course. The trainees received a small financial incentive from the state while undergoing training and establishing their centres. The total cost of the programme from December 2000 to October 2002 was approximately US$32 000. As discussed, additional income-generating or funding sources may be required if the income generated from the centres is inadequate.

Future Direction

The direction of the project will continue to be guided by careful ongoing evaluation conducted with the cooperation and involvement of all partners. The community and local NPO appear sufficiently empowered at present to play an increasingly active role in deciding future direction. It is anticipated that CMHS will withdraw from the programme within the coming year. This is in keeping with the philosophy of community development in which the primary partner withdraws once the community and other partners are sufficiently resourced and skilled to sustain the project.

Acknowledgements

Mrs Ingrid Daniels, Director, and Mrs Ekin Kench, Project Coordinator, Cape Mental Health Society, Private Bag X7, Observatory 7935, South Africa.

References

A report on the project by Kench E and Prinsloo E L is available from unpublished project reports and proposals, 2001–2002 at http://www.capementalhealth.co.za

. . . .

Facilitating Empowerment through Developing Capacities and Mutual Support

In this section we explore the role of peer support programmes in facilitating change by providing learning and growth opportunities through the medium of linking relationships, bridging the gap between one life phase and another during a critical life transition period. Learning comes from the linking relationship with other persons who provide peer support in the form of supportive and nourishing relationships with a peer. The mutual help model is seen as facilitating change through emphasising the value of other persons as helpers. The special mutuality in this relationship is seen as being particularly important. A mutual exchange takes place which involves people who share a common problem, which one of them has previously coped with successfully. The helping person has expertise based on personal experience in solving the particular problem. The effectiveness of peer support programmes is supported by research indicating positive benefits for both community members in receipt of, and community members delivering, the programmes. For example, based on a systematic review of studies evaluating the effectiveness of health promotion interventions, Cattan (2002) reports that self-help groups, bereavement support and counselling were all found to be effective in reducing social isolation and loneliness among older people. Wheeler et al (1998) also report on the positive effects on mental well-being for older people who volunteer and also the effectiveness of peer counselling in reducing depression for older people who receive support from an older volunteer. Moodie and Jenkins (2005) reference the 'Ageing Well UK Network', which is a national health promotion programme where trained volunteer peer mentors aged 55 years or older provide support, advice and information to their peers in order to promote positive physical and mental health

We will now examine a volunteer community programme concerned with bereavement support. The nature of bereavements and their inevitability, as pointed out by Raphael and Martinek (1998), means that bereavement cannot be prevented; however, it is possible to prepare people for bereavements and to promote coping strategies that will reduce the distress and pain that are often part of this life experience. Reviews of the literature (Stroebe & Stroebe 1993) have highlighted the potential negative impacts of bereavement including heightened risk of mortality, especially among younger people, men, and those who are socially isolated. Psychiatric morbidity studies also indicate the increased vulnerability to depressive episodes such as major depression following be-reavements (Jacobs 1993, Zisook et al 1995). For many people experiencing bereavement, effective help comes from family, friends and existing social sup-port networks. However, for those where this help is not available, mutual help programmes offer an effective and acceptable means of meeting the needs of the bereaved in a non-judgemental, accessible community context. Silverman's (1988) Widow-to-Widow programme is essentially a peer-support programme which values the experiential knowledge of community members and seeks to avoid any negative labelling that may be associated with receiving professional support.

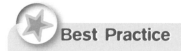 **Best Practice**

Widow-to-Widow: a Mutual Support Bereavement Programme

(Silverman 1986, 1988)

The Widow-to-Widow programme was developed by Silverman (1986) and has served as a model programme for the newly widowed since its inception. This is a volunteer community programme for recently widowed persons still experienc-ing bereavement and the problems of coping with the loss of a loved one. In this programme, other widowed persons are the primary helpers providing support to the newly widowed.

A community outreach service is provided which usually involves an unso-licited offer of help to the newly widowed by trained volunteer helpers. A very useful overview of the programme, including guidelines for its development and implementation, may be found in Chapter 14 of Price et al's 'Fourteen ounces of prevention: a casebook for practitioners' (1988). Here we provide a summary account of the programme and focus on the key implementation features of a mutual help model of community mental health promotion.

Programme Content

The programme sets out to identify the unmet needs of the newly widowed 6 weeks to 2 months after the death, and focuses on promoting people's ability to cope with their pain and to deal effectively with the changes in their lives. A mutual help model is employed which emphasises the value of other widowed people as helpers. On this basis an outreach programme staffed by volunteer widowed people is established in the community. Names are obtained from death notices and referrals from funeral directors and clergy. Contact is made by phone and home visits are made during the first year with group discussion and so-cial activities also offered to those who have been widowed longer. The outreach volunteers or helpers are seen as neighbours who contact the bereaved and offer support. The basis of the help is a widow-to-widow relationship, thereby reducing the potential stigma attached to accepting this kind of help.

The conceptual framework of the programme is that widowhood is viewed as a period of transition and the programme helps to move people from one phase of the transition to the next. In identifying the needs of the widowed, Silverman (1988) points to the fact that widowhood involves not only profound feelings of grief at the loss of a loved one but also a role shift involving changes in the way they live their lives resulting from the loss. The mutual help model is seen as facilitating change in the widowed through emphasising the value of other widowed persons as helpers. As the widow moves through the phases of transition, the help offered progresses from a one-to-one assistance to help through involvement in a new community. Finally, the widowed person has the opportunity to move from the role of recipient to that of helper. As Silverman points out 'The ability to shift roles in the system and the sharing of personal experiences are the fundamental factors that distinguish mutual help from other helping exchanges and, in large part, account for the success of this type of programme' (1988:183). In programmes developed subsequent to the initial trial, there have been many variations on these themes. Many programmes provide a progression of services from outreach to group discussion and social activities to becoming involved as helpers in turn. Some have developed telephone hotlines instead of outreach services.

Evaluation

Evaluation of the initial programme focused on demonstrating the feasibility of the mutual-help model and its acceptance by the newly widowed (Silverman 1986). This evaluation employed a qualitative, descriptive approach and, therefore, did not seek to establish the programme's effectiveness on protective and risk factors of the mental health of the widowed. The original research (Silverman 1986) demonstrated that the model of programme delivery did work and was feasible. The original programme continued for 2.5 years during which time the aides reached out to 300 women with 60% of them accepting the offer of help. The extension of the programme to older people, in addition to the newly widowed, had a 75% acceptance rate. Women with children at home were more likely to accept the offer of help.

Vachon et al replicated the programme in Toronto (Vachon 1979, Vachon et al 1980, 1982) and examined the impact of the programme in a randomised controlled study. The results of this study found that the intervention had a positive impact and significantly facilitated the process of adaptation to bereavement. They also reported that the programme was most effective with those who were at highest risk in terms of higher initial distress. In the Toronto replication newly widowed women were randomly assigned to control and experimental groups. The intervention programme commenced 1 month after the bereavement and involved a wide range of activities including supportive counselling. Widows who participated in the programme were found to have begun new relationships and activities and experienced less distress than women who were not in the programme. The programme was found to be most effective with those who experienced high levels of distress immediately after the death. The high distress participants who did not receive the intervention were found to have a higher level of psychological distress 24 months after the death. Vachon et al's (1982) findings supported the idea that widowhood may be a time of great stress and that social support can act as a protective factor against experiencing psychological distress, particularly where a prior history of mental health problems is present. It would appear that the quality of the support offered in the Widow-to-Widow programme is the discriminating factor and explains the power of the intervention. Many of those who refused the original programme and were managing well felt that they were already involved with others who were widowed and, therefore, the help offered was redundant. The findings support the original supposition on which the programme is based, i.e. that another widow is the most effective helper.

Many variations of the programme have developed subsequently in many different countries. The Widowed Person's Service sponsored by the American Association of Retired People, implemented over 200 affiliated programmes nationwide in the USA. As part of this initiative, training manuals for outreach volunteers and materials were developed to help with the organisation and operation of local groups. Professionals were involved in providing support to organisers and national trainers but did not themselves take on initiating new groups. All of the Widowed Person's Service trainers, organisers and outreach helpers served as volunteers. The programme involved ongoing recruitment of widowed volunteers as people moved in and out of the programme. A challenge identified in this initiative is how to involve widowers as helpers in the programme.

Focus on Programme Implementation

Establishing community outreach: In choosing a community to implement the programme, Silverman (1988) advises that a new outreach programme should choose a specific geographic area where there are clear possibilities of identifying the target population. To legitimate the service in the community, Silverman points out that a Community Advisory Board was established which was composed of representatives of the major religious and ethnic groups in the community. This board helped develop the criteria for choosing helpers and procedures for recruiting them. Important links were also established with local funeral directors and religious groups in helping to identify bereaved people in the community.

Recruiting helpers: The qualities of the helpers were identified as being crucial to the success of the programme. Among the desirable characteristics identified are:

- attractive, engaging people whom the newly widowed would want to invite into their homes
- people who saw the value in talking to other people about their grief
- people who had developed some perspective on their own grief so that they could share their experience in order to help others
- an ability to listen to other people's stories without getting unduly upset or needing to use the occasion to deal with their own grief at the time.

It is estimated that persons widowed for at least 2 years would have reached such a point. They would need to live in the community that they would be

117

working in. Recruitment in the original programme was by word of mouth through local community action programmes and through the local religious orders. Helpers took on the job title 'widow aide'. A small amount of pay was offered as it was found that it would be difficult to sustain in the longer term if full salaries were involved. All helpers were female in the initial programme; however, subsequent replications of the programme have included both male and female helpers on a strictly volunteer basis.

Role of professional support: As the initiator of the programme, Silverman (1988) reports that she initially served as a consultant to the programme providing weekly staff meetings with the aides in order to provide support and act as a sounding board for any difficulties they encountered. She reports that with time, as the aides became more experienced, they acted as consultant to each other. Interestingly she points out that for professionals to work successfully with this type of mutual-help programme, they need to be able to relinquish control and accept the value of experiential knowledge. The skills required extend beyond those employed in clinical work and call for the skills of consultant and facilitator together with an understanding of organisation development and process.

Procedures for reaching out: Contact with the new widow is made 2 months after the death. The helpers use designated stationery listing the members of the Community Advisory Board. The contact letter clearly states that the helper too is widowed and knows the value of meeting another widowed person. A time is given for a visit to the house, and a phone number in case this time needs to be changed. Once verbal contact is made, Silverman reports that even the most reluctant widows find talking to be very helpful. Contact was maintained about twice a month over the first year and most often this contact was on the phone. The aide was available at any time of the day or night. Social visits involved sharing meals, going to a movie and sometime taking the children out. Following initial one-to-one contact, group discussions were set up in the local churches or in people's homes to discuss common problems. An opportunity for recently widowed people to meet others and extend their social network and participation in social activities was provided.

Extending participation to the wider community: The mutual support model is identified by Silverman (1988) as a way of helping people to create more caring communities and break down social barriers. Through mutual help an environment is created that minimises barriers between people and legitimises people's needs for each other and their ability to use their experiences on each other's behalf.

Self-generating programme: The programme is in essence self-generating as some people who receive help from the programme go on to become involved as helpers. The bereaved do not have to remain in the role of recipient but are encouraged, once ready, to become involved as helpers, sharing their experience with another person. The helping relationship is not exclusive as the bereaved are introduced to other widows/ers and become involved in offering peer support. In this way, the programme generates the next generation of helpers.

Low-cost replicable bereavement support programme: The programme is staffed by community volunteers, it avoids professionalisation of the support offered and has the potential to be taken up by community groups with minimal resources. Specific standards for training and programme delivery were not established in the original programme, although training manuals were developed in subsequent versions of the programme. Silverman (1988) points out that the model allows for local groups to develop the programme to meet local needs with the resources available to them.

Recommendations

The Widow-to-Widow programme has demonstrated the benefits of a mutual support model in meeting the needs of the bereaved. The evaluation findings underscore the value of mutual help programmes and peer support in meeting the needs of the widowed. The programme has a universal focus and seeks to meet the needs of the bereaved in an accessible community context. Through sharing the expertise that people gain from their life experiences, the model highly values the role of experiential knowledge in mental health promotion and embeds the programme in the wider context of socially shared knowledge. As Silverman points out, the development and growth of the Widow-to-Widow programme 'has shown that mutual help generally has an advantage over professional help in that it does not treat people as ill and has an image-enhancing emphasis on learning from peers' (1988:186). As help is provided in the form of peer support, the programme avoids any negative labelling that may be associated with more targeted provision for those at 'higher risk' or deemed not to be coping successfully with their loss. Help is provided by neighbours who have gone through the same personal experience, thereby reducing any perceived stigma attached to receiving help. A range of organisations for dealing with bereavements in different groups have been established in different countries, e.g. CRUSE for widows and widowers in the UK, Compassionate Friends for parents who have lost a child, Parents of Murdered Children, Military Widows, Still-birth and Neonatal Death Support, SIDS and many others. However, few of these organisations have systematically evaluated the impact of their programmes and interventions. However, it would appear that the mutual help model employed in the Widow-to-Widow programme does have the potential for application to other interventions for the bereaved. It would be interesting to determine whether the model could be applied to programmes for other bereaved groups such as parents following the death of a child, children and young people following bereavements and the effects of traumatic incidents such as suicide.

Generic Principles Underpinning the Successful Implementation of Community Programmes

In this chapter we have showcased a number of model and innovative programmes which illustrate the effective translation of community mental health promotion principles into practice. While it is acknowledged that there is no one best way of implementing community programmes, on the basis of the reviewed literature a number of critical factors and conditions are identified that are needed to succeed. These key principles are now summarised.

Clarifying Boundaries of the Community

There are many different definitions and meanings of the term 'community', ranging from those that describe a geographically-based community such as a local neighbourhood, city or rural locality, to groups of people who share a common identity, e.g. communities based on sexual, ethnic or cultural identities, who may not be geographically based. The majority of definitions do, however, refer to such key features as a group of people sharing values and institutions, a sense of belonging or shared social meaning and social structures that serve to connect interdependent social groups (Rifkin et al 1988). As Israel et al (1994) point out, neighbourhoods, cities and catchment areas may be made up of unconnected people who have little sense of communality or shared identity. Indeed many of these larger geographical areas may be composed of numerous smaller communities. The initial task may be, therefore, to identify the appropriate unit of practice; be that social group, neighbourhood or regional level. As Bracht et al (1999) point out, clarity about community boundaries or sense of community is critical to effective programme planning and development.

Determining Community Readiness

Community readiness may be described as the extent to which the community is ready to take on its task; to work together across a range of sectors in addressing issues at the local level. One issue which may be relevant is whether the impetus for the project comes from within or outside the community, i.e. internal motivation to respond to local concerns or an approach from an external agency to work together on addressing an identified issue. In either case, issues of community ownership, prior history of collaboration and current ability to collaborate and avoid competition between and within partners is critical to determining the readiness of communities. Communities may be at different stages of readiness for implementing programmes and this readiness may be a key factor in determining the ultimate success of the programme. The Tri-Ethnic Center for Prevention Research at Colorado State University in the USA proposes a community readiness model as a practical tool to help communities mobilise for change. This model (Edwards et al 2000) defines nine stages of community readiness ranging from 'no awareness' through to 'professionalisation' of a health issue or problem in the community. Assessment of the stages of readiness is accomplished through key informant interviews with questions on six different dimensions of a community's readiness for change. The model provides a tool for communities to focus and direct their efforts and training methods based on the model are used to work with community teams.

Community readiness may have particular significance when addressing mental health promotion as communities may not feel empowered or willing to take on programmes promoting positive mental health for groups in the community. It may, therefore, be quite important not to rush into programme planning and implementation in advance of determining the degree of readiness in the community to engage with mental health issues locally. As Wolff (2001) points out, the most successful community coalitions take time to establish relationships, personally visit the key local players and build strong personal links and support in order to engage effectively with, and mobilise, the community.

Creating Clear Structures

The key feature of effective community-based programmes is successful collaborative working (Foster-Fishman et al 2001, Wolff 2001). Structures for planning and delivery will vary between projects but an agreed organisational structure is critical to effective community-based projects. Clear lines of communication are important and can be enhanced, for example, by detailed minutes of planning, review sessions, clearly defined roles and expectations and a good flow of information. Successful community coalitions and partnerships are characterised by a collaborative style of leadership, expanding leadership among members and delegating responsibility rather than relying on a single charismatic person.

Generating Community Participation

Community participation has been identified as one of the key mechanisms of enabling people to take control over their health and that of their community. As Bracht et al point out 'participation facilitates psychological empowerment by developing personal efficacy, developing a sense of group action, developing a critical understanding of social power relationships and developing a willingness to participate in collective action' (1999:87). Obtaining meaningful community participation is a major challenge. Practitioners need to be mindful that participation may occur in different ways and at different levels ranging from token involvement to real control of the process. The classic depiction of the degrees of participation in Arnstein's (1971) 'ladder of participation' and Brager and Specht's (1973) 'spectrum of participation' are useful reminders of the need to ensure maximal levels and degree of participation in the development of the community organisation process. As Kreuter et al (2000) point out, community participation is seen as mutually benefiting both the community and the success of the programme. The active involvement of community representatives enables the project to be more responsive to, and understanding of, local needs. Community participation also enhances acceptance for an initiative within a community and can lead to individual and community empowerment through building capacity locally, and enhancing perceived control of the local environment. New members may need to be recruited as the project develops and there is an ongoing need to build trust and positive relationships between diverse groups of people around a shared goal.

Translating Plans into Action

The importance of moving beyond the consultation and planning stages into concrete action is critical for success. Developing written action plans and realistic work plans, including measurable indicators of success, are important steps in translating key project aims and objectives into action. Feedback on the success and impact of project activities through process and interim evaluations can play an important role in motivating action or indeed changing the focus and direction of action. Action plans may need to be regularly reviewed in the light of evaluation findings and feedback from participants. Disseminating successes and media publicity of achievements play an important part in enhancing the motivation for change, increasing the visibility of the project and consolidating its role in the community.

Technical Assistance

The planning and implementation of community programmes is a highly complex task requiring a range of skills and expertise that may not be readily available within the group. In recognition of this, the provision of appropriate technical assistance, training and support for project members may be needed at various stages of programme delivery to enable members to fulfil the many functions and tasks that are involved. External technical assistance can be provided in relation to assisting with planning, conducting needs assessment, designing strategies, facilitating partnership, group process, managing conflicts, dealing with start up and sustainability and project evaluation.

Building Core Competencies and Capacities

Ongoing training and support in developing a range of skills is critical to the functioning of working community partnerships. Skills in communication, management, facilitation and evaluation are all examples of core capacities from which community projects can benefit. In this way programme sustainability will be ensured in terms of strengthening resources from within the project.

Sustaining Community Programmes

Sustainability is used here as a general term to refer to the process of project continuation. A distinction can be made, for example, with terms such as 'integration' or 'institutionalisation', which imply continuation or survival within an organisational structure. Sustainability may occur at levels other than at the organisational or institutional levels, including the individual and network levels. Here it is used as a broad term which indicates continuation without specifying or limiting the form that it may take. Among the operational indicators that are used in monitoring sustainability over time are maintenance of health benefits achieved through an initial programme, level of institutionalisation of the programme within an organisation and measures of capacity building in the recipient community.

What makes a programme sustainable? Akerlund (2000) defines a sustainable programme as one that is endurable, liveable, adaptable and supportable. The programme is replicable, and is of reasonable cost. Points that make a programme sustainable include:

- high quality – scheduled needs assessments, ongoing programme planning and adaptation, evaluation and staff training
- evaluation data documenting success
- strong administration with plans for continued funding – developing plans for survival beyond major project funding includes funding diversification and training in management and fundraising
- community-based and community-owned – support and involvement of the community add to the prospect of receiving funding from other sources
- meets funder priorities – balancing the meeting of the funders' goals with those of the community.

Shediac-Razallah and Bone (1998) present an organising framework for conceptualising and measuring sustainability and tentative guidelines to facilitate sustainability in community programmes. They emphasise that sustainability is a dynamic process, and that goals and strategies for achieving it must continuously adapt to changing environmental conditions. They highlight the following policy directions for future development:

- community programmes need to be driven by the needs of communities
- sound planning for sustainability dictates that programmes be designed with local capability in mind
- unless sufficient resources are available to yield initial success, long-term sustainability is unlikely
- allocating resources to cover the maintenance and recurrent costs of programmes with a track record.

Planning for sustainability should begin early in the life of the programme and not in the last year of funding. Long-range plans for receiving ongoing programme support should be developed including concrete funding goals and strategies for a diversified, broad and stable funding base. It may be useful to develop a timeline for seeking additional funds, identifying possible sources and when they become available. The success of the sustainability plan should be regularly reviewed. Programme integration with other service providers may also be considered along with support in kind, volunteer engagement, etc. If a programme does have to be ended then it is important that this should also be planned, signalled well in advance and carried out with sensitivity and due regard for the community members and organisations involved.

Comprehensive Evaluation

The complexity of multifaceted community programmes presents a particular challenge in terms of programme evaluation regarding both the methodologies applied and the role of the evaluator. Brown (1995) outlines the following challenges for evaluators of comprehensive community initiative:

- broad multiple goals dependent on an ongoing process of synergistic change
- programmes are purposively flexible and responsive to local needs and conditions
- the principles of community empowerment, participation and ownership are central to their mission
- recognise the nature of longer-term community change requiring longer time frames than more narrowly defined approaches
- produce impacts at different levels in different spheres.

More general discussions of methodological issues in evaluating community partnerships and comprehensive community initiatives may be found in the writings of Connell et al (1995), Kaftarian and Hansen (1994) and Rindskopf et al (1997).

Realistic evaluation (Pawson & Tilley 1997) has also been identified as a useful framework for evaluating community initiatives as this approach seeks to link the specific context of an initiative with the mechanisms of change, i.e.

how interventions achieve change over time in specific contexts. Judge and Bauld (2001) provide an interesting account of the practicalities of evaluating the community health improvement process, employing a realistic evaluation and theories of change approach, as part of a national evaluation of the Health Action Zones in the UK. At a more general level, Gabriel points out that in the spirit of a community approach, evaluators must become partners with practitioners and the community in '... adapting their designs, assessment techniques and reporting strategies to fit the local context and needs' (2000:340). This calls for a movement away from traditional evaluation approaches to one characterised by partnership with key players, which includes approaches such as empowerment evaluation (Fetterman et al 1996), participatory, collaborative and utilisation-focused evaluation. Israel et al (1994) advocate employing a participatory action research approach in order to identify outcome and process goals and objectives that are consistent with the community empowerment concept. A participatory action research approach implies that community members are involved in all aspects of the programme action and research in a collaborative and reflective process.

Process evaluation takes on a particularly important role in the context of community programmes, which typically constitute multifaceted interventions implemented with diverse target populations in complex settings. Detailed process evaluation is considered necessary to monitor implementation and to pinpoint effective components leading to desired outcomes. Community-based interventions require especially comprehensive process evaluation systems to track implementation and ensure adequate documentation of a wide range of activities and procedures (Cunningham et al 2000). As highlighted earlier in this chapter, the formulation of logic models provides a very useful opportunity for evaluators and practitioners to share their perspectives and expertise in formulating project design and sequential planning. Logic models also provide a useful blueprint for sharing perspectives in monitoring the process of programme implementation and collaboration. The practitioner and/or programme implementer has a key role to play in this process as data on programme implementation are collected as events occur. Data may be recorded in the form of activity logs, records of meetings, process reports together with critical observations and reflections. This detailing of the programme in action permits an accurate record of the programme as it unfolds and plays a crucial role in informing the detection of intermediate level changes leading to ultimate programme outcomes. Barry (2003) outlines the use of a logic model framework in guiding the evaluation of the Rural Mental Health Project, discussed earlier. The evaluation logic model provided a systematic framework for intervention monitoring and feedback on project activities and impacts, which was incorporated as an integral part of the planning and delivery of the project.

Drawing on lessons of the past decade on community partnerships and coalition evaluations, Gabriel (2000) offers guidance on the effective use of evaluation of community-based programmes. Among the lessons learned are the following:

* the traditionally detached and external role of the evaluator does not meet the needs of the dynamic and multifaceted community programmes.

Partnership between the evaluator and the programme better equips the evaluator to understand the actualities of programme activities and leads to a better informed assessment of programme processes and outcomes

- the use of logic models provides the critical connections between local community needs, the partnership/programme activities and intended intermediate and long-term outcomes
- greater energy must be directed toward the identification and systematic elimination of rival explanations to the evidence of positive change in these outcomes. This theory-based approach is offered as a viable alternative to the use of typically inadequate comparison or control groups for community-based programmes
- the reporting of evaluation results is most useful for programme improvement when done frequently and simply by the evaluator.

References

Akerlund K M 2000 Prevention program sustainability: the state's perspective. Journal of Community Psychology 28(3):353–362

Arnstein S R 1971 A ladder of citizen participation in the USA. Journal of the Royal Town Planning Institute 57:176–182

Arole R, Fuller B, Deutschman P 2005 Community development as a strategy for mental health promotion: lessons from rural India. In: Herrman H, Saxena S, Moodie R (eds) Promoting mental health: concepts, emerging evidence, practice. A report of the World Health Organization, Department of Mental Health and Substance Abuse in collaboration with the Victorian Health Promotion Foundation and University of Melbourne,WHO, Geneva:243–251

Barnes M, Bauld L, Benezeval M et al (eds) 2005 Health action zones: partnerships for health equity. Routledge, London

Barry M M 2003 Designing an evaluation framework from community mental health promotion. Journal of Mental Health Promotion 2(4):26–36

Barry M M 2005 The art, science and politics of creating a mentally healthy society: lessons from a cross border rural mental health project. Journal of Public Mental Health 4(1):30–34

Berkman L F, Glass T 2000 Social integration, social networks, social support and health. In Berkman L F, Kawach I (eds) Social

epidemiology. Oxford University Press, New York

Bracht N, Kingsbury L 1990 Community organization principles in health promotion: a five-stage model. In: Bracht N (ed) Health promotion at the community level. Sage, California:66–90

Bracht N, Kingsbury L, Rissel C 1999 A five-stage community organization model for health promotion: empowerment and partnership strategies. In: Bracht N (ed) Health promotion at the community level 2: new advances. Sage, California:83–117

Brager G, Specht H 1973 Community organizing. Columbia University Press, New York

Bronfenbrenner U 1979 The ecology of human development: experiments by nature and design. Harvard University Press, Cambridge, Massachusetts

Brown P 1995 The role of the evaluator in comprehensive community initiatives. In: Connell J P, Kubisch A C, Schorr L B et al (eds) New approaches to evaluating community initiatives: concepts, methods and contexts. Aspen University, Washington DC:201–225

Butterfoss F D, Goodman R M, Wandersman A 1993 Community coalitions for prevention and health promotion. Health Education Research: Theory and Practice 8(3):315–330

Cattan M 2002 Supporting older people to overcome social isolation and loneliness. Help the Aged, London

Chavis D M 2001 The paradoxes and promise of community coalitions. American Journal of Community Psychology 29(2):309–320

Connell J P, Kubisch A C, Schorr L B et al 1995 New approaches to evaluating community initiatives. The Aspen Institute, Washington DC

Cunningham L E, Michielutte R, Dignan M et al 2000 The value of process evaluation in a community-based cancer control program. Evaluation and Program Planning 23:13–25

Dalgard O S, Tambs K 1997 Urban environment and mental health: a longitudinal study. British Journal of Psychiatry 171:530–536

Davey Smith G, Whitely E, Dorling D et al 2001 Area based measures of social and economic circumstances: cause specific mortality patterns depend on the choice of index. Journal of Epidemiology and Community Health 55:149–150

Durkheim E 1897 Suicide: a study in sociology. (ed. G Simpson and tr. J A Spaulding and G Simpson 1951) Free Press, New York

Edwards R W, Jumper-Thurman P, Plested B A et al 2000 Community readiness: research to practice. Journal of Community Psychology 28(3):291–307

Fawcett S, Sterling T, Paine-Andrews A et al 1995 Evaluating community efforts to prevent cardiovascular disease. Center for Disease Control, Atlanta

Fetterman D M, Kaftarian S J, Wandersman A 1996 Empowerment evaluation: knowledge and tools for self assessment and accountability. Sage, California

Florin P, Wandersman A 1990 An introduction to citizen participation, voluntary organizations, and community development: insights for empowerment through research. American Journal of Community Psychology 18:41–54

Flynn B S 1995 Measuring community leaders' perceived ownership of health education programs: initial tests of reliability and validity. Health Education Research 10:27–36

Foster-Fishman P G, Berkowitz S L, Lounsbury D W et al 2001 Building collaborative capacity in community coalitions: a review and integrative framework. American Journal of Community Psychology 29(2):241–261

Gabriel R M 2000 Methodological challenges in evaluating community partnerships and coalitions: still crazy after all these years. Journal of Community Psychology 28(3):339–352

Gillies P 1998 Effectiveness of alliances and partnerships for health promotion. Health Promotion International 13(2):99–120

Goodman R M 2000 Bridging the gap in effective program implementation: from concept to application. Journal of Community Psychology 28(3):309–321

Goodman R M, Wandersman A, Chinman M et al 1996 An ecological assessment of community-based intervention for prevention and health promotion: approaches to measuring coalitions. American Journal of Community Psychology 24(1):33–61

Goodman R M, Speers M A, McLeroy K et al 1998 An attempt to identify and define the dimensions of community capacity to provide a basis for measurement. Health Education and Behavior 25:258–278

Green L W, Kreuter M W 1991 Health promotion planning: an educational and environmental approach, 2nd edn. Mayfield, Mountain View, California

Greiger H J 1993 The undeserving poor in US health and social policies. Presentation at the Annual Meeting of American Public Health Association, San Francisco, 26 October

Harachi T W, Ayers C D, Hawkins J D et al 1996 Empowering communities to prevent adolescent substance abuse: process evaluation results from a risk- and protection-focused community mobilization effort. The Journal of Primary Prevention 16(3):233–254

Harachi Manger T, Hawkins D, Haggerty K P et al 1992 Mobilizing communities to reduce risks for drug abuse: lessons on using research to guide prevention practice. The Journal of Primary Prevention 13(1):3–22

Hauf A M, Bond L A 2002 Community-based collaboration in prevention and mental health promotion: benefiting from and building the resources of partnership. International Journal of Mental Health Promotion 4(3):41–54

Hawkins J D 1999 Preventing crime and violence through communities that care. European Journal on Criminal Policy and Research 7:443–458

Hawkins J D, Catalano R F, Arthur M W 2002 Promoting science-based prevention in communities. Addictive Behaviors 27(6):951–976

Henderson S, Whiteford H 2003 Social capital and mental health. Lancet 362:505–506

Himmelman A T 2001 On coalitions and the transformation of power relations: collaborative betterment and collaborative empowerment. American Journal of Community Psychology 29(2):277–284

House J S, Landis K R, Umberson D 1988 Social relationships and health. Science 214:540–545

Israel B A, Checkoway B, Schulz A et al 1994 Health education and community empowerment: conceptualizing and measuring perceptions of individual, organizational and community control. Health Education Quarterly 21(2):149–170

Jackson T, Mitchell S, Wright M 1989 The community development continuum. Community Health Studies 8:66–73

Jacobs S C 1993 Pathologic grief: maladaptation to loss. American Psychiatric Press, Washington DC

Johnson C A, Pentz M A, Weber M D et al 1990 The relative effectiveness of comprehensive community programming for drug abuse prevention with high risk and low risk adolescents. Journal of Consulting and Clinical Psychology 58:4047–4056

Johnson Z, Molloy B 1995 The Community Mothers Programme: empowerment of parents by parents. Children and Society 9(2):73–85

Judge K, Bauld L 2001 Strong theory, flexible methods: evaluating complex community-based initiatives. Critical Public Health 11(1):19–38

Kaftarian S J, Hansen W B 1994 Improving methodologies for the evaluation of community-based substance abuse prevention programs. Journal of Community Psychology, CSAP special issue:3–5

Kar S B, Pascual C A, Chickering K L 1999 Empowerment of women for health promotion: a meta-analysis. Social Science and Medicine 49:1431–1460

Kawachi I, Kennedy B 1997 Socioeconomic determinants of health: health and social cohesion. Why care about income inequality? British Medical Journal 314:1037–1040

Kaye G 1997 Improving and mobilizing the grassroots. In: Kaye G, Wolff T (eds) From the ground up: a workbook on coalition building and community development. AHEC/Community Partners, Amherst, Massachusetts:99–122

Kreuter M, Lezin N, Young L 2000 Evaluating community based collaborative mechanisms: implications for practitioners. Health Promotion Practice 1(1):49–63

Kumpfer K L, Turner C, Hopkins R et al 1993 Leadership and team effectiveness in community coalitions for the prevention of alcohol and other drug abuse. Health Education Research 8(3):359–374

Labonté R 1989 Community empowerment: the need for political analysis. Canadian Journal of Public Health 8:87–89

Labonté R 1990 Empowerment: notes on professional and community dimensions. Canadian Review of Social Policy 26:1–12

Labonté R 1993 Community development and partnerships. Canadian Journal of Public Health 84(4):237–240

Lewin K 1951 Field theory in social science. Harper, New York

McKinney M M 1993 Consortium approaches to the delivery of HIV services under the Ryan White CARE Act. AIDS and Public Policy Journal 8:115–25

Matarasso F 1997 Use or ornament? The social impact of participation in the arts. Comedia, Stroud. Cited in Mentality 2003 Making it effective: a guide to evidence based mental health promotion. Radical mentalities – briefing paper 1. Mentality, London

Mentality 2003 Making it effective: a guide to evidence based mental health promotion. Radical mentalities – briefing paper 1. Mentality, London

Miller M 1985 Turning problems into accountable issues. Organise Training Center, San Francisco

Minkler M 1994 Ten commitments for community health education. Health Education Research: Theory and Practice 9(4):527–534

Moodie R, Jenkins R 2005 "I'm from the government and you want me to invest in mental health promotion. Well why should I?" Promotion and Education Suppl2:37–41

Narayan D, Petesch P 2002 Voices of the poor: from many lands. Oxford University Press, New York

Nazroo J Y 1998 Rethinking the relationship between ethnicity and mental health. Journal of Social Psychiatry and Psychiatry Epidemiology 33:145–148

Nazroo J Y, Karlsen S 2001 Ethnic inequalities in health: social class, racism and identity. ESRC research findings no. 10 from the

Health Variations Programme, Lancaster University, Lancaster

Norris T 2001 America's communities movement: investing in the civic landscape. American Journal of Community Psychology 29(2):301–307

OECD (Organization for Economic Co-operation and Development) 2001 The well-being of nationals. The role of human and social capital, education and skills. OECD, Centre for Educational Research and Innovation, Paris

OJJDP (Office of Juvenile Justice and Delinquency Prevention) 1997 Report to congress, title V: Incentive grants for local delinquency prevention programs. OJJDP, Washington DC

Orford J 1992 Community psychology: theory and practice. John Wiley, Chichester

Patel V 2005 Poverty, gender and mental health promotion in a global society. Promotion and Education Suppl2:26–29

Patel V, Swartz L, Cohen A 2005 The evidence for mental health promotion in developing countries. In: Herrman H, Saxena S, Moodie R (eds) Promoting mental health: concepts, emerging evidence, practice. A report of the World Health Organization, Department of Mental Health and Substance Abuse in collaboration with the Victorian Health Promotion Foundation and University of Melbourne,WHO, Geneva:189–201

Pawson R, Tilley K 1997 Realistic evaluation. Sage, London

Pentz MA, Anderson CA, Dwyer JH, MacKinnon DM, Hansen WB, Flay BR 1989. A comprehensive community approach to adolescent drug abuse prevention: effects on cardiovascular disease risk behaviors. Annals of medicine, 21: 219–222

Pentz M A, Trebow E A, Hansen W B et al 1990 Effects of program implementation on adolescent drug use behavior: the Midwestern Prevention Project (MPP). Evaluation Review 14(3):264–289

Pentz M A, Mihalic S F, Grotpeter J K 1997 Blueprints for violence prevention. Book one: The Midwestern prevention project. Center for the Study and Prevention of Violence, Institute of Behavioural Science, University of Colorado, Boulder, Colorado

Potapchuk W R, Crocker J, Schechter H 1997 Systems reform and local government: improving outcomes for children, families and neighbourhoods – a working paper. Annie E Casey Foundation, Baltimore

Price R H, Cowen E L, Lorion R P et al 1988 Fourteen ounces of prevention: a casebook for practitioners. American Psychological Association, Washington DC

Putnam RD 2000 Bowling alone. Simon & Schuster, New York

Putnam R 2001 Social capital: measurement and consequences. Canadian Journal of Policy Research Spring:41–51

Raeburn J 2001 Community approaches to mental health promotion. International Journal of Mental Health Promotion 3(1):13–19

Raphael B, Martinek N 1998 Bereavements and trauma. In: Jenkins R, Usten T B (eds) Preventing mental illness: mental health promotion in primary care. John Wiley, Chicester:353–378

Rappaport J 1985 The power of empowerment language. Social Policy 16:15–21

Rifkin S B, Muller F, Bichmann 1988 Primary health care: on measuring participation. Social Science and Medicine 26:931–940

Rindskopf D, Livert D, Saxe L et al 1997 From theory to practice: design and analysis of community-based programs using Multi-Level Models. Graduate Center, City University of New York, New York

Robertson A, Minkler M 1994 New health promotion movement: a critical examination. Health Education Quarterly 21(3):295–312

Robinson K L, Elliott S J 2000 The practice of community development approaches in heart health promotion. Health Education Research 15(2):219–231

Scheirer M A 1996 A user's guide to program templates: a new tool for evaluating program content. New Directions for Evaluation 72:61–80

Shediac-Razallah M C, Bone L R 1998 Planning for the sustainability of community-based health programs: conceptual frameworks and future directions for research, practice and policy. Health Education Research: Theory and Practice 13(1):87–108

Silverman P R 1986 Widow-to-widow. Springer, New York

Silverman P R 1988 Widow-to-widow: a mutual help program for the widowed. In Price R H, Cowen E L, Lorion R P et al (eds) Fourteen ounces of prevention: a casebook for practitioners. American Psychological Association, Washington DC, Chapter 14:175–186

Stokols D, Allen J, Bellingham R L 1996 The social ecology of health promotion: implications for research and practice. American Journal of Health Promotion 10:247–251

Stroebe W, Stroebe M S 1993 The impact of spousal bereavement on older widows and widowers. In: Stroebe M, Stroebe W, Hansson R O (eds) Handbook of bereavement. Cambridge University Press, New York:208–226

Thompson B, Kinne S 1999 Social change theory: applications to community health. In: Bracht N (ed) Health promotion at the community level, new advances, 2nd edn. Sage, California:29–46

Thomson H, Petticrew M, Douglas M 2003 Health impact assessment of housing improvements: incorporating research evidence. Journal of Epidemiology and Community Health 57:11–16

Tones K, Tilford S 2001 Health promotion: effectiveness, efficiency and equity, 3rd edition. Nelson Thomas, Cheltenham

Vachon M L 1979 Identity change over the first two years of bereavement: social relationships and social support in widowhood. Unpublished doctoral dissertation. York University, Toronto

Vachon M L, Lyall W A, Rodgers J et al 1980 A controlled study of self-help interventions for widows. American Journal of Psychiatry 137:1380–1384

Vachon M L, Sheldon A R, Lancee W J et al 1982 Correlates of enduring distress patterns following bereavement: social network, life situation and personality. Psychological Medicine 12:783–788

VicHealth 2002 Maryborough mental health promotion project: rural mental health in Australia. The Victorian Health Promotion Foundation, Carlton South, Victoria

VicHealth 2004a Sports and active recreation program. The Victorian Health Promotion Foundation, Carlton South, Victoria. Online. Available: http://www.vichealth.vic.gov.au/ publications/physical activity October 2005

VicHealth 2004b The partnership analysis tool: for partners in health promotion. The Victorian Health Promotion Foundation, Carlton South, Victoria

VicHealth 2005 Mental health and well-being research summary sheets, no.2. Social inclusion as a determinant of mental health and wellbeing. The Victorian Health Promotion Foundation, Carlton South, Victoria

Wallack L, Dorfman L, Jernigan D et al 1993 Media advocacy and public health: power for prevention. Sage, Newbury Park, California

Wallerstein N 1992 Powerlessness, empowerment and health: implications for health promotion programs. American Journal of Health Promotion 6:197–205

Weiss E S, Miller Anderson R, Lasker R D 2002 Making the most of collaboration: exploring the relationship between partnership synergy and partnership functioning. Health Education and Behavior 29(6):683–698

Wheeler J A, Gorey K M, Greenblatt B 1998 The beneficial effects of volunteering for older volunteers and the people they serve: a meta-analysis. International Journal of Aging and Human Development 47:69–79

Whiteford H, Cullen M, Baingana F 2005 Social capital and mental health. In: Herrman H, Saxena S, Moodie R (eds) Promoting mental health: concepts, emerging evidence, practice. A report of the World Health Organization, Department of Mental Health and Substance Abuse in collaboration with the Victorian Health Promotion Foundation and University of Melbourne,WHO, Geneva

WHO (World Health Organization) 1986 The Ottawa Charter for health promotion. WHO, Geneva

WHO Regional Office for Europe 1997 Twenty steps to develop a Healthy Cities project, 3rd edition. WHO regional Office for Europe, Copenhagen. Online. Available: http://www. euro.who.int/healthy-cities October 2005

Wilkinson R G 1996 Unhealthy societies: the afflictions of inequality. Routledge, London

Wilkinson R G, Marmot M 2003 Social determinants of health: the solid facts, 2nd edition. WHO Regional Office for Europe, Copenhagen

Wittig M A 1996 An introduction to social psychological perspectives on grassroots organizing. Journal of Social Issues 52(1):3–14

Wolff T 2001 Community coalition building – contemporary practice and research: introduction. American Journal of Community Psychology 29(2):165–191

Zisook S, Shuchter S R, Summers J 1995 Bereavement risk and preventing intervention. In: Raphael B, Burrows G (eds) Handbook of studies on preventive psychiatry. Elsevier, Amsterdam

Mental Health Promotion in the Home for Children and Families

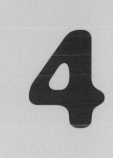

Introduction

The early years of life are recognised as a crucial period in human development, as they lay the foundations for healthy development and good mental health throughout the lifecycle. The importance of investing in the early years has been highlighted in terms of supporting families and children in reaching their full potential and reducing the risk of behavioural problems and poor mental health. There is a strong case for investing in early years. Substantial social and economic benefits have been shown to accrue from high quality early childhood interventions (Karoly et al 1998). A review of the effectiveness of programmes in this area prepared for the European Commission concluded that 'there is strong evidence that the early years of life have a crucial impact on mental health throughout the life cycle. The development of strategies to promote the mental health of young children is therefore of fundamental importance' (Mental Health Europe 1999). The earlier family interventions are put in place, the better the mental health outcomes for the child. Key transition points in the life of families include the period around birth (the first year), the pre-school period and transition to and from school. Selective interventions involving intensive home visits and educational pre-school programmes have been effective in promoting positive outcomes and modifying a wide range of risk factors for mental health problems. However, once-off interventions are of limited effectiveness and there is a need for follow up and integrated approaches in order to promote long-term maternal and child functioning (Barnes & Freude-Lagevardi 2003).

In this chapter we examine a number of different approaches designed to improve parenting, family functioning and children's mental and social development. A selected number of model programmes are examined in order to highlight details of their successful implementation and the critical factors which contribute to their success. Case studies of programme development and their replication are also included in order to examine the realities of implementing programmes outside of controlled research conditions.

Rationale for Promoting the Mental Health of Children and Families

A healthy start to life is critical to a child's overall functioning and development throughout the lifecycle. The importance of the early years in providing a foundation for good mental health is clearly recognised. Developmental theorists have highlighted the importance of early attachment, a supportive family, a secure and safe home environment and informal sources of support in the local community as protective factors for a child's positive psychosocial development (Cowen & Work 1988, Rutter 1987). Children's mental health and well-being are influenced by their interaction with their caregivers, families and local communities. Ecological models of human development (Bronfenbrenner 1979) highlight how children are influenced by multiple interacting systems including the social context in which they live such as neighbourhoods, physical environments, culture and society (Lerner 1995, Sampson 1997). Poverty, racial segregation, crime and violence, common to many low-income communities may, however, hinder the ability of families to protect themselves and their children (McLoyd 1998). Poverty influences on the local community may impact on children directly through poor housing, and through a lack of resources such as safe playgrounds, recreational centres and positive role models. At a broader level, children may be affected indirectly by influences from the larger society that impact on their family's financial, emotional and physical health status. Therefore, multi-layered strategies are required at the level of policies, communities and families in order to secure the health and well-being of children. A wide range of policy measures are required to fully address the determinants of childhood poverty and disadvantage, including those to reduce health inequalities. Integrated approaches are needed where interagency interaction and cross-sectoral partnerships are put in place. It is, therefore, important that programmes seek to enhance supportive environments as well as promote individual skills and competencies. Programmes need to take account of the broader environmental context and the values, culture and norms of the community, in their efforts to enhance children's well-being.

Families serve as a critical link between children and other aspects of their environment. There is much evidence that family relationships have a strong association with later emotional development and positive mental health (Resnick et al 1997). Poor mental health in children such as behavioural problems, anxiety and depression, is a significant risk factor for poor school outcomes, poor physical health, poor social skills and suicidal behaviour (Mental Health

Foundation 1999). Mental health promotion interventions are aimed at enhancing protective factors and reducing risk factors. Positive parenting and family support can serve to protect against the negative effects of socioenvironmental factors on mental health, especially those relating to poverty, violence and conflict (Jané-Llopis et al 2005). A number of interventions have been developed to promote positive mental health in the early years of life through empowering parents, and enhancing resilience and competence in both children and parents. Such interventions have been found to produce positive outcomes for both children and their parents and have been found to be especially effective for families at higher risk and those living in disadvantaged communities (Olds et al 1997, 2004).

Children in low-income and disadvantaged families are at higher risk of mental health and adjustment problems including delinquency, substance misuse, teenage pregnancy, violence and school failure (Dryfoos 1990, Wilson 1987). These behaviours do not usually occur in isolation; in fact, they frequently co-occur and have common risk factors (Jessor 1993, Lerner 1995) including poor coping skills, lack of nurturance and support and family violence. Risk factors can accrue cumulatively to place children at greater risk of poor health outcomes and poorer adjustment. The value of early intervention approaches lies not only in their ability to reduce these risk factors for negative developmental outcomes, but also in their potential to enhance positive child and family functioning through promoting competence, positive relationships and supportive environments for development. The protective factors identified include a sense of positive connection, a cohesive family, good communication, intimacy and confiding, self-esteem, good school performance and adaptive coping skills (Cowen & Work 1988, Rutter 1987). Social support from at least one caring adult has been found to be protective in relation to a wide range of adversities (Wolkow & Ferguson 2001).

Titterton et al (2002) reviewed the evidence base for interventions in the early years. This review identified a range of characteristics associated with successful interventions and best practice (Box 4.1). This report highlighted the importance of programmes beginning early and being directed at risk factors and risk processes. Outcomes were found to be affected by not only type of

Box 4.1

Characteristics of effective programmes identified by Titterton et al (2002)

- programmes that are long-term in nature
- programmes sustained by committed funding
- programmes that are part of a wider range of public policy measures, including those to reduce health inequalities
- integrated approaches where multidisciplinary and multi-agency interaction is encouraged, such as partnership with the voluntary sector

intervention but also the manner and location of delivery. The review by the Mental Health Foundation (1999) also highlights the importance of community participation, local interventions, effective assessment of needs and the need for long-term security for programmes, including stable funding.

Early interventions, therefore, have an important role to play not only in terms of preventing problems and their potential secondary effects, but also in their positive impact on enhancing family and community resilience via cultivating positive relationships and environments, which in turn fosters coping mechanisms. In contrast to the 'risk and prevention' perspective, the 'enhancement and coping' approach is also likely to be less stigmatising or threatening and more acceptable to participants which may encourage greater programme participation (Barnes & Freude-Lagevardi 2003).

Implementing Programmes for Children and Families

Interventions that provide quality family support programmes, quality pre-school programmes and enhance parenting skills have the potential to achieve long-term mental health benefits for both the child and the parents. In terms of family support programmes, these entail specially trained community members or professionals providing ongoing support to families during pregnancy, infancy and early childhood with the goal of empowering parents and their children. Programmes focus variously on enhancing nurturing and attentive parenting, developing parents' personal development and well-being and enhancing healthy child development. Parenting programmes have shown increased positive attitudes towards children, better knowledge about child behaviours, a more stimulating and safer environment for children and a more healthy, psychosocial and physical environment. In terms of the under fives, parenting support programmes, home visiting and pre-school or early childhood education programmes will be focused on in this chapter.

Parenting

Parenting programmes have an important role to play in the promotion of mental health. Such programmes show a direct effect on the mental health of mothers through the development of participants' skills, understanding and self-confidence and, through these changes, enhance the lives and mental health development of their children. Hoghughi (1998) found that parenting is the single largest variable contributing to positive health outcomes for children, including accident rates, teenage pregnancy, substance misuse, truancy, school exclusion and under-achievement, child abuse, juvenile crime and mental health problems. Pugh et al (1995) point out that absence of childcare, lack of transport and programmes' failure to be tailored towards need all contribute to the exclusion of parents in greatest need. They also point out that it is unlikely that one approach will always be best for all parents and the type of programme offered should reflect the needs of individual parents.

The Triple P programme (Sanders 1999) is a population-based parenting programme which aims to enhance the knowledge, skills and confidence of parents and promotes nurturing, safe, engaging, non-violent and low-conflict environments for children, thereby reducing behavioural, emotional and developmental problems. The Triple P programme has been found to be an effective parenting intervention in a range of controlled randomised trials (Dean et al 2003, Sanders 1999, Sanders et al 2000). A group version of Triple P is also available which focuses on the application of parenting skills to a broad range of behaviours (Turner et al 1998). Dean et al (2003) evaluated a community-wide implementation of the group programme in south-eastern Sydney in partnership with a range of public health service agencies and community agencies. Parental evaluations demonstrated an increase in parents' knowledge and use of positive parenting practices, which in turn resulted in improvements in their children's behaviour, e.g. reduction in disruptive child behaviour, lower levels of dysfunctional parenting, reduction in conflict between parents over child rearing and gains in parental mental health. These gains were maintained at 6 and 12 months' follow up. The project demonstrated that it is possible to take an evidence-based intervention programme such as Triple P, which has been developed and evaluated within controlled research settings, and successfully incorporate it into service delivery in a range of health and community services. Dean et al 2003 identified the following factors as contributing to the success of the programme:

- all services were provided with free training and resources in order to increase participation levels
- a project coordinator was made available to assist the group facilitators
- programme training, accreditation and ongoing workshops were conducted throughout the project for group facilitators who came from a range of professional backgrounds and levels of experience in addressing parenting issues
- ongoing support was provided to group facilitators during project delivery
- to ensure sustainability, project coordinators worked with local service management in order to establish local systems of administration and planning from Triple P group programmes.

Different formats and techniques have been found to be effective in parenting programmes. For example, the 'Incredible Years' series (Webster-Stratton et al 2001), which is a comprehensive training programme for parents, teachers and children aimed at preventing and reducing behavioural and emotional problems in children aged 2–8 years, employs a combination of techniques. The parent training programmes utilise a collaborative training process of group discussion guided by trained facilitators and programme materials such as videotapes, parent books, audiotapes, modelling and home activities (Webster-Stratton 1982). Findings from six randomised trials show that the parent programme is effective in reducing conduct problems and increasing positive affect and compliance with parental commands (Webster-Stratton 1990, 1999, Webster-Stratton et al 2001). It is interesting to note, however, that guidelines based on the findings from this programme caution against the use of parent-training programmes with families under stress, and argue that it is only by addressing the broader ecological needs of families that we can begin to reach the 30–50% of families that fail to benefit from the traditional parent-training approaches (Webster-Stratton & Hammond 1990).

A systematic review of the effectiveness of group-based parenting programmes in improving maternal psychosocial health by Barlow et al (2001) concludes that parenting programmes can be cost-effective in improving a range of psychosocial outcomes in mothers of children between the ages of 3 and 10 years. Based on a meta-analysis of a sub-sample of 17 programmes, they conclude that there is clear evidence of the short-term effectiveness of parenting programmes in improving self-esteem, anxiety/stress, depression and relationships with spouse/marital adjustment. Similar results were obtained from different types of parenting programmes and it is indicated that process factors are important in influencing the outcome for parents. However, little research is available on the quality of programme delivery or other process factors that may be influential in producing positive outcomes. However, it seems likely that the group facilitator/leader has an important role to play in creating an atmosphere of trust and openness between the participating parents and in helping parents to feel respected, understood and supported. The lack of data on process factors in these studies does not allow conclusions to be drawn concerning whether it is the content of the programme or its delivery which is crucial to successful outcomes. Most likely, it is the interaction of the two that makes the difference and accounts for positive change.

Good practice parenting support initiatives have been found to include the following characteristics:

* adopt empowerment approaches aimed at raising parents' confidence and self-esteem
* broad-based content
* focus on individual and family interpersonal issues
* focus on specific parenting skills
* accessible to those most at risk.

Home Visiting Programmes

The most common type of early years interventions are intensive home visiting programmes and centre-based support. Home visiting programmes may have a variety of goals and service elements; however, they all share a focus on the importance of children's early years, the pivotal role of parents in shaping children's lives and the importance of the home as a place or setting for promoting positive mental health (Box 4.2). As a strategy for delivery, home visiting programmes bring services and the programme to the family home rather than expecting families to seek assistance through their community services.

A shared assumption of home visiting programmes is that children's earliest experiences play a fundamental role in shaping their life opportunities and

> ## Box 4.2
>
> ## Goals of home visiting programmes
> (Gomby et al 1999)
>
> - promotion of enhanced parental knowledge, attitudes and behaviour to child rearing
> - promotion of children's health
> - promotion of children's development
> - prevention of child abuse and neglect
> - enhancement of maternal well-being and life course

parental care-giving is the most important of these earliest experiences (Olds et al 2000). Most of the programmes assume that vulnerable families/parents need both additional information and community resources to promote their children's development more effectively. They also assume that a strong relationship between parents and the home visitor is crucial to the success of these programmes (Gomby et al 1999). Home visitors see the environments that families live in and can, therefore, gain a better understanding of the families' needs in order to tailor services to meet those needs.

By definition, home visiting programmes are delivered into the homes of families with young children and seek to improve the lives of the children by encouraging changes in the attitudes, knowledge and/or behaviour of parents. Most of the programmes provide both social support and practical assistance to parents, in many cases linking families with other community services, child development, education and parenting programmes. Programmes may, however, differ in their specific goals. While most programmes focus on improving parenting skills to promote healthy child development, in addition many seek to prevent child abuse and neglect and/or to improve the lives of parents through encouraging mothers to find jobs, return to education and to plan subsequent pregnancies. Many programmes also seek to promote the use and take-up of preventive services such as prenatal care, immunisations or well-baby check ups. Programmes differ in terms of their onset; during pregnancy or after the birth of the child, last from 2 to 5 years and scheduled visits range from weekly to monthly. Staffing and training requirements also vary. Home visiting programmes can be provided by trained health care professionals such as health visitors/ nurses (e.g. Olds (1997) 'Prenatal and Infancy Home Visitation by Nurses' programme), social workers, psychologists and also by trained community volunteers, e.g. in the 'Community Mothers Programme' (Johnson & Molloy 1995). The effective delivery of home visiting programmes by trained health visitors in the Jamaican home visiting programme (Powell & Grantham-McGregor 1989) and by trained community workers in a pilot programme in South Africa (Cooper et al 2002) demonstrate the feasibility of such programmes in low-income settings.

There is strong evidence to suggest that intensive home visiting and centre-based support is successful in enhancing resilience and competence in both children and parents, which in turn helps prevent mental health problems (Jané-Llopis et al 2005). However, to be successful such interventions must begin early, be sustained in the long term and target risk and protective factors (Mental Health Foundation 1999, Titterton et al 2002). It is also recognised that families often in most need of such programmes are least likely to avail of them, therefore, community-based initiatives with the opportunity for local participation are more likely to be successful in reaching families at higher risk. Building partnerships with parents is recognised as an essential strategy for promoting children's healthy development. Partnerships in themselves can help create a context that promotes and sustains mental health among children, adults and communities at large (Bond 1999). This is particularly important when working with vulnerable children and families living in disadvantaged communities, as the parents' own development and empowerment may be key to supporting their abilities to create and sustain conditions that are supportive of their children's mental health and development. Programmes adopting a competence enhancement approach, carried out in partnership with parents, families, local communities and services are, therefore, more likely to be successful in reaching those who need them most.

As home visiting programmes often deal with the most vulnerable families, such as those living in socially and economically disadvantaged communities and often experiencing high levels of stress and increased risk, we need to have realistic expectations about how much such programmes can achieve. These programmes typically consist of 20–40 hours of contact per year and seek to impact on complex problems such as child abuse, neglect and the negative effects of poverty. Intervention programmes tend to focus primarily on parents and children, and as such can not address the wider structural factors such as poor, disorganised or violent communities. By themselves such programmes are insufficient to alleviate the effects of poverty on child development and family functioning. As such they are necessary but not sufficient, and should not be judged against their ability to impact on problems that are societal or community-wide in nature. If families live in communities where poverty is entrenched, programmes that focus solely on individual change rather than broader policy solutions may have limited impact. As Weiss cautions, 'home visits in the early years to enhance parents and help families should not be viewed as a lone silver bullet or panacea' (1993:121).

We will now examine a model programme that has been tested, refined and replicated across multiple sites and rigorously evaluated; the 'Prenatal and Infancy Home Visitation by Nurses' programme (Olds 1997, Olds et al 1997, 1998b), also known as the 'Nurse Home Visitation' programme. This programme, which has been developed over the last 25 years, is a theory-driven, research-based model programme delivered to disadvantaged mothers and their babies by trained nurse home visitors. We will then go on to examine, via case studies, two further programmes; the 'Community Mothers' and the 'Mothers Inform Mothers' programmes, which illustrate an empowerment-based model of parenting delivered by trained community mothers living in disadvantaged communities. The 'Home-Start' programme, which is an initiative based on a voluntary organisation dealing with families under stress, is also described in Chapter 7.

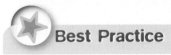

Best Practice

Prenatal and Infancy Home Visitation by Nurses

(Olds 1997, Olds et al 1997, Olds et al 1998b)

The Prenatal and Infancy Home Visitation by Nurses programme is a cost-effective, intensive and comprehensive programme developed by David Olds and his colleagues (Olds 1988, Olds & Korfmacher 1997), designed to improve three aspects of maternal and child functioning:

1. prenatal health and the outcomes of pregnancy
2. care provided to infants and toddlers in an effort to improve the children's health and development
3. the mother's personal development, particularly with regards to family planning, educational achievement, and participation in the workforce.

The programme is designed to serve low-income, unmarried and adolescent pregnant women having their first child. Comprehensive evaluation indicates that this programme is most effective with women bearing their first child as the women have not yet developed established ways of caring for themselves and their children during pregnancy. Low-income parents experience more than their share of life challenges and, without help, they and their children are more likely to experience compromised development.

The findings from three randomised controlled trials indicate that the programme is effective in the short term and even more so in the long term. Results show that the nurse home visitation programme can promote healthy maternal and child functioning early in life (Olds et al 1988). At 15 years follow up there are clear signs of less child abuse or neglect, completed family size, less welfare dependence, fewer behavioural problems due to substance abuse and less criminal behaviour on the part of low-income, unmarried mothers who participated in the programme (Olds et al 1997). Karoly et al (1998) report that by the time children from high-risk families reach age 15, the cost savings are four times the original investment because of reductions in crime, welfare and health care costs and as a result of taxes paid by the working parents. A detailed account of the implementation of this programme may be found in book seven of the 'Blueprints for violence prevention' series (Olds et al 1998b), to which the reader is advised to refer.

Programme Content

The programme is based around a trained nurse visiting a woman at home during her first pregnancy and the subsequent 2 years after the child's birth. One nurse visitor is assigned to each family for the duration of the programme; this is important, as process studies have shown that programme effectiveness declines if families are assisted by more than one nurse over the course of the programme. The nurse visits the family once a week for the first month after registration, and then every other week through delivery. After delivery, the visits are scheduled for once a week, and gradually phased out to once a month until 24 months postpartum. Visits typically last 60–90 minutes. The nurse may visit the family more frequently if the family exhibits crises that would warrant more intensive support, e.g. health problems associated with the pregnancy or adverse domestic conditions. The nurse follows a strict protocol that focuses on the mother's personal health, environmental health, quality of care-giving for the infant and toddler and the mother's own personal development, i.e. practising birth control, finding work or returning to education. The protocols, which have been developed and tested over a 20-year period, provide guidance to the nurses on a day-by-day basis and may be subtly adapted to meet the individual needs of each family.

Research suggests that the comprehensiveness of this programme is responsible for its success. The content of the programme focuses on the care and development of the child including the physical care of the child, promotion of the child's socioemotional and cognitive development and providing a positive and safe home environment. In addition the programme focuses on the promotion of the mothers' self-efficacy with respect to their health-related behaviours, completing their education, participating in the workforce and planning future pregnancies. The integration of these two elements is seen as being critical to maximising the opportunities for creating and sustaining change (Olds et al 1994). Also critical to the programme is the close working relationship that nurses develop with the mothers, identifying small achievable objectives in order to build the mothers' confidence and pave the way for setting and reaching life goals. Home visitation is used in conjunction with family, friends and various statutory and voluntary health and human services in order to enable families to develop their strengths and achieve their goals.

The following key programme components have been identified by Olds et al (1998c):

* focus on low-income first-time mothers
* trained experienced mature nurses with good interpersonal skills make the home visits
* home visits begin during pregnancy and continue for 2 years after a child is born
* home visitors see families at home every 1–2 weeks
* home visitors focus simultaneously on the mother's personal health and development, environmental health and quality of care-giving for the infant and toddler
* family members and friends are involved in the programme and help families use other community support services when needed
* each full-time nurse home visitor carries a maximum caseload of 25 families
* a nursing supervisor provides supportive guidance and oversees programme implementation
* detailed assessments and records are kept on families and their needs, services provided, family progress and outcomes; this is also important for the monitoring and evaluation of the programme.

Evaluation Findings

Trials of the programme have been conducted in several US states with participants from a number of cultural backgrounds in both urban and rural settings. It has also been replicated in various 'demonstration site' communities to determine how to develop the programme, e.g. high-crime urban areas or delivering the programme with paraprofessionals instead of registered nurses. The findings from the three main randomised controlled trials (Elmira, New York; Memphis, Tennessee; and Denver, Colorado) will now be summarised.

The first trial of the programme was held in Elmira, New York (Olds et al 1986, 1988, 1994, 1997). A sample of 400 women were recruited during pregnancy and followed through the child's 15th birthday. Anyone bearing their first child was permitted to participate; however, some 85% of enrolled women were either low-income, unmarried or teenaged and none had previous live births. A randomised control design was used, stratifying for demographics, and women were randomly assigned to receive either home visitation services (intervention group) or comparison services (control group). Impressive results were demonstrated in relation to prenatal conditions, child development and maternal life course at the end of the programme. In comparison to the control group, the mothers in the intervention group exhibited the following positive outcomes: an improved diet, fewer kidney infections, greater social support and made better use of formal community services. Among the women who smoked, the intervention mothers showed a 25% decrease in smoking rates during pregnancy, had 75% fewer pre-term deliveries and, for the young adolescents, had babies with higher birth weights. With regards to child development, the effect on child abuse and neglect approached significance ($p = 0.07$), there were fewer child injuries and ingestions, and the children had developmental quotients that were higher than their counterparts in the control group (Olds et al 1986). Finally, in terms of maternal life course, women in the intervention group experienced a reduced number of subsequent pregnancies.

A follow-up study of the Elmira trial assessed the impact of the programme during the child's 3rd and 4th years of life (Olds et al 1994). No enduring effects were found on the rates of child abuse and neglect or on the children's level of intellectual functioning. However, the evaluation did report several lasting programme effects on household safety: 35% fewer instances of the child visiting the emergency department; 40% fewer child injuries and ingestions; 45% fewer child behavioural/parental coping problems; and an increased quality of care which low-income, unmarried teenagers provided to their children (Olds et al 1994). The follow-up study also demonstrated that women in the intervention group were more likely to participate in the workforce (increased by 83%) and to delay subsequent pregnancies (reduced by 42%) during the first 4 years after delivery as compared to the control group (Olds et al 1988).

A follow up of the Elmira study at 15 years confirmed additional significant enduring effects on child development and maternal life course (Olds 1997, Olds et al 1997). In relation to primarily white families, the following findings were reported for the first-born child of mothers in the intervention group: 79%

fewer verified reports of abuse and neglect; 60% fewer instances of running away; 56% fewer arrests; 81% fewer convictions of violations of probation; 63% fewer lifetime sex partners; 56% fewer days of alcohol consumption; and 40% fewer cigarettes smoked per day. Maternal life course results were also encouraging, as women who had participated in the programme achieved an average of 2+ years' interval between first child and second child, 69% fewer maternal arrests, increased workforce participation, 44% fewer maternal problems due to alcohol and drug abuse and 30 months less in receipt of social welfare. It is of interest to note that these positive effects were found not for the whole sample, but were specific to higher risk families, i.e. poor unmarried women and their children who participated in the programme.

A second evaluation of the programme took place in the city of Memphis, Tennessee (Kitzman et al 1997). The sample consisted of 1139 low-income, primarily African-American unmarried women, randomly assigned to intervention and control groups. Again, notable results were demonstrated in relation to prenatal conditions, child development and maternal life course. In comparison to the control group, the women in the programme had greater use of community services, they were more likely to be employed ($p = 0.06$) and they exhibited fewer instances of pregnancy-induced hypertension. The first-born child had fewer injuries and ingestions, fewer days hospitalised due to injuries and ingestions and lived in a home more conducive to child development. Finally, the mothers themselves had fewer subsequent pregnancies and fewer months in receipt of social welfare. A follow up when the children were 6 years old (Olds et al 2004) demonstrated the continuing positive impact of the programme. Mothers in the intervention group were in receipt of less social welfare support and had better family planning skills, while children had higher behavioural and educational outcomes.

A third randomised controlled study of this programme in Denver, Colorado, conducted with 1178 pregnant women, examined the unique contributions that nurses and lay community health visitors might make when both were trained in the prescribed programme model. Results indicated that the paraprofessionals produced effects that rarely achieved statistical or clinical significance while the nurses made significant impacts on a wide rage of maternal and child outcomes (Olds et al 2002). There has, however, been some debate as to whether this result is generalisable to other contexts (Guterman et al 2003) and this requires further investigation.

The programme cost an estimated $3200 per family per year during the start-up phase (i.e. for the first 3 years) and $2800 per family per year thereafter once nurses are completely trained and working at full capacity (Olds et al 1998c). A report from the Rand Corporation estimated that by the time children from high-risk families reach age 15, the cost savings are four times the original investment due to reductions in crime, welfare and health care costs and as a result of taxes paid by the working parents (Karoly et al 1998). The replication of this programme has been underway since 1997 and includes over 200 sites in 23 states in the US. As such, there is a wealth of experience to draw upon in identifying essential elements that make the programme work, and in building on the lessons learned in informing the development and dissemination of best practice programmes.

Programme Implementation Features

The programme has been refined and adapted over the last 25 years. Research of the dissemination process and experience (Olds et al 1998b, Racine 2000, 2002) have indicated the following key features of the planning and implementation of this programme:

Model based on theoretical foundations: The programme is grounded on the integration of three well-established theories of human development and change. In terms of self-efficacy (Bandura 1977), the content of the programme focuses on developing the mothers' confidence in their abilities as parents, helping mothers plan for themselves and their babies and through setting short-term achievable goals to gradually assist mothers in gaining a sense of control over the direction of their lives. Human attachment theory (Ainsworth & Bowlby 1991, Bowlby 1977) highlights the importance of the child's level of attachment to a caregiver for their healthy emotional and social development. The programme focuses on the formation of the mother–child relationship and teaches mothers how to recognise and respond to the child's emotional needs. Human ecology theory (Bronfenbrenner 1992) emphasises the importance of the social context such as other family members, social networks and the wider community on human development. This theory focuses the programme on the parent–child relationship in the context of other family and community relationships and the need to manage such relationships so that they are supportive of positive development.

Recruitment and retention of target population: This programme has been found to be most effective with women who are unmarried and from low-income households. The programme is based on voluntary participation, and women's interest in participating will be affected by their desire to have questions answered about their pregnancy, the health of the baby, and the need to find resources in the community. Eligible women are typically identified through referrals from health clinics, hospitals, doctor's offices, schools and facilities serving low-income women. In randomised trials, 80–95% of the women who were offered the opportunity to participate accepted (Olds et al 1998b). Many families are difficult to engage, however, for a number of reasons, e.g. distrust of the nurse visitor or the inability to manage competing time commitments (Gomby et al 1999). Therefore, the programme model takes the position that unless a mother explicitly asks to be dropped from the programme she is retained on the programme caseload. While this may border on being intrusive, evaluation proves that many mothers thank the nurses for persisting with them during their crises or through the early days of distrust.

Staffing: The successful selection of home nurse visitors and supervisors is critical to successful implementation, as the home visitor is the embodiment of the programme for families (Gomby et al 1999). The programme model recommends full-time female nurses who have a recognised qualification, previous relevant experience and strong interpersonal skills. Past experience with the programme has proven the importance of recruiting nurses who have knowledge or a clear understanding of home visiting, low-income pregnant women and parents of young children. Thorough training, supervision and solid clinical decision-making skills are also necessary to implement the programme. A full-time nurse visitor should carry a caseload of no more than 25 families, due to the intensity of intervention. The nursing supervisor is responsible for overseeing implementation and assuring clinical supervision on a regular basis so that participating nurses may discuss cases and obtain feedback. Supervisors play a vital role in collaborative relationships with ancillary service providers upon whom the programme depends for multidisciplinary support. A full-time supervisor should support no more than eight home visitor nurses.

Training and technical assistance: Staff training for this programme includes an initial 1-week session for nurses and their supervisor in Denver, Colorado, followed by a 3-day and 2-day follow-up training on site to coincide with the nurses' need to begin using the infancy and then toddler protocols with the families (Olds et al 1998b). Provisions for training new staff within an existing community are being developed.

Key community contacts: Communities must decide what organisation will take the lead for administering the programme; in the US, this role has been filled generally by a local health department. The programme's success depends on strong local leadership and commitment to effective implementation in order to target services and ensure programme integrity. A local multidisciplinary planning group or task force, including national and/or local directors of health and social services, should help to determine which agencies should be involved in developing the programme. Once in operation, the programme relies on coordination and cooperation among a variety of statutory and voluntary service providers and such commitment must be made evident from the outset to ensure integration into current health and social service systems.

Interagency collaboration: Though nurses are the primary providers of this programme, they do not have the capability to manage all types of physical, mental and social health, particularly in high-risk families. The programme requires active multidisciplinary support. As nurses will have to refer mothers and families to various health and social service providers, the nurses themselves must understand and have a working relationship with those other services. Agreements may need to be established with certain agencies and primary care providers to contract services to the programme.

Funding and resources: In 1997, it was estimated that the programme cost $3200 per family per year during the start-up phase (first 3 years of implementation) and $2800 per family per year once nurses are trained and working to full capacity. Communities in the US retained a variety of local, regional and governmental funding to support the programme. When the programme focuses on low-income women, the costs to fund the programme are recovered by the time the first child reaches age 4 (Olds et al 1998c). It is reported that by the time children from high-risk families reach age 15, the cost savings are four times the original investment because of reductions in crime, welfare and health care costs and as a result of taxes paid by the working parents (Karoly et al 1998). When implementing this programme outside of the US, funding will need to be considered in the light of each individual country's funding for health and social services. Several resources are important for the implementation of this programme. A single administrative home for the programme will centralise communications and act as a home base for the visiting nurses. The nursing staff must have relevant training, as well as copies of the programme protocols and record keeping forms. Finally, the nurses will require standard treatment tools, e.g. blood pressure cuffs and baby scales.

Programme modifications in response to family needs: Although there are specific protocols to guide each nurse visit, the protocols are designed to be adapted to the individual needs of each mother and her family. For example, the nurse will need to concentrate more on smoking cessation and the consequences of prenatal cigarette smoking for women who smoke. Specific educational and behavioural change approaches are set in motion on the basis of the nurses' individualised assessments. The programme has also been modified to meet the needs of populations with greater ethnic and racial diversity.

Key Recommendations for Replication

Integrate the programme into existing health services: The adaptation of the programme to local conditions may require the involvement of professionals from different disciplines and different agencies to implement the programme effectively. A particular challenge may be integrating the programme into a health system that already has existing programmes for young families whose funding may by threatened by the financial support demands of implementing this model (Olds et al 1998b). In addition, local and national public policy support is paramount for the eventual upscaling of this programme in order to give both credibility and necessary resources (Racine 2002).

Foster community support: Community support and positive relationships are vital to this programme's success. Indeed, a study by McGuigan et al (2003) suggests that families are more likely to drop out of the programme if they come from certain communities, e.g. with high levels of violence, even when confounding influences on attrition were controlled for, such as nurses' empathy, educational background and the mother's marital status. Given the strong evidence of this programme's effectiveness, communities may have to make difficult choices such as elimination or transformation of certain programmes that evidence suggests do not work. In doing this, programme implementers must be cognisant of minimising damage to professional relationships and enhancing the strength of community service delivery systems for families.

Monitor implementation and gradual dissemination: Formative evaluation, as prescribed, will monitor programme fidelity and highlight the features of successful implementation. According to David Racine, who has been involved in replicating and upscaling the programme, the fidelity to the purpose of the programme ('functional fidelity') and the fidelity to its components ('structural fidelity') are crucial to reproducing the positive outcomes of the clinical trials (Racine 2002). It is imperative that programme implementers prevent this intervention from becoming diluted and compromised in the process of development. It is particularly noted that the programme should not be rolled out on a large scale in a short period of time. Systematic monitoring and evaluation of the process of implementation will help ensure that the programme's fidelity is maintained. Rapid dissemination without sufficient planning and capacity building will compromise the quality of programme implementation and effectiveness (Olds et al 1998b).

Adapt the programme to fit cultural context: Thus far, this programme has been rolled out and evaluated in the US. It is expected that certain alterations will need to be made in order to adapt the programme to another country and culture. Programme implementers will need to set up a local advisory committee to review the programme content and materials and thus ensure relevance and sensitivity to the new populations served (Olds et al 1998b). All nurses should undertake relevant training regarding racial and ethnic diversity, e.g. with regards to working with ethnic minority groups and asylum seekers. Engaging family members and friends of the mother participating in the programme will help integrate programme delivery with respect to cultural and situational circumstances. Continuous process evaluation will help to fine tune programme components to suit the local context.

. . . .

Next we examine the 'Community Mothers' programme (Johnson & Molloy 1995, Johnson et al 1993), which is a good example of a low-cost and highly effective programme which promotes parenting skills and child development, employing an empowerment model of parenting. This parent support programme involves experienced volunteer mothers in disadvantaged areas, who give support and encouragement to parents in child rearing. Of interest is the fact that the programme can be delivered effectively by non-professionals, themselves mothers living in disadvantaged areas. The Community Mothers programme has gained an international reputation and various models are in operation across Ireland, the Netherlands, the UK, Australia and USA. Replications include the Mothers Inform Mothers Programme in the Netherlands, which has also been evaluated and provides supportive findings of the effectiveness of this model of promoting positive parenting. Given its structure, this programme has the potential to be applied in low-income countries and settings with relatively few adaptations to programme structure and materials used. Case studies by the author of the original programme and its adaptation in the Netherlands will now be examined.

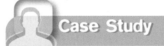

Case Study

Community Mothers Programme

. . . .

Brenda Molloy

Introduction

The Community Mothers Programme (CMP) is a support programme for first-time and some second-time parents of children aged from birth to 24 months who live in mainly disadvantaged areas. This includes lone parents, teenage parents, 'travellers', asylum seekers and refugees. Following pilot phases, the CMP was formally launched in the former Eastern Health Board (now known as the Health Service Executive – Eastern Region), Republic of Ireland, in 1988. The programme is delivered to nearly 2000 parents each year (Molloy 2002).

The programme aims to support and aid the development of parenting skills, thereby enhancing parents' confidence and self-esteem. Non-professional volunteer mothers known as 'community mothers', who are recruited, trained and supported by specially trained public health nurses known as 'family development nurses', deliver it. Each family development nurse supports 15–20 community mothers who each in turn support between five and 15 families. Each nurse works with up to 100 families at any one time. The community mothers visit parents in their own homes once a month and use a specially designed child development programme, which focuses on health care, nutritional improvement and overall development. The programme model is one of parent enablement and empowerment (Johnson & Molloy 1995). Participation is voluntary.

In 1990 the programme was evaluated by a randomised controlled trial when programme children were 1 year old (Johnson et al 1993) and was found to have significant beneficial effects for both mothers and children. Children in the intervention group scored better in terms of immunisation, cognitive stimulation and nutrition, and their mothers scored better in terms of nutrition and self-esteem than those in the control group. At that time the programme was aimed only at first-time parents during the first 12 months of the child's life; parents received a maximum of 12 visits, usually one per month, each lasting approximately 1 hour. In 1997–1998 a 7-year follow-up study (Johnson et al 2000) was undertaken to find out whether the benefits of the programme had been sustained over the intervening period, by which time the children were 8 years of age. Approximately one third of the mothers who had been in the original intervention and control groups were located and asked for details on the child's health, the diet of both mother and child, the development of the child and the mother's parenting skills and feelings of self-esteem. In a nutshell, the findings were very positive; intervention mothers were more likely to check their child's homework every night and to disagree with the statement, 'Children should be smacked for persistently bad behaviour'. Mothers in the intervention group demonstrated higher self-esteem and greater enthusiasm for motherhood, intervention children were less likely to have an accident (although more likely to have been hospitalised for an illness), and subsequent children of the intervention mothers were more likely to have completed their primary immunisation programme.

The conclusion is that the CMP has a beneficial impact on parenting skills and maternal self-esteem that is sustained over time and which is carried through to subsequent children. In order to enhance these effects even further, and as a direct result of continuing and regular evaluation, the programme has been extended to the first 24 months of the child's life. A study carried out on the programme in 2003 showed that the programme aided the development of parent–child bonds and attachment (McGuire-Schwartz 2003). The impact of the programme on the community mothers (Conroy 2001, Molloy 1992, Molloy 2005) and the travelling community (Fitzpatrick et al 1997) has also been evaluated with very positive results. The success of the programme in recent years has led to the development of peer-led interventions based on the idea of the CMP in other health service regions in Ireland, as well as in the UK, the Netherlands, Sweden and Australia. These programmes have not, to date, been evaluated by randomised controlled trials and it is thus difficult to compare them with CMP.

Programme Implementation and Recommendations

The CMP evolved from a child development programme based in the UK (Barker 1987). The public health nurses who implemented the pilot project had many other commitments to existing prevention and treatment activities in the community at large and were not able to continue implementing the visiting programme. It was, therefore, decided by the health board to pilot a community-based programme using experienced mothers as non-professionals to visit and support other mothers.

The first couple of years of the programme were quite difficult as it was a new experience for everyone involved and there were many difficulties to overcome. The nurse managers, the local public health nurses and, indeed, health board management were very anxious about 'ordinary' mothers getting involved in primary relationships with families; nothing like this had ever been done before and there were no precedents to follow. It was a case of trial and error, learning by doing and adapting as necessary. Many of the community mothers were worried about whether they would be accepted or not, but gradually they overcame their doubts as the parents they were visiting let them know that they were happy to be visited by a community mother. They stated that they felt that they were people they could trust and because they came from their local areas, they saw this as an advantage as they could have a better understanding of their problems and also the difficulties of rearing children in those communities, especially if they were lacking in facilities.

The CMP is essentially based in the community as well as being dependent on a formal organisation and, to a large extent, firmly part of the formal system. Most of the problems in the early years revolved around keeping a balance between these formal and informal worlds. The CMP can be seen as an attempt to bring together the public world of the bureaucrat with the private world of mothers, which can, and has, led to tensions. Overall, the success of the CMP has shown that the two need not be antithetical, but great care is needed to interweave the two systems in a way that avoids incorporation of the informal by the formal. The aim is to enable the statutory services to interweave their help so as to use and strengthen the help already given, to overcome existing limitations and to facilitate a process of empowerment in the community. It is not a question of plugging the gaps, but of working with society to close the gaps.

Key Factors that Made the Programme Possible and Ensured its Successful Planning and Delivery

Experience has shown that the CMP works because it is based on the following key elements:

- programme visiting is essentially focused on parent empowerment. The home visit is the catalyst that sparks the process of empowerment, which in turn has an impact on the women's social and mental well-being. Parents are empowered to believe in their own capabilities for parenting without being dependent on professionals

- a clearly structured format
- a one-to-one relationship between the community mother and the parent being visited
- a fundamental equality between the community mother and the parent being visited
- the use of illustrated materials to provide easy, non-threatening and relevant information for parents
- the programme is delivered not by health care personnel, but instead by experienced mothers. The community mothers relate to the parent as an 'ordinary mother' and not as a mini professional. Community mothers are empowered through this process because they recognise and value their worth as women and mothers
- a key aspect of the recruitment policy is that community mothers reflect the ethos of the community they intend to visit and they are paid nominal expenses for each visit. This is seen as necessary as the programme is operating in working class communities and the small payments enable the community mothers to participate
- a successful reorientation for the family development nurses enables them to 'de-role' and abandon attitudes that they have received through training in the biomedical model of health, and commit themselves to working with the disadvantaged in a spirit of equality and in a participatory process with the community mothers. The family development nurses are empowered because they are no longer confined by their profession and are enabled to see health in its holistic sense of social and mental well-being (Lang 1991)
- the programme is situated within the health services. The community mothers do not belong to an autonomous voluntary organisation. The health service executive recognises the enlightened nature of the programme. Accordingly the programme is somewhat autonomous but still remains a structure within the health service executive. This has enabled the programme to grow
- the educational content and process reflects the needs of the community mothers in their work of home visiting
- everything is done in the community, for example, the visits and the training of the community mothers
- the programme has continually evaluated its methods and adapted them with the findings, as well as the changing circumstances in society.

The key factors outlined above would need to be considered for programme replication.

The Future

The results of the follow-up study have shown that the benefits of the CMP have been sustained for both mothers and children. The positive effects were sustained; they were not 'washed out'. Of equal importance is the fact that it has shown that it is possible to develop, implement and maintain, even within the confines of a health bureaucracy, a programme that contains within it empowering processes directed at human development, contributing to both health and well-being.

The CMP has received international acclaim and has undergone external evaluation (Mental Health Europe 2000). An evidence-based programme delivered by non-professional volunteer mothers in partnership with 'de-roled' professionals, it provides benefits and advantages to families and future generations.

The programme could be further developed both nationally and internationally. The challenge would be our ability to maintain the essence of the programme while at the same time transferring the concept.

References

Barker W 1987 Seeking client needs or empowering parents? THS Health Summary Vol IV(VI):1–3

Conroy P 2001 Volunteering and the organisation. Ralaheen Ltd., Dublin

Fitzpatrick P, Molloy B, Johnson Z 1997 Community Mothers Programme: extension to the travelling community in Ireland. Journal of Epidemiology and Community Health 51:299–303

Johnson Z, Molloy B 1995 The Community Mothers Programme: empowerment of parents by parents. Children and Society 9(2):73–85

Johnson Z, Howell F, Molloy B 1993 Community Mothers Programme: randomised controlled trial of non-professional intervention in parenting. British Medical Journal 306:1449–1452

Johnson Z, Molloy B, Scallon E et al 2000 Community Mothers Programme: seven year follow-up of a randomised controlled trial of non-professional intervention in parenting. Journal of Public Health Medicine 22(3):337–342

Lang G 1991 Primary health care as an educational framework for the empowerment

of communities. Unpublished thesis, University of Manchester

McGuire-Schwartz 2003 An exploration of the relationships between family and social support and parent–child attachment: multicultural perspectives in the United States and Ireland. Unpublished PhD thesis, University of Massachusetts

Mental Health Europe 2000 Health promotion for children up to six years. Mental Health Europe, Brussels

Molloy B 1992 Effects of providers participating in a parent support programme. Unpublished thesis, Trinity College, Dublin

Molloy B 2002 Still going strong: a tracer study of the Community Mothers Programme, Dublin Ireland. Early Childhood Development: Practice and Reflections No. 17. Bernard van Leer Foundation, The Hague

Molloy M 2005 Volunteering – a pathway to lifelong learning: a study of volunteers in the Community Mothers Programme. Unpublished BEd thesis, University of Dublin in association with St Catherine's College of Education for Home Economics

Case Study

Mothers Inform Mothers

Bert Prinsen, Mieke Vergeer, Yvonne de Graaf

This case study concerns the development, implementation and evaluation of the 'Mothers Inform Mothers' (MIM) programme in the context of the Dutch child health care system.

Introduction

The MIM programme is an early childhood care and development programme. It is based on a synthesis of nursing, pedagogical and health-promotional knowledge and theories. The programme is part of the regular child health care services and it aims to support young parents with parenting, helping them to cope, staying abreast of their child's development and preventing child-rearing problems. The MIM programme supports the aim of enhancing the ability of women to cope with their newborn baby, of encouraging them to adapt their behaviour after receiving health educational information, increasing the number of women breastfeeding and enabling women to feel in control of their lives. The main goal is focused on mothers by trying to reinforce their sense of self-esteem and thereby improving their ability to act as a self-supporting parent. The core of MIM is (Hanrahan & Prinsen 1997a, b, Vergeer et al 2003):

- educational and social support for inexperienced parents
- experienced mothers visit the young mother (programme mother) with a first baby in her own home with a minimum of 18 home visits over an 18-month period
- the experienced visiting mother uses two aids; the chat paper – a home-visiting checklist to set the agenda of the visit, and the programme sequence of cartoons
- a community nurse is the coach and facilitator of the visiting mothers.

The Philosophy of MIM

MIM is connected to the philosophy of primary health care by characteristics such as promoting the ability to cope for oneself, participation and the joint responsibility for health and welfare. Another core notion is that mothers themselves are knowledgeable about their own child and they learn to rely more on their intuition. Mothers get the feeling of 'being master of their own existence'. In this way the concept of empowerment takes shape as the heart of MIM.

Innovation: Start Small, Embedding in Child Health Care

The original project of local nursing agency Thuiszorg Breda and the Netherlands Institute for Care and Welfare/NIZW was an example of innovating the method of parenting support. The first objective was to develop an application for the Netherlands based on a translation of the Irish 'Community Mothers Programme' considering the quality guidelines which were set for home visits within the 'Early Childhood Development Programme' (Barker 1992). This adaptation took place in the context of the well-baby clinic. The home visits were to be made by volunteers with the mentoring of child health care nurses. After the development of the programme in Breda, MIM became available for dissemination in the Netherlands. The innovation approach was experiment at a small scale, evaluation, designing the MIM manual, standardisation of the method of the programme and preparing for dissemination.

The History of Innovation: Development and Implementation of MIM

The development of the MIM programme took place in three important steps:

Phase 1: the development (1991–1994): This phase is characterised by the adaptation of the English–Irish Community Mothers Programme (Barker 1992, Johnson et al 1993). In two districts of the city of Breda child health nurses and a pedagogue experiment with the programme. The NIZW takes care of the programme description and the evaluation. A cultural adaptation is the next step after the translation of the Irish programme. The volunteers have a decisive vote, especially about the instruments: the cartoons and the chat paper. The development of the method at local scale and the participation of the visiting mothers is the breakthrough to a useful and applicable Dutch version (Wolf 1995). Evaluative research in this phase yields that:

- the ability of the participants to cope for themselves increases and they have more conscious attention to the development of their child
- the volunteers are coping better for themselves, which reflects in increased participation in education and volunteer work
- participants, volunteers and professionals evaluate the programme positively
- the theoretical foundation of the programme and the MIM method is finished and the instruments are applicable; the implementation can start.

Phase 2: first diffusion and further standardisation (1994–1996) Backed by private funding (Bernard van Leer Foundation, Fonds Kinderpostzegels Nederland, Juliana Welzijn Fonds, VSB Fund) the standardisation of the programme is the priority in the second phase as well as the diffusion among early adopting organisations. In the period 1994–1996 the MIM Cooperative is established, in which four nursing agencies – the early adoptors – and the NIZW jointly aim the implementation of MIM. The manual of the programme is finished and a video of the programme is made. An intervision group is started and individual learning for nurses is established. Once the MIM Cooperative has sufficient solidity, the phase of larger scale implementation dawns.

Phase 3: the implementation path of MIM (1996–2005): The implementation takes place in two steps. In the first step in 1996–2000 two objectives are prioritised; prepare the programme in all its parts for dissemination and for embedding in the infrastructure of child health care. In the next step in 2000–2005, the emphasis is on evaluative research and supporting the implementation within organisations on a larger scale. Initially all energy was focused on the dissemination of the programme. In this period the programme manual is published and the training for coordinators is developed. The quality of the professionals gets an incentive from the intervision platform and a series of annual working visits. Organisations have access to the 'Toolkit of MIM', which they can use to draft a project plan for MIM on their own. Because the actual dissemination does not take place fast enough, the MIM Cooperative explicitly reconsiders its implementation strategy in 1997. Analysis leads to the initiative to position parenting support more firmly as a basic task of child health care. In the meantime, the conclusion from an international working conference in Amsterdam in 1997 is that MIM in the Netherlands shares the quality features of a useful and potentially effective home visitation programme for the support of inexperienced mothers living in high-risk circumstances, comparable with programmes in Ireland, England and the US (Hanrahan & Prinsen 1997a). This provides a stimulus for taking charge of both the implementation within organisations and researching the effects of the Dutch programme next to the embedding of the programme in child health care policy.

Since 1999, a lot of attention has been devoted to the implementation of MIM. The 'Toolkit of MIM' facilitates organisations in formulating a local version for the local implementation of MIM. In total 18 newsletters find their way in the child health care system. MIM is present at every important manifestation and conference. Future coordinators receive tailor-made support; individually and 'in-company'. All programme materials are brought together in the MIM Programme Package in early 2003.

Participating Mothers

The percentage of the numbers of first borns as compared to the total numbers of newly borns in the MIM sites varies from 13–49%. Sites that have worked with MIM for a number of years reach on average 24% of the mothers of first borns. In the year 2002, 600 mothers participate in the MIM programme; 59% of the mothers are Dutch natives and 41% have a variety of ethnic backgrounds; 11% of the participating mothers raise their children without the help of a partner. The age of the programme mothers is 20–30 years old (49%) or 30–40 years old (45%). Mothers under 20 years old can be found at six sites.

After 18 months the programme stops; 60% of the participants have completed this MIM cycle. Reasons to stop are starting to work, no more interest and moving. About 280 visiting mothers – 83% of these volunteers are native Dutch and 17% are from 17 different ethnic backgrounds – do voluntary work with the MIM programme.

Dissemination

From the very beginning the intent has been to implement MIM in the entire Dutch child health care system with the perspective of a stronger policy on parenting support. With that goal in mind a number of activities have been carried out. Obviously such an innovation – adaptation of a new programme – in the Netherlands cannot succeed without a correct description of the method based on a thorough evaluation of practical experiences with the programme. Important stakeholders including the mothers, volunteers, nurses and nursing agencies, the Ministry of Health and Welfare, NIZW, municipalities and foundations have determined the implementation strategy (Hanrahan-Cahuzak 2002). Until now the main parts have been played by the professional organisations, the volunteers, the nurses and the NIZW.

Research

In 1998 an evaluation study is started at the University of Wageningen based on the design of the randomised community trial. The results of this evaluation are:

- participating mothers can increase their self-confidence and competence in raising children
- participation in MIM had no significant effect on the mental health of the mother
- on the satisfaction with the well-baby clinic, mothers participating in MIM scored significantly negative before starting the programme. This negative difference with the control groups decreased during the programme. MIM mothers equalled the satisfaction of mothers in the two control groups
- on health variables, MIM does not show significant effects with parents or children; nonetheless, the general health of the babies of MIM mothers post-measurement was on average higher than pre-measurement, whereas the general health of babies in the control groups had decreased
- about 38% of the mothers that breastfed did so for more than 3 months and 23% did so for more than 6 months; these percentages exceed the national average
- babies of the participating mothers consume more protein as a source of energy than fat compared to babies of the control groups. No significant differences were observed between the three groups for switching from feeding by bottle to feeding by cup.

These results are consistent with findings from previous international research (Barker 1992, Clinton 2001, Johnson et al 1993, Molloy 2002, Olds et al 1997), but they do not confirm every result. The decrease in child abuse could not be measured because of non-registration. The increase in vaccination rate was not expected, because of the current high rate in the Netherlands. In summary, Hanrahan-Cahuzak (2002) concludes that MIM represents a theoretically founded and, in practice, well applicable programme with promising effectiveness.

Innovation

In assessing the development and implementation of MIM in the Netherlands against criteria of effective innovation (De Caluwé en Vermaak 1999, Grol en Wensing 2001), we can identify the following success and failure factors in the innovation process.

Success factors:

- the appeal to use the basic human capacities of parents: empowerment
- the mix of bottom-up and top-down innovation strategies within nursing agencies and within the child health care system
- joint and shared cooperation between professionals (nurses) and parents (experienced and inexperienced mothers), supported by private funding

154

- from the perspective of quality, the requirement of 'community action' in cconnection with a professional organisation
- close connection between the innovation in practice and the embedding of that innovation in policy
- the programmatic approach developed as a multi-year continued project, which has resulted in continuity of innovation over many years
- the contribution to the professional development of nurses by task-enlargement and task-enrichment
- the considerable reinforcement of the social participation of mothers
- increasing political and public attention in relation to child raising and family. Parenting is nowadays on the Dutch agenda.

Failure factors:

- a partially missed connection to the revision of legislation and recent renewal of national policy on child health care
- imperfect programming of parenting support in child health care, at both the policy level and the professional level and research
- the unstable continuity of public financing of the programme
- the tendency towards specialisation and, therefore, isolation of the MIM coordinators within their nursing agency
- the small scale of evaluation and a deficient national research tradition in parenting support.

The question as to whether MIM will be part of the parenting support and health promotion policy of the Dutch child health care services in the next decade is open. MIM certainly has the potential and will succeed if:

- parenting support will be a major public health issue
- the quality of MIM raises from promising to effective
- parenting support, including home visiting programmes like MIM, become the core business of preventive youth policies at local level.

References

Barker W 1992 Child protection: the impact of the Child Development Programme. Early Childhood Development Unit, School of Applied Social Studies, University of Bristol

Clinton B 2001 MIHOW: the Maternal Infant Health Outreach Worker Program. Bernard van Leer Foundation, Den Haag

De Caluwé en Vermaak L H 1999 Leren veranderen. Samsom, Alphen aan de Rijn

Grol en Wensing B 2001 Implementatie. Effectieve verandering in de patiëntenzorg. Elsevier, Maarssen

Hanrahan M, Prinsen B (eds) 1997a Community health, community care, community support. NIZW/MIM Cooperative, Utrecht

Hanrahan M, Prinsen B 1997b Let's talk. NIZW/MIM Cooperative, Utrecht

Hanrahan-Cahuzak M H 2002 Mum to mum. An evaluation of a comunity-based health promotion programme for first-time mothers in the Netherlands. Wageningen University, Wageningen

Johnson Z, Howell F, Molloy B 1993 Community Mothers Programme: randomised controlled trial of non-professional intervention in parenting. British Medical Journal 306:1449–1452

Molloy B 2002 Still going strong. A tracer study of the Community Mothers Programme, Dublin, Ireland. Bernard van Leer Foundation, Den Haag

Olds D L, Eckenrode J, Henderson C R et al 1997 Long term effects of home visitation on maternal life course and child abuse and neglect. Journal of the American Medical Association 278(8):637–643

Vergeer M, Prinsen B, de Graaf Y 2003 MIM Program Package. NIZW, Utrecht

Wolf E J R M 1995 Met steun van een moeder: actiebegeleidend onderzoek van het programma MIM. NIZW, Utrecht

Pre-School Programmes

Early childhood or pre-school education programmes aim to provide children under 5 years with the knowledge, skills and social competence required for normal development and successful adjustment in school. Pre-school programmes promote cognitive and social skills that enhance school readiness and promote better school adjustment and performance, which is recognised as a protective factor for behavioural problems such as delinquency (Schweinhart & Weikart 1988) (Box 4.3). Many pre-school programmes also include extensive contact with parents as well as teachers, including home visits. These programmes seek to engage parents in their children's education and enhance parental competence and involvement in their children's development. The programmes impact on parents' behaviour and foster more positive expectations of the child's performance in school, of the school itself and of the teachers. Therefore, programmes that focus on both children and their socialising environments appear to produce the most enduring gains (Weissberg et al 1989). Such programmes promote multiple competencies and are capable of producing positive effects on many risk and protective factors for diverse problem behaviours. Research findings from the 'High/Scope Perry Preschool Programme' (Schweinhart & Weikart 1988) and the Consortium for Longitudinal Studies (Lazar et al 1982) show that high quality pre-school programmes can produce positive enduring changes in children's social and behavioural functioning.

Impressive long-term results have been achieved by programmes that address pre-school development such as enhancing language, cognitive and social skills. Positive cognitive and emotional benefits for younger children have been found for parent–child interaction, with interaction through use of story books playing an important role in the development of literacy (Baker et al 1997, Mentality 2003). Shure and Spivack (1988) developed the 'Interpersonal Cognitive Problem-Solving' (ICPS) programme for pre-schoolers and kindergartens. The ICPS programme is designed to teach children to consider alternative solutions and consequences to problems and solution–consequence pairing. Using scripts, games and exercises, the programme develops interpersonal cognitive problem-solving skills to support adaptive problem-solving efforts through improved communication around problem situations in the home and pre-school. The findings from the evaluation of this programme with pre-school children indicate that ICPS skills lead to improved positive behaviours, e.g. concern for others, and decreases in negative behaviour such as aggression and impatience in children. Training in cognitive problem-solving skills was found to be related to children's social adjustment and interpersonal

Box 4.3

Characteristics of high quality pre-school programmes
(Schweinhart & Weikart 1988, Weissberg et al 1991)

- a developmentally appropriate curriculum
- based on child-initiated activities
- teaching teams that are knowledgeable in early childhood development
- receiving ongoing training and supervision
- class sizes limited to fewer than twenty 3–5-year-olds with at least two teachers
- administrative leadership that includes support from the programme
- systematic efforts to involve parents in their child's education
- sensitivity to the non-educational needs of the child and family
- evaluation procedures that are developmentally appropriate

competences, with gains being maintained up to 2 years after programme participation (Shure and Spivack 1988). However, the more comprehensive programmes, which combine elements of home visits with day care, high quality education programmes and parent support appear to be the most effective.

A pioneering and highly effective project for children living in poverty is the High/Scope Perry Preschool project. This project was developed along the same lines as the 'Head Start' initiative, which was started in 1965 as part of the US government's 'war on poverty'. The Head Start project (see www.acf.dhhs.gov/programs/hsb) addressed the child's health, mental health and pre-school education and offered a comprehensive array of services to the child and family. Likewise, the Perry Preschool project works with children and families from low-income homes who are deemed to be at risk of school failure because of environmental factors and low IQ scores. Both the Perry Preschool project and Head Start programmes aim to improve the academic success of low-income children and to promote their mental and social development. We will now examine the High/Scope Perry Preschool project in more detail in order to highlight the key factors that contributed to its successful implementation and impressive long-term positive outcomes some 40 years after the programme was first implemented.

157

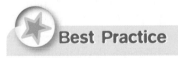 **Best Practice**

High/Scope Perry Preschool Programme

(Schweinhart & Weikart 1988, Schweinhart et al 2005)

The High/Scope Perry Preschool Programme (HSPPP) is a community-based, pre-school education intervention designed to promote intellectual and social development in children aged 3 and 4 years from disadvantaged backgrounds. The HSPPP uses an active learning approach, imparting cognitive and learning skills and encouraging independent and intuitive thinking that will support children's development through school and into young adulthood. The programme aims to improve the academic success of low-income children and assist parents in providing the necessary support for their children to develop intellectually, socially and mentally. It also aims to reduce the risk of underprivileged children becoming delinquent and continuing a life of poverty, by improving their chances of finishing school and thus attaining greater economic and social wealth.

The rationale behind the programme is that low intelligence and poor school performance have been associated with continued cycles of poverty, dependence on welfare and anti-social behaviour (Schweinhart & Weikart 1988). The programme developers believed that employing a comprehensive programme for early childhood education could positively affect the progression from childhood poverty to subsequent related adult problems (Schweinhart & Weikart 1988). Children aged 3 and 4 years were targeted as research indicates that an early childhood programme in the year or two prior to school entry is the best to develop a child's skills and dispositions for the school setting and subsequent life changes (Schweinhart & Weikart 1988).

The HSPPP was initiated in 1962 in Ypsilanti, Michigan, USA. The original HSPPP followed 123 disadvantaged African-American children over 40 years, from the age of three and four years through adulthood in order to assess longitudinal effects of the programme. Positive results were reported at all follow-up periods. Findings confirm that a high-quality, early childhood programme can achieve a significant impact on the life course of disadvantaged 3- and 4-year-olds. The longitudinal design of the evaluation also indicated the duration of such intervention in altering behaviour into adulthood (Weikart 1998). A benefit–cost analysis of the programme by Barnett (1993), based on findings from a 25 year follow-up, indicated that there was a seven to eight fold return on the initial investment in the programme, estimated at $1000 per child, due to decreased schooling costs, welfare and justice costs and higher earnings due to improved academic and social outcomes of the programme participants.

Programme Content

The programme content focuses on academic achievement, social and emotional competence, and parental involvement. The programme seeks to develop the reasoning, cognitive and social cooperation skills needed to prepare children for school. It also focuses on independent thinking, initiative, creativity and imagination in an environment that promotes investigation, problem solving and decision making. Parents are engaged in their children's development and facilitated in extending classroom learning at home. The programme incorporates five strategies about how children learn and develop:

1. active learning – children learn best from activities that they plan and carry out themselves
2. adult–child interaction – teachers interact with children and encourage each child's initiative and learning activities

3. creating an effective learning environment – the classroom is arranged so that children can use materials needed to carry out their chosen activities
4. maintaining daily routine – a daily schedule of events that is predictable and consistent
5. daily observational assessments – recorded notes can assist in planning children's growth and development.

Children attend 3-hour classes on weekday mornings 5 days a week for 7 months a year, from October through to May. The day is spent engaging in a number of activities, which are unique to the HSPPP in comparison with other pre-school programmes. One is the idea of 'key experiences' which includes exposing children to concepts of music, space, time, social relations, classification and language. The 'plan-do-review' routine is another major component of the programme in which children are encouraged to plan an activity they will complete, including the area and materials they will use, carry out the activity according to plan, and review their work and obtain feedback from the teacher and the class. This helps to give children a sense of control and responsible independence (Weikart & Schweinhart 1997).

Once a week, on a weekday afternoon, the teacher visits the home of each mother and child for a 1.5-hour appointment. Home visits provide an open framework of educational practice, where teachers can join parents as partners in the education and natural development of their children. Through home visits, a teacher can build a partnership with parents, explain child development principles and show parents how to assist their children, e.g. read stories aloud and demonstrate positive regard for books (Schweinhart & Weikart 1988).

Teachers regularly record assessments of each child's activities, knowledge and interests. The teacher uses these assessments to plan specific interventions that will encourage the child's growth and development (SAMHSA 2004). Members from each teaching team challenge themselves by observing fellow teachers' performance and mutually supporting each other (Weikart & Schweinhart 1997).

Programme Features

- a well defined classroom programme
- developmentally appropriate curriculum that encourages child-initiated learning activities
- emphasis on language, literacy (cognitive), social relations, initiative, movement, music, classification, space and time
- small groups to build good relationships between the teacher and the child
- circle time
- highly trained staff
- supportive teachers and parents
- a child-to-staff ratio of no more that 10 children per adult
- consistent staff supervision and training.

High/Scope publishes more than 300 titles in print, video, audiocassette and CD formats on programme resources and materials which are designed to support teachers, parents and researchers. Further details are available from www.highscope.org.

Evaluation Findings

The original 1962 HSPPP has been monitored for over 40 years (Schweinhart 2002a, 2003a, Schweinhart & Weikart 1988, Schweinhart et al 2005, Weikart 1998, Weikart & Schweinhart 1997). The evaluation research employed a randomised controlled design involving 123 'high-risk' African-American children aged 3 or 4 years, 'high-risk' meaning the children were from low socioeconomic backgrounds and of low intellectual performance with IQ scores between 70 and 85 (borderline mental impairment). From this group of children, 58 were randomly assigned to the programme group (participants) and 65 were chosen to remain at home within the family without a programme (non-participants). The groups were stratified according to IQ and sociodemographics to ensure proportional representation. Researchers collected data annually up to age 10, and then when the children were aged 14/15 (high school entry), 19 (after high school), 27 (family formation and job entry pattern), and most recently at ages 39–41. Longitudinal follow ups had very little missing data, e.g. at ages 39–41, 95% of the original study group were interviewed, minimising attrition as a source of bias (Schweinhart 2002a).

Since 1970, the High/Scope Foundation has published six comprehensive monographs on the study detailing the effects of the programme. The main findings from these evaluations will now be examined.

Effects on school success: The children who participated in the HSPPP were found to have lower participation in special education (8% of the intervention group versus 37% of the control group). Throughout secondary school, students in the HSPPP had better marks and fewer failing grades than non-participants (Schweinhart & Weikart 1988). The participant group had significantly higher achievement scores at age 14 and literacy scores at age 19 (Schweinhart 2002a). They also expressed a more favourable attitude towards high school than the non-participants. At 27 years old, 71% of participants had graduated from regular or adult high school or achieved General Educational Development certification, compared with 54% of the non-participants (Schweinhart 2002a, 2003a, Weikart 1998).

Effects on socioeconomic success: By the age of 19, those who had participated in the HSPPP had higher employment rates, better jobs, higher earnings and job satisfaction than their non-participant counterparts (Schweinhart & Weikart 1988); at age 40, significantly more participants (76%) were employed than non-participants (62%) (Schweinhart et al 2005). Participants were also more likely to be able to support themselves on their own salary (Schweinhart & Weikart 1988). At age 27, 29% of participants earned at least $2000 a month while only 7% of the non-participants reported such earnings (Schweinhart 2003a); similar trends were reported at age 40 (Schweinhart et al 2005). At age 27, more participants were home owners (36% versus 13% of non-participants) and more participants owned second cars (30% versus 13% of non-participants) (Schweinhart 2003a); again, similar trends were reported at age 40 (Schweinhart et al 2005). Finally, at age 27, significantly fewer participants were in receipt of social service benefits (59% versus 80% of non-participants) (Schweinhart 2002a, 2003a). While this trend was also reported at age 40, the difference was not significant (Schweinhart et al 2005).

Effects on social responsibility: Crime prevention is perhaps the strongest and most significant long-term impact of this programme on individuals. At age 27, those who had participated in the HSPPP had significantly fewer arrests, including arrests for drug making or dealing (Schweinhart & Weikart 1988). Only 7% of adult participants had been arrested five or more times, compared with 35% of the non-participants (Schweinhart 2002a, 2003a). These trends continued and remained significant when participants were aged 40 (Schweinhart et al 2005).

Effects on marriage and single parenthood: At age 19, women in the participant group reported fewer pregnancies and births than the non-participant group (Schweinhart & Weikart 1988). At age 27, there were significantly fewer single mothers in the participant group than in the non-participant group (57% of births in the participant group were by single mothers versus 83% of births in the non-participant group). At age 27, women who had participated in the intervention were five times more likely to be married, and wedded participant group males were married nearly twice as long as the married non-participant males (Weikart 1998). Finally, at age 40, more of the programme than the non-programme group said they were getting along very well with their families: 75% versus 64% non-participants (Schweinhart et al 2005).

Cost–benefit analysis on the data when the children were aged 27 revealed that the programme returned $7.16 to the public for every dollar invested in the programme, and overall savings to the government are much higher than the costs at approximately $25 000 versus $12 000 for each participating family (Barnett 1996, Karoly et al 1998, Schweinhart 2003a). This reflects that the programme appears to be an extremely good economic investment.

It must, however, be noted that these findings apply to a single group followed over time, namely African-American children living in poverty at a high risk of school failure. Therefore, findings may not be generalisable across all circumstances. There is less evidence of pre-school programme effectiveness for children who are not poor or otherwise at risk of school failure (Schweinhart & Weikart 1988). It is important to note that all evaluation studies to date have been conducted by the High/Scope Educational Research Foundation, the original designers and founders of the programme.

Programme Implementation Features

Use of an educational model to guide implementation and roll out: The High/Scope educational approach, which views the child as an active learner, is based on the principles of the developmental psychologist Jean Piaget (Schweinhart 2003a). The model emphasises children's intellectual and social development, as well as decision-making and problem-solving capacities, before the child enters a formal school environment (Weikart 1998).

A well defined and consistent classroom programme/routine: By adhering to the set curriculum and maintaining a consistent routine in the classroom, the child develops a sense of control and responsibility while honing skills to foster respectful independence (Weikart & Schweinhart 1997). The High/Scope approach advocates specific periods in the day for small group times, large group times and children to play independently. Surprises, such as field trips or special visitors, are not introduced as a consistent routine helps children develop a sense of responsibility.

Interactive teacher–child relationship: The High/Scope approach stresses that teachers should not use one-way instruction, but should interact with the children and encourage play to become meaningful. Often the role of the High/Scope teacher is to actively observe the children and set up problem-solving situations for the children to work out logically. The teacher employs a style of questioning the youngster in an open-ended way, encouraging answers beyond 'yes' or 'no' and allowing free conversation to flow (Weikart & Schweinhart 1997).

Training provision: Programme implementation requires that teachers be properly trained through systematic in-service curriculum training (Schweinhart 2003a) to promote programme quality. The training must be on site and model focused, though carefully adapted to the actual work settings of the group of children involved (Schwenihart 2003b). The High/Scope Foundation offers a 7-week Training of Trainers programme to prepare teachers on the curriculum (Weikart & Schweinhart 1997). Indeed, teachers trained in the subject scored significantly higher than untrained teachers in their understanding of the High/Scope model and actual implementation of the approach (Epstein 1993). Beyond the formal training, however, it is also important to include informal reflective practice and group discussions with fellow teachers in order to set objectives, plan and implement interventions.

Multidisciplinary support: Throughout implementation, teachers require support from a number of sources including researchers, curriculum specialists and a designated supervisor (Frede 1995). In the planning stage, researchers must arrange the tools and means of evaluating the impact of the programme after it has been implemented in a community. Curriculum specialists help the teacher plan implementation procedures, and also provide the most up-to-date knowledge and skills from High/Scope programmes around the globe. A programme administrator is necessary to provide individual teachers with equipment and resources, hire qualified staff to existing programmes and allocate staff time for daily planning and monthly in-service training. The supervisor also supports and encourages participating teachers to attend early childhood conferences in order to stay on top of the field (Schweinhart & Weikart 1988).

Parental involvement: Involving the parents is central to the HSPPP. Teachers can help parents improve their skills through home visits and establish a collaborative relationship with parents to share knowledge about the child from both the home and classroom perspectives (Frede 1995). This dual nature of information flow is key, particularly so that the teacher gets a better idea of the child's and family's culture, language and goals (Schweinhart 2003b).

Key Recommendations for Replication

The HSPPP has been replicated throughout the US and in a range of other countries such as Indonesia and Ireland. The following recommendations for successful replication are highlighted by the programme developers.

Adhere to model principles: The principles and practices of the HSPPP are unique and should be adhered to in order to replicate positive results found in the original programme (Schweinhart 2002b). For example, the aforementioned concepts of 'key experiences' and 'plan-do-review' are major components of this learning model, and leaving out such key aspects can jeopardise the scale and intensity of programme effects (Frede 1995). The High/Scope curriculum is not strict in terms of laying out exactly what teachers must do in terms of day-to-day instruction, but is open to allow small variations due to external circumstances such as culture or geographic location. It is important to refrain from adding new components to the programme as well. The curriculum purposefully does not contain a number of standard pre-school components, i.e. the teacher does not use workbooks or study guides to train mathematical or alphabet skills and the teacher does not set up projects for the children to undertake (Weikart & Schweinhart 1997). Such activities impose authority and impede independent decision making on the part of the children, and introducing such activities may impede positive results of the programme.

Ensure internal consistency: In replicating this programme, internal consistency should be maintained, such that the model's programme practices, curriculum content, assessment tools and staff training are all consistent with the programme's goals (Schweinhart 2002b). The lead organisation must agree on aims and objectives for the programme and how it will be implemented in the cultural and sociodemographic context for which it is proposed. Following this, programme leaders can use practices and principles of the HSPPP to tailor the individual programme content, tools and training to meet those specific goals in a consistent fashion.

Foster teacher–parent relationship: The home visiting component of the HSPPP is important for its success. Teachers and mothers, coming from different backgrounds, may have to overcome a certain hesitation about participating in such home visits, particularly during the first few visits (Weikart & Schweinhart 1997). The details of the home visiting component should be made clear to parents before enrolling their child in the course.

Limit children to staff ratio: This programme encourages small class sizes and low child-to-teacher ratios. This is important as it allows teachers to spend more time with individual children and to know more about their learning interests and also creates a more comfortable environment for children who may be shy or reserved (Frede 1995). The original HSPPP had a ratio of 1 teacher for every 5.7 children; however, further research on the programme determined that the programme could be highly effective with 8 children per staff member thus reducing the programme cost (Weikart & Schweinhart 1997). However, a National Day Care study (Ruopp et al 1979) found that programme effectiveness declines when the number of children per staff member exceeds 10.

Teacher training: Training and supervision are integral to the programme and are aimed at improving the effectiveness of the programme and supporting the teachers. A trained curriculum specialist provides teachers with hands-on workshops, observation and feedback. The High/Scope Foundation has a nationwide certified trainers programme and each trainer works with an average of 25 teachers.

Policy support: While simple replication of the various components of this model may lead to positive outcomes, widespread dissemination will rely on local, regional and national policy support in order to ensure high standards of programme quality and effectiveness on a larger scale (Schweinhart 2002b). Without such high standards, the quality may become diluted and potentially be a waste of time, effort and money.

Sensitivity to non-educational needs: Teachers leading the HSPPP should be sensitive to the external needs of children and their parents, particularly keeping in mind the circumstances of culture and environment in which the programme is replicated. Children and families living in poverty have certain non-educational needs that may need to be addressed, i.e. the teacher may need to recommend social service agencies to the parents (Schweinhart & Weikart 1988). As another example, working parents may have childminders to care for their children during the day; in this case, it is beneficial for teaching staff to get to know childcare providers, as these individuals are in frequent daily contact with the children (Schweinhart & Weikart 1988).

Drawing on the findings from the impressive long-term results of the HSPPP, the following common elements have been identified as being critical to the long-term effectiveness of pre-school programmes (Frede 1995):

* small class sizes with low ratios of children to teachers
* teachers who received training and support to reflect on and improve their teaching practices
* close relationships with parents
* a concentration on long-lasting interventions and curricula that serve as a bridge between home and school.

However, it should be noted that while pre-school programmes have the potential to produce findings such as that found in the HSPPP, as Zigler and Styfco (2001) caution, 'A year or two of attending pre-school is not an inoculation against all past and future developmental risk imposed by living in poverty'. Pre-school programmes need to be seen as part of a wide range of measures required to fully address the determinants of childhood poverty and disadvantage.

Generic Principles of Effective Programme Implementation in Working with Families and Young Children

This chapter has examined a number of programmes that promote the mental health of young children and their parents. There is substantial evidence to indicate that high quality comprehensive programmes carried out in collaboration with families, schools and communities can produce lasting positive benefits for young people and their parents. When these programmes are implemented effectively they lead to improvements not only in the mental health of children and their parents but also improved social functioning, academic and work performance and general health behaviour. The effects are especially evident in relation to the most vulnerable families from disadvantaged backgrounds and, therefore, investment in such initiatives is well spent and cost-effective. The critical issue is ensuring that the programmes are of high quality and are implemented effectively and are sustained for enduring effects. Based on the existing research and the programmes reviewed in this chapter, we will now outline the key generic principles underpinning good practice and successful programme implementation in working with families and young children. In particular, guidelines based on the Barnes and Freude-Lagevardi (2003) report commissioned by the Mental Health Foundation, and key points from a paper by Black and Krishnakumar (1998) on mental health promotion interventions for children in low-income urban settings, are incorporated.

- Undertake a needs assessment to establish the characteristics and wishes of the population who are intended to receive the programme; assess the social context and family circumstances and ensure that programmes are matched to participants' needs.
- Develop programmes based on a strong theoretical framework.
- Interventions that include at least two generations, i.e. both parents and children, appear to be most likely to lead to improvement. Group interventions for parents appear to be cost-effective and acceptable.
- Programmes should start prenatally, be of long duration and of high intensity. Prenatal programmes followed by comprehensive postnatal services over the first year appear to be most effective. Offering a small number of high intensity services to a family is likely to be more effective than a large number of low intensity programmes.
- Interventions with first-time parents have the clearest positive effects because the development of adaptive parenting styles can be carried forward to later-born children. Where there are limited resources this type of intervention is recommended.
- Programmes targeting families from disadvantaged backgrounds such as high levels of poverty, single or adolescent parents, produce greater benefits.
- Programmes need to be delivered in a non-stigmatising way and in a style that is acceptable to the families. Build programmes with community participation and collaborate with families and communities to ensure cultural relevance and programme sustainability. High-risk families will benefit from lay workers and professionals working together, sharing the decision making. Combine cultural and developmental sensitivity into intervention programmes.
- Programmes that adopt a systems or ecological perspective will address factors that influence family functioning in terms of their everyday contexts including linkages with the community, external services and wider peer support.
- Multi-method interventions which combine multiple delivery formats such as books, added services, home visits and day centres, may enhance benefits rather than using a single method approach. No single approach will have

all the answers. Understanding the level of risk of children and their parents and developing shared understanding of goals is likely to be more important than any specific perspective.

- A positive relationship between parents and the programme implementers, based on mutual trust and respect, can instil a sense of control and worth in participant parents and address the needs of both the parent and the child.
- Ensure that intervention programmes are accessible to children and families; offer incentives such as meals or free transport and aim to reduce barriers to access by means of e.g. flexible settings or hours.
- Provide staff training and support for programme providers. Service providers need to be sensitive to the cultural and social traditions of their community such as family structures, local neighbourhood attitudes, power relations, poverty and the politics of welfare services. Both professionals and lay workers have been found to have positive outcomes and relative efficacy in terms of programme delivery.
- Conduct early intervention evaluation research to improve the programme quality and implementation. Carefully monitor and document activities during the programme planning and implementation phases and collect process evaluation data so that more informed judgements can be made about which elements are contributing or detracting from the positive outcomes.
- Prepare for policy recommendations by incorporating accountability and cost analysis into intervention programmes.
- Several studies have been found to have sleeper effects, which suggest that a positive outcome will only become apparent at a later stage. Plan for longitudinal follow up to capture positive intervention effects.

References

Ainsworth M D, Bowlby J 1991 An ethological approach to personality development. American Psychologist 46(4):333–341

Baker L, Scher D, Mackler K 1997 Home and family influences on motivations for reading. Educational Psychologist 32:69–82

Bandura A 1977 Self-efficacy: toward a unifying theory of behavioural change. Psychological Review 84:191–215

Barlow J, Coren E, Stewart-Brown S 2001 Systemic review of the effectiveness of parenting programmes in improving maternal psychosocial health. Health Services Research Unit, University of Oxford

Barnes J, Freude-Lagevardi A 2003 From pregnancy to early childhood: early interventions to enhance the mental health of children and families. The Mental Health Foundation, London

Barnett W S 1993 Benefit–cost analysis of pre-school education: findings form a 25-year follow-up. American Journal of Orthopsychiatry 63(4):500–508

Barnett W S 1996 Lives in the balance: age 27 benefit–cost analysis of the High/Scope Perry Preschool Programme. Monographs of the High/Scope Educational Research Foundation, 11. High/Scope Press, Ypsilanti, Michigan

Black M M, Krishnakumar A 1998 Children in low-income, urban settings: interventions to promote mental health and well-being. American Psychologist 53(6):635–646

Bond L A 1999 Partnerships with parents to promote healthy development. International Journal of Mental Health Promotion 1(4):4–13

Bowlby J 1977 The making and breaking of affectional bonds. British Journal of Psychiatry 130:201–210

Bronfenbrenner U 1979 The ecology of human development: experiments by nature and design. Harvard University Press, Cambridge, Massachusetts

Brofenbrenner U 1992 The process-person-context model in developmental research principles, applications and implications. Unpublished manuscript, Cornell University, Ithaca, New York

Cooper P J, Landman M, Tomlinson M et al 2002 Impact of a mother–infant intervention in an indigent peri-urban South African context: pilot study. British Journal of Psychiatry 180:76–81

Cowen E L, Work W C 1988 Resilient children, psychological wellness and primary prevention. American Journal of Community Psychology 16(4):591–607

Dean C, Myors K, Evans E 2003 Community-wide implementation of a parenting programme: the south east Sydney positive parenting project. Australian e-Journal for the Advancement of Mental Health 2(3):1–12

Dryfoos J G 1990 Adolescents at risk: prevalence and prevention. Oxford University Press, New York

Epstein A S 1993 Training for quality: improving early childhood programmes through systematic in-service training. Monographs of the High/Scope Educational Research Foundation, 9. High/Scope Press, Ypsilanti, Michigan

Frede E C 1995 The role of programme quality in producing early childhood programme benefits. The Future of Children 5(3):115–132

Gomby D S, Culross P L, Behrman R E 1999 Home visiting: recent programme evaluations – analysis and recommendations. The Future of Children 9(1):4–26

Guterman N B, Anisfield E, McCord M 2003 Home visiting. Pediatrics 111(6):1491–1494

Hoghughi M 1998 The importance of parenting in child health. British Medical Journal 316:1545–1550

Jané-Llopis E, Barry M, Hosman C et al 2005 What works in mental health promotion. Promotion and Education Suppl2:9–25

Jessor R 1993 Successful adolescent development among youth in high-risk settings. American Psychologist 48:117–126

Johnson Z, Molloy B 1995 The Community Mothers Programme: empowerment of parents by parents. Children and Society 9(2):73–85

Johnson Z, Howell F, Molloy B 1993 Community Mothers Programme: randomised controlled trial of non-professional intervention in parenting. British Medical Journal 306:1449–1452

Johnson Z, Molloy B, Scallon E et al 2000 Community Mothers Programme: seven-year follow-up of a randomised controlled trial of non-professional intervention in parenting. Journal of Public Health Medicine 22(3):337–342

Karoly L A, Greenwood P W, Everingham S S et al 1998 Investing in our children: what we know and don't know about the costs and benefits of early childhood interventions. Rand Publications, California

Kitzman H, Olds D L, Henderson C R et al 1997 Effect of prenatal and infancy home visitation by nurses on pregnancy outcomes, childhood injuries, and repeated childbearing: a randomised controlled trial. The Journal of the American Medical Association 278:644–652

Lazar I, Darlington R, Murray H et al 1982 Lasting effects of early education: a report from the Consortium for Longitudinal Studies. Monographs of the Society for Research and Child Development 47:2–3, Serial no 195

Lerner R M 1995 America's youth in crisis: challenges and options for programmes and policies. Sage, California

McGuigan W M, Katzev A R, Pratt C C 2003 Multi-level determinants of retention in a home visiting child abuse prevention programme. Child Abuse and Neglect 26(4):363–380

McLoyd V C 1998 Socioeconomic disadvantage and child development. American Psychologist 53:185–204

Mental Health Europe 1999 Mental health promotion for children up to six years: directory of projects in the European Union. Mental Health Europe, Brussels

Mental Health Foundation 1999 Bright futures: promoting children and young peoples' mental health. Mental Health Foundation, London

Mentality 2003 Making it effective: a guide to evidence based mental health promotion. Radical mentalities – briefing paper 1. Mentality, London

Molloy B 1992 Effects of providers participating in a parent support programme. Thesis, Trinity College Dublin, Dublin

Molloy B 2002 Still going strong: a tracer study of the Community Mothers Programme, Dublin, Ireland. Early Childhood Development Practice and Reflections No. 17. Bernard van Leer Foundation, The Hague

Olds D L 1988 The prenatal/early infancy project. In: Price R H, Cowen E L, Lorion R P et al (eds) Fourteen ounces of prevention: a casebook for practitioners. American Psychological Association, Washington DC

Olds D L 1997 The prenatal/early infancy project: fifteen years later. In: Albee G W, Gullotta T P (eds) Primary prevention works, vol 6: issues in children's and families' lives. Sage, London:41–67

Olds D L, Korfmacher J 1997 Maternal psychological characteristics as influences on home visitation contact. Journal of Community Psychology 26:23–36

Olds D L, Henderson C R, Chamberlain R et al 1986 Preventing child abuse and neglect: a randomized trial of nurse home visitation. Pediatrics 78:65–78

Olds D L, Henderson C R, Tatelbaum R et al 1988 Improving the life course development of socially disadvantaged mothers; a randomized trial of nurse home visitation. American Journal of Public Health 78(11):1436–1445

Olds D L, Henderson C R, Kitzman H 1994 Does prenatal and infancy home visitation have enduring effects on qualities of parental care giving and child health at 25 to 50 months of life? Pediatrics 93(1):89–98

Olds D L, Eckenrode J, Henderson C R et al 1997 Long term effects of home visitation on maternal life course and child abuse and neglect: fifteen year follow up of a randomised trial. Journal of the American Medical Association 278(8):637–643

Olds D L, Henderson C R, Kitzman H et al 1998a The promise of home visitation: results of two randomised trials. Journal of Community Psychology 26(1):5–21

Olds D L, Hill P L, Mihalic S F et al 1998b Blueprints for violence prevention. Book seven: prenatal and infancy home visitation by nurses. Center for the Study and Prevention of Violence, Institute of Behavioural Science, University of Colorado, Boulder, Colorado

Olds D L, Hill P, Rumsey E 1998c Prenatal and early childhood nurse home visitation. Office of Juvenile Justice and Delinquency Prevention, Washington DC

Olds D L, Hill P, Robinson J et al 2000 Update on home visiting for pregnant women and parents of young children. Current Problems in Pediatric and Adolescent Health Care 30:109–141

Olds D L, Robinson J, O'Brien R et al 2002 Home visiting by paraprofessionals and by nurses: a randomized, controlled design. Pediatrics 110(3):486–496

Olds D L, Kitzman H, Cole R et al 2004 Effects of nurse home-visiting on maternal life course and child development: age 6 follow-up results of a randomised trial. Pediatrics 114(6):1550–1559

Powell C, Grantham-McGregor S 1989 Home visiting of varying frequency and child development. Pediatrics 84(1):157–164

Pugh G, De'Ath E, Smith C 1995 Confident parents, confident children: policy and practice in parent education and support. The National Children's Bureau, London

Racine D P 2000 Investing in what works. Replication and Programme Strategies, Philadelphia

Racine D P 2002 Scaling up the nurse–family partnership. In: The Second World Conference: the Promotion of Mental Health and Prevention of Mental and Behavioural Disorders. Developing Partnerships: Science, Policy and Programmes. The Clifford Beers Foundation, London

Resnick M D, Bearman P S, Blum R W et al 1997 Protecting adolescents from harm: findings from the National Longitudinal Study on Adolescent Health. Journal of the American Medical Association 278(10):823–832

Ruopp R, Travers J, Glantz F et al 1979 Children at the centre: summary findings and their implications. Abt Associates, Cambridge, Massachusetts

Rutter M 1987 Psychosocial resilience and protective mechanisms. American Journal of Orthopsychiatry 57:316–331

SAMHSA (Substance Abuse and Mental Health Service Administration) 2004 High/Scope Perry Pre-school Programme. SAMHSA Model Programmes. Online. Available: http:// modelprograms.samhsa.gov/ 11 October 2005

Sampson R J 1997 The embeddedness of child and adolescent development: a community level perspective on urban violence. In: McCord J (ed) Violence and childhood in the inner city. Cambridge University Press, New York

Sanders M 1999 The Triple P-positive parenting programme: towards an empirically validated multilevel parenting and family support strategy for the prevention of behaviour and emotional problems in children. Clinical Child and Family Psychology Review 2(2):71–90

Sanders M, Markie-Dadds C, Tully L et al 2000 The Triple P-positive parenting programme: a comparison of enhanced, standard and self-directed behavioural family intervention from parents of children with early onset conduct problems. Journal of Consulting and Clinical Psychology 68(4):624–640

Schweinhart L J 2002a How the High/Scope Perry Preschool study grew: a researcher's tale. Online. Available: http://www.highscope.org/Research/PerryProject/tale.htm 13 October 2005

Schweinhart L J 2002b Making validated educational models central in pre-school standards. Working paper for the National Institute for Early Education Research. Online. Available: http://nieer.org/resources/research/schweinhart.pdf 13 October 2005

Schweinhart L J 2003a Benefits, costs and explanation of the High/Scope Perry Pre-school Programme. Conference Proceedings, presented at the Meeting of the Society for Research in Child Development, Tampa, Florida, 26 April

Schweinhart L J 2003b Validity of the High/Scope Preschool education model. Online. Available: http://highscope.org/Research/preschoolvalidity.pdf 13 October 2005

Schweinhart L J, Weikart D B 1988 The High/Scope Perry Preschool Programme. In: Price R H, Cowen E L, Lorion R P et al (eds) Fourteen ounces of prevention: a casebook for practitioners. American Psychological Association, Washington DC:53–65

Schweinhart L J, Montie J, Xiang Z et al 2005 Lifetime effects: The High/Scope Perry Pre-school Study through age 40. Monographs of the High/Scope Educational Research Foundation, 14. High/Scope Press, Ypsilanti, Michigan. Online. Available: http://www.highscope.org/Research/PerryProject/PerryAge40SumWeb.pdf 13 October 2005

Shure M B, Spivack G 1988 Interpersonal cognitive problem solving. In: Price R H, Cowen E L, Lorion R P et al (eds) Fourteen ounces of prevention: a casebook for practitioners. American Psychological Association, Washington DC:69–82

Titterton M, Smart H, Hill M 2002 Mental health promotion and the early years: the evidence base for interventions. Journal of Mental Health Promotion 1(4):10–24

Turner KM, Markie-Dadds C, Sanders M R 1998 Facilitators' manual for group Triple P. Families International Publishing, Brisbane

Webster-Stratton C 1982 Teaching mothers through videotape modelling to change their children's behaviour. Journal of Pediatric Psychology 7(3):279–294

Webster-Stratton C 1990 Long-term follow-up of families with young conduct-problem children: from pre-school to grade school. Journal of Clinical Child Psychology 19(2):144–149

Webster-Stratton C 1999 Researching the impact of parent training programmes in child conduct problems. In: Lloyd E (ed) Parenting matters: what works in parent education. Barnardos, Ilford

Webster-Stratton C, Hammond M 1990 Predictors of treatment outcomes in parent training for families with conduct-problem children. Behaviour Therapy 21:319–337

Webster-Stratton C, Mihalic S, Fagan A et al 2001 Blueprints for violence prevention. Book 11: The Incredible Years: parent, teacher and child training series. Center for the Study and Prevention of Violence, Institute of Behavioral Science, University of Colorado, Boulder

Weikart D P 1998 Changing early childhood development through educational intervention. Preventive Medicine 27(2):233–237

Weikart D P, Schweinhart L J 1997 High/Scope Perry Pre-school Programme. In: Albee G W, Gullotta T P (eds) Primary prevention works, vol 6: issues in children's and families' lives. Sage, London:146–166

Weiss H B 1993 Home visits: necessary but not sufficient. The Future of Children 3(3):113–128

Weissberg R P, Caplan M Z, Sivo P J 1989 A new conceptual framework for establishing school-based social competence promotion programmes. In: Bond L A, Compas B E (eds) Primary prevention and promotion in the schools. Sage, Newbury Park, California:255–296

Weissberg R P, Caplan M, Harwood R L 1991 Promoting competent young people in competence enhancing environments: a systems-based perspective on primary prevention. Journal of Consulting and Clinical Psychology 59(6):830–841

Wilson W J 1987 The truly disadvantaged: the inner city, the underclass and public policy. University of Chicago Press, Chicago

Wolkow K E, Ferguson H B 2001 Community factors in the development of resiliency: considerations and future directions. Community Mental Health 37(6):489–498

Zigler E, Styfco S J 2001 Extended childhood intervention prepares children for school and beyond. Journal of the Medical American Association 285(18):2336–2338

Mental Health Promotion in Schools

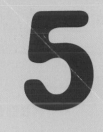

5

Chapter contents

Introduction

Schools have become one of the most important settings for promoting the mental health of young people (WHO 2001). The school setting provides an opportunity to reach many young people during their formative years of cognitive, emotional and social development. As most young people spend a large proportion of their time in school, there are few other settings where large numbers of young people can be reached. The school environment is not only a place of learning, it is also an important source of friends, social networks and adult role models. As such, schools provide a socialising context that has a significant influence on the development of young people. There is a long tradition of health education in schools in many countries. However, in more recent times, with the influence of the WHO Health Promoting Schools initiative (WHO 1998), the emphasis has changed from a focus on curriculum and knowledge-based approaches to more comprehensive programmes. These more holistic programmes seek to promote generic life skills and supportive environments that foster positive youth development and a sense of connectedness with the family, community and broader social context of young people's lives (Rowling et al 2002). The importance of the school as a setting for mental health promotion is reflected in the increasing number of programmes that successfully promote academic, social and emotional competence and significantly reduce school drop-out rates and a range of negative health and social outcomes (Jané-Llopis et al 2005). In this chapter we will overview a range of approaches including skills training, whole school approaches and targeted programmes that have been used in promoting mental health in the school setting. A number of international programmes and case studies are profiled to illustrate the key elements which contribute to successful programme implementation.

Rationale for Promoting Mental Health in Schools

The school system offers a very efficient and systematic means of promoting the psychological, social and physical health of school-aged children and adolescents. Attendance at school is compulsory in many countries and schools have sustained contact with most children during their formative years of development (Rutter et al 1979). There is increasing recognition that enhancing children's mental and physical health will improve their ability to learn and to achieve academically as well as their capacity to become responsible citizens and productive workers (Weissberg et al 1991, Zins et al 2004). Schools have an important function in nurturing children's social–emotional development as well as their academic and cognitive development. Elias et al (1997) suggest that schools will be most successful when they integrate their educational mission with efforts to promote social and emotional learning of young people as well as academic learning. In their book 'Building academic success on social and emotional learning' Zins et al (2004) make a compelling case, based on existing theory and evidence, for linking social emotional learning to improved school attitudes, behaviour and performance.

There is a high prevalence of mental health problems in young people (20–30%) (Stephens et al 1999) and many experience multiple problems, which often go undetected and remain untreated (Offord et al 1999). Changing economic, social and cultural conditions have sharply increased young people's vulnerability to negative life outcomes (Dryfoos 1998). Weare (2000) points to the growing social pressures on young people and cites reports from the UK that one third of younger teenagers report feeling currently 'stressed' or 'depressed' (Gordon & Grant 1977), while in the US, 60% of girls and 40% of boys have experienced 'depressive episodes' by the time they reach their older teens. Globally the number of suicides among young men has risen steadily over the last 20 years, while attempted suicides have increased among girls (Coleman 1997). Suicide rates show a large variation across countries; however, studies have shown a significant increase in rates of suicidal behaviour among young people aged 15–25 years (Apter 2001). While it is generally recognised that the factors linked to youth suicide are many and complex, international research suggests that up to 90% of young people who commit suicide have evidence of serious mental health problems before their death, with depression being one of the most common (Beautrais et al 1996).

Schools are being seen as a key setting, along with the home and the community, in tackling these issues and promoting positive youth development.

Poor performance and achievement in school are recognised as risk factors for a range of social and health problems such as substance misuse, unwanted teenage pregnancy, conduct problems and involvement in crime (Dryfoos 1997, Rutter & Smith 1995, Wells et al 2001). A sense of connectedness with family and school is a recognised protective factor for youth mental health. A positive educational experience and a good level of academic achievement can contribute significantly to enhancing self-esteem and confidence, better employment, life opportunities and social support (Mentality 2003). Schools, therefore, have an important role in strengthening young people's mental health and their ability to cope with change, challenges and stress.

Schools are social places as well as places of learning and the influence of peers, teachers, families and communities are important dimensions that need to be considered when addressing the broader context of young people's development and growth. This holistic approach is captured in the concept of the health promoting school. As defined by the WHO, a health promoting school 'can be characterised as a school constantly strengthening its capacity as a healthy setting for living, learning and working' (WHO 1997). Components of the health promoting schools approach include improving the school ethos and environment, curriculum approaches and involving families and the local community. A systematic review of the effectiveness of the health promoting schools approach, conducted by Lister-Sharp et al (1999), found that while the available evidence was limited it was nonetheless promising, particularly in relation to evidence of the positive impact on areas of emotional and social well-being such as self-esteem and bullying. A number of studies suggest that traditional topic based approaches to health education are of limited value and that the more successful programmes are those that involve parents and the wider community, strengthen school connectedness and address the ethos and culture of the school as a whole (Mentality 2003). This is referred to as adopting a whole school approach. Readers are referred to Katherine Weare's (2000) book, 'Promoting mental, emotional and social health: a whole school approach' for a more detailed account of this approach.

Evidence of Effectiveness

There is substantial evidence that mental health promotion programmes in schools, when implemented effectively, can produce long-term benefits for young people including emotional and social functioning and improved academic performance (Durlak & Wells 1997, Greenberg et al 2001a, Harden et al 2001, Hodgson & Abbasi 1995, Lister-Sharp et al 1999, Tilford et al 1997, Wells et al 2001, 2003). An overview of the evidence from systematic reviews highlights that comprehensive programmes that target multiple health outcomes in the context of a coordinated whole school approach are the most consistently effective strategies (Jané-Llopis et al 2005). Browne et al (2004) suggest that the enhancement of protective factors and the promotion of competencies may be more readily achieveable with comprehensive multi-modal initiatives. Green et al (2005) reviewed the evidence base on the effectiveness of school-based programmes for primary school-aged children. Synthesising the results of a number of reviews, Green et al report that despite variations in populations and methods, school-based mental health promotion programmes can be effective (Box 5.1). For example, in a systematic review of universal approaches (i.e. provided to all children) to mental health promotion in schools, Wells et al (2003) found positive evidence of effectiveness from programmes that adopted a whole school approach, were implemented continuously for more than a year and were aimed at the promotion of mental health as opposed to the prevention of mental disorder. They also concluded that long-term interventions promoting the positive mental health of all pupils, and involving changes to the school environment, are likely to be more successful than brief class-based prevention programmes. A number of high quality successful programmes have been developed and implemented in collaboration with families, schools and communities in order to produce long lasting positive mental health and social outcomes. Reviewers recommend that a combination of universal and targeted programmes would be required to cater for the needs of all children in a school (CASEL 2003, Hodgson et al 1996, Tilford et al 1997).

Box 5.1

Characteristics of programmes associated with effective outcomes identified by Green et al 2005

(adapted with permission of The Clifford Beers Foundation)

- aimed at the promotion of mental health rather than the prevention of mental health problems (Wells et al 2001)
- implemented continuously and long term in nature, i.e. more than a year (Wells et al 2001)
- included changes to the school climate rather than brief class-based prevention programmes (Wells et al 2001)
- went beyond the classroom and provided opportunities for applying the learned skill (CASEL 2003)
- replicated positive behavioural implementations in different sites and sustained them over time (CASEL 2003)
- adopted a health-promoting schools approach focusing on aspects of the social and physical environment of the school, family and community links with the school, the school curriculum and pupils' knowledge (Lister-Sharp et al 1999)
- directed at school-aged children in high-risk groups to enhance coping skills and the development of social skills and good peer relationships (Hodgson et al 1996)
- focused on improving self-esteem (Haney & Durlak 1998), self-concept and coping skills as a general approach as well as those focusing on specific life events (Tilford et al 1997)

Implementing School-Based Programmes

The implementation of school-based programmes is not without its challenges, as programmes are competing for time and space in an increasingly crowded school curriculum. Likewise, teachers may be hesitant about addressing mental health issues in the classroom and a high level of support and training may be required. Most of the evidence-based programmes have been developed under controlled research conditions. Ensuring effective implementation of interventions across a variety of school settings is an important challenge. A variety of contextual factors such as leadership, the school organisation and management, teacher training and support have been found to influence both the level and quality of programme implementation (Greenberg et al 2001b). The school management and staff need to be aware of the importance of mental health and be convinced of the value of the intervention for their school and the students. Guided by a conceptual model of implementation for school-based programmes, Greenberg et al (2001b) outline useful strategies for practitioners and school personnel to facilitate effective programme delivery. These strategies are linked to each of the three stages of programme implementation as follows:

1. Pre-Adoption Phase

This phase refers to the planned intervention which includes the programme model (content, structure, etc.), quality of delivery, target audience and participant responsiveness. In addition to the actual intervention, the implementation support system also needs to be planned including the quality of materials, extent and quality of technical support and assessment of implementer readiness. In particular, Greenberg et al 2001b recommend paying attention to the following points:

- involve key stakeholders such as administrators, teachers, parents and students, in the decision-making process
- assess the programme fit in relation to the existing needs, resources and the philosophy and organisational capacity of the school
- appoint a project coordinator to ensure successful implementation and programme evaluation
- provide training for the implementers so that they are knowledgeable and confident in their abilities
- create a supportive and problem-solving atmosphere that allows for discussion and resolution of difficulties.

2. Delivery Phase

Monitor the actual implementation of the intervention and the support system as delivered, i.e. as opposed to what was planned. This includes details of the programme as actually delivered such as the amount, frequency, quality of delivery and level of student engagement. Attention also needs to be paid to the contextual factors operating external to the programme at the level of the classroom, school, district and community. At the classroom level, this includes the influence of implementer characteristics, classroom climate and peer relations. At the school and district levels, the level of administrative stability, leadership and support, awareness of student needs, school goals, climate and communication may also influence actual delivery. At the community level, the importance of school–family and school–community relations together with community support and readiness for the programme should not be overlooked. Therefore, careful monitoring of the programme quality as delivered, and the support and response of key stakeholders, is required on an ongoing basis. Providing sustained support to implementers and maintaining open communication and a positive school atmosphere will all assist with successful delivery.

3. Post-Delivery Phase

Based on findings from the programme evaluation, decisions will be made about the programme in terms of overall quality, viability and sustainability. Feedback to and from implementers regarding the programme and the factors that affected its implementation will play an important role in making these decisions. If the programme is found to be successful, steps will need to be taken to integrate the programme into the school structure and ensure its sustainability.

Approaches to Implementing School-Based Programmes

There are a number of approaches or strategies for promoting mental health in the school setting. These may be divided into three groupings as follows:

1. classroom-based skills training – the teaching of life skills and social competencies that promote adjustment through delivering a specific curriculum in the classroom
2. a whole school approach – concerned with modifying the classroom and changing the school environment and ethos, including involving the parents and the community, in order to improve outcomes and provide a supportive context within the school
3. targeted interventions – interventions for students at higher risk aimed at strengthening their coping skills and reducing the risk of negative mental health outcomes, including suicide.

Each of these different approaches will now be examined and examples of successful programmes will be described in order to highlight principles of good practice.

Classroom-Based Skills Training

Skills training programmes are designed to teach and model such skills as effective communication, peer pressure resistance, assertiveness, problem-solving, relationship and coping skills. These classroom-based programmes usually involve methods of role playing, rehearsal, modelling and peer instruction and can be applied to a range of social situations (Rhodes & Englund 1993). While many of the early skills-based programmes were topic specific, e.g. a focus on substance misuse, these programmes have been expanded to promote more general social competencies and adopt a broad-based approach. The value of a social competence approach, which focuses on generic skills designed to increase resilience, promote self-esteem and enhance protective factors for health, is supported by the evidence (Lister-Sharp et al 1999, Mentality 2003, Tilford et al 1997).

A variety of classroom-based programmes have been evaluated including those that emphasise generic personal and social skills training. Research suggests that knowledge-only programmes have minimal effects on young people's behaviour (Botvin & Tortu 1988) and that programmes that teach generic broad-based competencies such as self-control, coping skills, etc., produce significant positive outcomes (Elias et al 1986, Shure & Spivack 1988, Tilford et al 1997). Research also indicates that multiple years of classroom-based skills training may be required to produce long-term gains (Weissberg et al 1991). Educational theories of learning suggest that learning is most effective when students are active participants in their own learning rather than the passive recipients of information delivered didactically. Teaching methodologies which engage young people in experiential, activity-based learning, including the use of techniques such as role play, reflection and group discussion, are therefore encouraged. Elias et al (1997) advocate that students derive more benefit from programmes which they help to design, plan and implement and where they have meaningful influence and participation in the process.

A number of successful school-based programmes targeting all pupils have employed cognitive skills training in promoting social and emotional competencies. These include the 'I Can Problem Solve' programme (Shure & Spivack 1988) which improves problem-solving abilities, and the 'Improving Social Awareness-Social Problem Solving' (ISA-SPS) programme (Bruene-Butler et al 1997) which leads to long-term improvements in coping with stressors. The 'Promoting Alternative Thinking Strategies' (PATHS) also employs cognitive training and leads to improved emotional understanding, reduced conduct problems and impulsivity (Greenberg et al 1995, Greenberg et al 2001a). This programme, which has been evaluated using randomised controlled trials, has been replicated with a wide range of children in different school settings across the US. Programmes such as the 'Resolving Conflict Creatively' programme (Aber et al 1998) and the 'Good Behavior Game' (Kellam et al 1994) have been found to lead to reduced levels of aggression in the classroom and improved interpersonal negotiating skills.

Generic social competence programmes have also applied skills training to specific topics such as substance misuse. Examples include the 'Positive Youth Development' programme (Caplan et al 1992) and the 'Life Skills Training' programme (Botvin & Tortu 1988, Botvin et al 1998), both of which apply generic self-control and social skills to alcohol and drug use. The Life Skills Training programme will now be examined in detail. This programme is included as one of the model programmes in the 'Blueprints for violence prevention' series and readers are referred to 'Book Five: Life Skills Training' (Botvin et al 1998) for further details of its implementation and replication across sites.

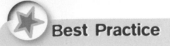

Best Practice

Life Skills Training

(Botvin & Tortu 1988, Botvin et al 1998)

Life Skills Training (LST) is a 3-year programme designed to provide general life skills training and social resistance skills primarily aimed at preventing drug use, i.e. tobacco, alcohol and marijuana. This programme is targeted at students aged 12–14 and provides them with personal self-management skills, social skills, drug-related information and prevention skills, e.g. resisting drug use influences. The rationale for the LST programme was that substance abuse was of major growing concern in the US and around the world and that many of the prevention approaches had proven ineffective (Botvin et al 1998). The original developers of the LST programme took a new angle on the traditional prevention approaches, hypothesising that a more useful procedure was to examine and address specific risk factors for drug use and hone in on preventing the consumption of 'gateway' substances such as tobacco, alcohol and marijuana (Botvin et al 1998). The 12–14-year-old age group targeted is due to the transitional nature of these years in terms of psychosocial changes, as well as the increasing importance of peer group and resulting peer pressure. In addition, experts have found that young people typically start experimenting with 'gateway' drugs at this age (Botvin et al 1998). Evaluation of the Life Skills Training programme by its developers has indicated that it is highly effective, in that it has been found to reduce alcohol, cigarette, and marijuana intake among young people by 50–70% (Botvin et al 1998). The positive effects on reducing smoking and heavy alcohol consumption have been sustained through the end of secondary school, as the programme reduced intake of illegal drugs by 66% and pack-a-day smoking by 25%.

Programme Content

The LST programme is comprised of 12 units, and the first year of the course is delivered over 15 sessions, usually taught in school by the classroom teacher. Each session lasts an average of 45 minutes, and can be delivered either once a week for 15 weeks or in a more frequent succession as an intensive short course. The three major themes in the course are as follows:

1. personal self-management skills – this component contains materials to help young people develop decision-making skills, identify and analyse media influences, learn basic principles of change and self-improvement and develop coping and stress management skills
2. social skills – this component is designed to influence and enhance students' general social competence; for example, it helps young people learn communication and conversation skills, assertiveness and how to overcome shyness
3. drug-related information and prevention skills – students are made aware of consequences of drug use, how to decline the social acceptability of drug

use, how to 'say no' and how the media can promote drugs as well as ways to resist media influences.

The primary 15-session course is followed up by a 2-year booster intervention, with supplementary sessions in year 2 and five booster sessions in year 3. The booster sessions are designed to reinforce the primary material taught in the first year, with continued development of the personal and social skills as well as the opportunity to practise these skills through group work and individual homework.

Curriculum materials include a teachers' manual with detailed lesson plans and appropriate activities as well as a students' guide containing reference materials, class exercises, homework and a 'self-improvement project' (Botvin et al 1998).

Evaluation Findings

Over the last 20 years, researchers at the Cornell University Medical College in New York have undertaken 12 major evaluation studies regarding the effectiveness of the LST programme as a drug abuse prevention programme. Positive effects were noted on a number of issues:

Cigarette smoking: In a study of the pilot LST programme (Botvin et al 1980), New York suburban students (n = 281) were randomly assigned either to receive the programme intervention (intervention group) or to not receive the intervention (control group). Results indicated that the intervention group had a 75% reduction in the number of new cigarette smokers at the completion of the programme and a 67% reduction in new smoking at 3 months' follow up ($p < 0.01$) as compared to the control group. A large-scale study of the programme determined that programme participants had significantly less cigarette smoking than controls at 28 months' follow up (Botvin et al 1990a).

Alcohol abuse: A randomised controlled study was carried out in New York City schools (n = 239) to measure the impact of the programme on alcohol use (Botvin et al 1984a). The study found that, although there was no significant impact at the end of the course, programme effects emerged at 6 months' follow up: in the intervention group as compared to the control group, 54% fewer students reported drinking in the last month ($p < 0.02$), 73% fewer reported heavy drinking ($p < 0.04$) and 79% fewer reported getting drunk at least once a month ($p < 0.01$). A larger study undertaken to replicate these results (Botvin et al 1984b) also found that students who participated in the programme drank significantly less alcohol per drinking session and were drunk less often as compared to the control group. This trend continued at 1 year follow up (Botvin et al 1990b).

Marijuana abuse: The larger study mentioned above (Botvin et al 1984b) also studied the programme effects on marijuana consumption and found a significant impact: intervention group students reported 71% less experimental marijuana use and 83% less regular marijuana use. This trend continued 1 year post-intervention, with 47% fewer intervention group students reporting experimental marijuana use (Botvin et al 1990b) and a large-scale study determined these effects continue at 40 months' follow up (Botvin et al 1990a).

Other illicit drug use: The LST programme has been found to reduce the use of illicit drugs. In one programme study (Botvin et al 2000) researchers analysed data collected from a random sub-sample of intervention and control group students (n = 447) involved in a long-term follow-up study of the LST programme (Botvin et al 1995). Results at 6.5 years post-intervention indicated that intervention group students reported levels of illicit drug use that were 25% lower than control group students. By individual drug category, there were significantly lower levels of use with regards to marijuana ($p < 0.029$), inhalants ($p < 0.012$), hallucinogens ($p < 0.015$), and heroin and other narcotics ($p < 0.033$). However, it should be noted that the overall sample for this study was from a white middle-class population, and further research is necessary to determine if similar effects are achievable in disadvantaged and high-risk populations.

Risky driving: A recent study examined the effects of the LST programme on adolescent risky driving (Griffin et al 2004). Controlling for gender and alcohol use, logistic regression analysis of the data indicated that the students who participated in the LST programme in school were less likely to have motor violations (OR = 0.75, 95% CI 0.61–0.94) and penalty points (OR = 0.75, 95% CI 0.60–0.94) on their driving record as compared to non-participant students. Findings also indicated that the more negative attitude towards drinking alcohol among participant students was significantly predictive of fewer driving violations in the final year of secondary school ($p < 0.05$).

Booster effects: Certain studies of this programme investigated the impact of booster sessions on programme impact. One study in New York schools (Botvin et al 1983) found that the student group receiving booster sessions had 50% fewer regular smokers than the group of students not receiving booster sessions. This effect continued at 1.5 years' follow up, demonstrating that booster sessions maintain and perhaps improve the overall positive effects of the LST programme.

Long-term effectiveness: A study of the long-term effectiveness of this programme (Botvin et al 1995) followed students (baseline n = 3597) from the 7th grade (age 12–13) through their final year in secondary school (age 17–18). Results indicated that there were fewer smokers, heavy drinkers or marijuana users among those students in the programme group as compared to the control group. At the end of secondary school, there were 66% fewer intervention group students than control group students who used tobacco, alcohol or marijuana one or more times per week. Strongest prevention effects were evident in those students who received the most complete implementation of the prevention programme.

Impact on other populations: Several studies of the programme dealt with assessing the impact of the programme on high-risk student populations, based on social and academic risk factors such as poor school performance. One such study (Griffin et al 2003) found that the LST programme had a significant effect on several outcome measures at 1 year follow up, whereby programme participants had lower levels of cigarette smoking ($p < 0.006$), alcohol use ($p < 0.008$), inhalant use ($p < 0.043$) and polydrug use ($p < 0.004$). A recent study (Botvin et al 2003) assessed the effectiveness of the programme when implemented among elementary school students, aged 8 through 12 (n = 1090). Analyses at 3 months post-intervention confirmed that the programme was successful in that intervention students reported less smoking in the past year ($p < 0.038$), high anti-drugs attitudes ($p < 0.044$), and lower normative expectations for peer smoking ($p < 0.019$) and alcohol use ($p < 0.001$) as well as higher self-esteem (p < 0.006) when compared to control students. These findings indicate that the LST programme produces prevention effects with a younger population, though further research is necessary to determine longer-term impacts and comparisons to the original programme targeting middle school students.

Evaluation in other countries: In 1995, the LST programme was implemented in primary schools in the north of England, and named 'Project Charlie'. Long-term follow up of the programme (Hurry & Lloyd 1997) determined several significant positive effects of the programme including lower tobacco use and lower illicit drug use. Project Charlie had no long-term effects on students' knowledge, but did have an impact on attitudes whereby participating students expressed more negative attitudes towards illicit drug use than non-participating students did. The sample sizes, however, were small and the authors emphasised that such findings must be replicated with larger samples and followed up over longer periods of time (Hurry & Lloyd 1997, Lloyd et al 2000).

Rural communities: An independent evaluation of the LST programme was conducted using a rural Midwestern sample (Trudeau et al 2003). The results were positive, as the programme was proven to reduce the number of students taking up smoking, alcohol and other drug use and increased students' intentions to refuse taking such substances. Another evaluation of the programme in rural communities is being conducted with nine rural school districts in Pennsylvania, assessing the impact of the LST programme as well as the impact of a slightly modified LST programme on students (Smith et al 2004). Data have been collected on five occasions: pre-implementation, post-intervention, and at 1, 2 and 3 years later. Thus far, the research team has analysed data at 2 years post-intervention. The evidence indicates that the LST programme initially had a moderate positive influence on participating females, but by the end of the second year the effects were almost non-existent. There was no programme impact on male participants. Such evidence demonstrates that programme effects may not be replicated when the programme is implemented in new communities; further research and evaluation of this programme is essential.

There have been a number of critiques of the evaluation of this programme, most notably by Gorman (2005) who states that there has been very little critical evidence pertaining to the LST programme. Gorman (2005) stresses that most of the research relating to this intervention has been carried out by a single research team, and calls for the evaluation studies to be critically examined by external researchers in order to validate their support and dissemination in terms of drug prevention policy.

Programme Implementation Features

Theoretical basis: The theoretical foundations of the LST programme are based on the cognitive-behavioural psychological models, particularly social learning theory and problem behaviour theory (Botvin & Tortu 1988), suggesting that substance use is a learned behaviour that is instigated and sustained by certain environmental factors and stimulus controls, i.e. peer pressure and/or disadvantaged background (Waldron & Kaminer 2004). The use of drugs may be stimulated by certain triggers such as attending a party where others are using drugs, and cognitive-behavioural strategies aim to equip individuals with skills to successfully identify and resist such triggers. Likewise, the aim of the LST programme is to develop students' personal and social skills to resist drug use and reduce potential motivations to use various drugs (Griffin et al 2003).

Staffing and supervision: A qualified programme provider should teach the LST programme; such an individual does not necessarily have to be a teacher but can also be, for example, a health professional or an older student trained in peer guidance. Indeed, some programme evaluation studies indicate that a peer-led programme may be more effective than one that is teacher led (Botvin et al 1998). It requires considerable effort to upskill and maintain peer leaders over time, however, and teachers are the logical choice as they have general classroom management experience and can include this programme as part of the overall school curriculum (Botvin et al 1998). The selection of course providers should hinge on their interest in the course materials, their image as a positive role model, and their willingness to follow the programme guidelines.

Teacher training and support: LST teachers are trained through either a 1 or 2 day workshop, with 2 day training as the preferred approach. Formal training helps to familiarise course providers with the programme content, rationale and evaluation results as well as to give them an opportunity to practise the skills necessary to implement the programme effectively (Botvin et al 1998). Ongoing teacher support is necessary to provide feedback on a teacher's performance and facilitate a forum for teachers to discuss their concerns and increase their self-efficacy in administering the programme (Botvin & Tortu 1988).

Programme setting: While the LST programme was designed to be implemented in the classroom, successful interventions have also been carried out in community centres and housing projects. The programme is flexible in that it can be implemented in any setting involving youth, as the most important point is that it reaches as large a number of children and adolescents as possible. In general, however, the school setting is considered the most convenient.

Flexible programme schedule: The LST programme is carried out over 15 sessions in the first year, 10 sessions in the second year and five sessions in the third year. The schedule has some flexibility, in that the programme can be put into practice in one of two ways:

1. scheduled once per week, such that the first year programme spans 15 weeks in total
2. scheduled on consecutive days as a mini-course, such that the first year programme spans 15 days.

Programme evaluation indicates that both methods of implementation are effective, though one study demonstrated that the more intensive mini-course model may produce slightly better results (Botvin et al 1998). The programme is also flexible in that it can be implemented through a number of different curriculum subjects such as science, social studies, health education and physical education. No clear evidence exists as to which subject area is most conducive to implementing the programme (Botvin et al 1998), though recent studies suggest that implementing during physical education was negatively related to student participation (−0.23) as students felt they were losing their 'free time' (Fagan & Mihalic 2003).

Monitoring implementation: Evaluation of the LST programme demonstrates a clear relationship between implementation fidelity and programme effectiveness (Botvin et al 1998). Therefore, for the programme to be effective it must be implemented carefully and comprehensively. Process evaluation forms, standardised by the original programme developers, are used to measure the degree to which the programme is implemented faithfully. These forms are also useful for teachers as an evaluation check to remind them to implement the programme completely.

Cost: The LST programme costs, as reported in the later 1990s, ranged from $5 to $10 per student per year, including the cost of materials and training (Botvin et al 1998). The developers point out that if several schools in an area work together to purchase material in bulk and obtain teacher training together, the cost can be significantly reduced. Those planning to implement the programme must decide where the funding will come from. It is useful to note that the cost of a preventive programme like this is extremely inexpensive when compared to the high costs associated with treatment or imprisonment due to drug abuse later in life.

Key Recommendations for Replication

Replicating this programme is relatively easy, as there are comprehensive printed materials for both teacher and student as well as a formal teacher training course to provide skills training and implementation planning. In addition, the extensive evaluation of the programme and the subsequent positive results, coupled with a growing concern in most communities regarding drug use, should facilitate a high level of community support for this programme (Botvin et al 1998).

Comprehensive programme planning: As with any new intervention, it is important to plan all stages of implementation well in advance. Several elements will have to be considered: Who will fund the programme? Who will teach the programme? How and where will the programme be implemented in the existing school curriculum? How will the programme be evaluated? In particular, the evaluation of the programme should be carefully considered, identifying appropriate outcome measures such as self-reported student questionnaires or even physical measures such as the collection of confidential carbon monoxide samples to determine actual drug use (Botvin et al 1998). Planning ahead is also important to ensure implementation fidelity as, for example, studies show that high fidelity may be more difficult in urban school settings than in suburban school settings (Griffin et al 2003).

Foster administration enthusiasm: Recent replications of the LST programme determined that a key factor which influenced the success of implementation was the cooperation and enthusiasm of key programme leaders (Fagan & Mihalic 2003). Initial and sustained commitment was necessary on a number of levels, particularly with programme coordinators and school administrators. In particular, schools which had a strong and committed programme coordinator tended to experience fewer problems during implementation and enjoyed better results. Teacher support, while important, did not appear to have as much of an effect on outcomes, as the measure of teacher commitment was uncorrelated with programme success (Fagan & Mihalic 2003). Faculty support is particularly important for programme success as one study found the most frequent obstacle in implementing the LST programme was that teachers and administrators did not want to take time away from 'core' academic subjects (Fagan & Mihalic 2003).

Involve parents and communities: In order to fully implement the LST programme as intended, it is important to generate support from a number of different sources including the school district, the local community, the programme administrators and parents (Botvin et al 1998). Programmes that involve parents in school drug education appear to be more effective (Lloyd et al 2000). As the LST programme attempts to influence students' behaviours and cognitive appraisals, parents should try to reinforce programme components in the home. A parent manual has been published in order to inform parents of how to reinforce the LST programme at home, though it is not a compulsory element of the LST school programme.

Replication fidelity: The most significant implementation problems in previous replications had to do with a partial or incomplete implementation of the programme (Botvin et al 1998). Studies indicate that the strongest long-term preventive programme effects are found in students who receive the most complete implementation of the LST programme (Botvin et al 1995). In addition, in other school-based substance abuse prevention programmes the effects decay over time and some authors posit this may be because they do not provide adequate booster sessions and they are implemented inadequately (Resnicow & Botvin 1993). The provision of booster sessions in the LST programme helps to maintain the overall positive programme effects over time.

Comprehensive teacher training: Teacher training is particularly important, and studies have shown that teachers who attend formal training and receive ongoing support produce a stronger impact on students than teachers who only view a training videotape and receive ongoing support (Botvin et al 1995). A recent replication of the programme confirmed that the effectiveness of the teacher-training workshop influenced the success of implementation; schools were encouraged to schedule training at times that would assure full teacher attendance (Fagan & Mihalic 2003). In addition, some sources have suggested that teacher training in the LST curriculum be integrated into initial teacher training courses (Lloyd et al 2000). This will help to disseminate and sustain the programme nationwide.

Replication in new populations: The LST programme has been implemented and proven both appropriate and beneficial with several different populations in the US; urban, suburban and rural communities as well as ethnic minorities, i.e. African-Americans and Hispanics (Botvin et al 1998). However, it is important to be aware of any cultural sensitivities when this programme is implemented in a new population, and modifications of the language, examples and activities may be necessary in order to engage the new population, i.e. if the population is from a disadvantaged background, the reading level of the student materials may need to be adjusted. It is interesting to note that Botvin et al (1998) state that the LST programme has the potential to be applied in youth settings other than the school, e.g. community-based youth centres and to areas other than substance misuse such as delinquency, violence reduction, teenage pregnancy, AIDS, etc. However, additional research is needed in order to demonstrate the usefulness of this approach in these areas. That said, as there is a clustering of protective and risk factors for a range of youth health and social well-being, this potential application of the programme is one that warrants further investigation.

The success of skills training programmes such as the LST may depend on their attention to changing socialisation patterns and supports in the school setting as well as specific programme delivery (Elias & Weissberg 1989). Ecologically oriented programmes stress the need for better integration between school-based training and community-based interventions, the mass media and other influences outside of the school setting. Multi-component interventions that coordinate the multiple socialising influences of peers, parents, community and opinion leaders, may be needed to produce long-term sustainable gains. Perry et al (1989) and Pentz et al (1989) have demonstrated the effectiveness of multi-level, multi-component programmes that involve parents, peers and community leaders as well as schools in promoting mental health and preventing substance misuse. An account of the multi-component community programme developed by Pentz et al (1989) is provided in Chapter 3.

A number of skills training programmes have also employed peer-led approaches where peers are involved in delivering the intervention. The 'Peer Coping Skills' training programme by Prinz et al (1994) works with teams of 6–9-year-olds in modifying pro-social coping skills. This 22 week programme, which includes both aggressive and non-aggressive young people, has resulted in significant reductions in teacher-rated levels of aggression and improved pro-social coping skills. Systematic reviews also point to some evidence for the effectiveness of peer-led approaches in schools (Durlak & Wells 1997, Lister-Sharp et al 1999). Also of interest is a growing evidence base on the value of mentoring programmes, which can be effective tools for enhancing positive youth development, especially for young people from disadvantaged backgrounds (DuBois et al 2002). An example of a successful mentoring programme is the 'Big Brothers Big Sisters of America', which has over 500 affiliate agencies throughout the US (McGill 1998). A one-to-one relationship is established between a matched pair of a volunteer adult and young person aged from 6–18 years of age. Evaluation of the Big Brothers Big Sisters programme has been found to lead to improved peer and family relationships, better school achievement and reduced substance use and aggression problems (Grossman & Tierney 1998). A research briefing paper by Jekielek et al (2002) highlights that in order for mentoring programmes to produce positive outcomes they need to be structured, planned, supported by training, driven by the needs of the young people and based on sustained relationships of longer duration. Both peer-led and mentoring programmes can also be applied beyond the confines of the school and implemented in community-based settings, thereby linking in with other important contexts for youth development.

Whole School Approach

A whole school approach moves beyond a focus on the classroom curriculum to consider the broader, more holistic aspects of the school setting such as the organisational structures and social environment, and provides opportunities for promoting the mental health of young people. This approach adopts a more eco-logical perspective and aims to include all relevant stakeholders including pupils, teachers, school administrators, parents and community members in fostering a positive school environment, ethos and sense of connectedness for pupils and staff. Programmes such as the 'Child Development Project' (Battistich et al 1996) focus on changing the learning environment by creating a 'caring community of learn-ers'. This programme strengthens students' sense of community which in turn fosters improved social and emotional learning and reduced problem behaviours. The 'School Transitional Environmental Project' (STEP) by Felner and Adam (1988) and Felner et al (1993) restructures the school environment in modifying the stress of moving to a new school. A 5 year follow up of this programme reports better adjustment to school change, lower dropout rates and better school grades among participating students. Programmes such as the 'Linking the Interests of Families and Teachers' (Reid et al 1999), the 'Seattle Social Development Project' (Hawkins et al 1991) and 'Promoting Action Through Holistic Education' (Project PATHE by Gottfredson 1990) have successfully involved parents and linked with the home environment in supporting the implementation of school programmes, including those focused on pro-social development and reducing aggressive behaviour.

The WHO health promoting schools initiative (WHO 1998), as described earlier, provides a useful framework to guide the development of a whole school approach. This framework addresses issues of school ethos and environment, policy and prac-tices and developing partnerships with parents, community groups, health agen-cies and services (Sheehan et al 2002). The whole school approach brings attention to school policies, codes of conduct and values, e.g. in dealing with bullying, con-flict resolution and issues of diversity. The concern with school ethos and environ-ment focuses attention on the relationships between people in the school, and the opportunities for participation by pupils and parents. The quality of the physical environment of the school, class sizes and the provision of services are also taken into account. The focus on the development of partnerships with parents, commu-nity groups and services links the school with the broader social context and also ensures that there is access to services for students needing additional support. Weare (2000) outlines the following critical features of the whole school approach:

- positive staff–pupil relationships
- staff development and education
- strong leadership and clear disciplinary policies
- teamwork
- focus on skills, attitudes and values rather than facts and information
- active involvement of parents, local community and key local agencies.

The Australian 'MindMatters' programme draws on the health promoting schools framework in developing a comprehensive approach to mental health in schools (Wynn et al 2000). This programme, which has been implemented on a country-wide level in Australia, is based on the three key components of a health promoting school:

1. curriculum teaching and learning
2. organisation, ethos and environment
3. partnership and services.

The MindMatters programme provides a guided and structured approach to implementing mental health promotion in schools, includes a range of innovative and high quality mental health materials and the provision of extensive training and development resources. The case study by Rowling and Mason outlines the development of the programme to date and highlights the key features of programme implementation, evaluation and dissemination.

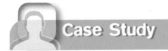

Case Study

MindMatters

Louise Rowling, Jo Mason

Background

In 1995/6, as part of the first National Mental Health Plan (Australian Health Ministers 1992), the Australian Commonwealth Department of Health funded research to identify the readiness of schools to adopt mental health promotion programmes. Lack of teacher confidence to teach about mental health, lack of appropriate classroom curriculum resources, the crowded curriculum with health being a low priority, teacher stress and low morale and stigma associated with the term mental health were found to be important influencing factors (Sheehan et al 2002, Youth Research Centre and Centre for Social Health 1996).

MindMatters is underpinned by research-based conceptual frameworks (Wynn et al 1999) that schools can use to promote mental health. It builds on educational research regarding effective school programme implementation and is grounded in the understanding that the professional development of teachers is fundamental to the success of any innovation. The approach taken by MindMatters, focusing on protective factors that promote connectedness, recognises the importance of the organisational structures, the social environment and the individual within this context. MindMatters can be distinguished from prior single topic health education projects because it places mental health within the core educational business of schools rather than identifying it as a health topic (Sheehan et al 2002). It also provides a framework for the selective inclusion of other targeted programmes and initiatives that address specific aspects of mental health and mental ill health. The MindMatters approach marks a significant shift away from mental health interventions that emphasise individual deficits of young people, and individually focused behaviour change models.

Programme Implementation and Recommendations

The unique approach in MindMatters provides a guided, structured strategy for generating health promoting schools which promote young people's mental health and well-being through all dimensions of the school environment. It is a universal approach using the school as a setting for intervention rather than a site where an intervention occurs.

The 'content' of MindMatters consists of materials for review and planning for school improvement, now published as SchoolMatters (Sheehan et al 2000). This includes practical tools for auditing, planning and managing mental health, and is targeted at school principals and teachers in positions of leadership. Curriculum and whole school change strategies for selected topics such as bullying and harassment, resilience, stress and coping, help seeking, loss and grief, and mental illness are other components. All these materials are available on the MindMatters website (www.curriculum.edu.au/mindmatters). Community Matters was added in 2002 to provide for the community context, specific groups of students with high needs and gathering the student voice. A Community Matters DVD was developed later to support this booklet's content along with the whole school and classroom approaches.

The pilot was conducted in 24 schools across Australia during 1998. The evidence from the pilot project demonstrated that the process and the materials worked in vastly different school contexts, thus maximising the conditions for transferability to school settings around Australia. The pilot identified quality practice criteria involving:

- the need for attention to professional development for teachers because of stigma and fear, the perception that mental health is not the core business of schools and the uncertainty about what constitutes good teaching practice in relation to mental health promotion
- careful use of language because of misinterpretation of mental health as mental illness and because of the importance of forming links to the school's core business around student welfare and pastoral care
- the development of materials and processes that match school practice conditions that are realistic and sustainable
- collaborative practices within the schools and between schools, agencies and parents
- the importance of developing and enhancing leadership for mental health at various levels within the school community
- contact with other schools engaged in similar work and allocation of a budget
- the acknowledgement of the critical role of the local school context including building on initiatives already underway in the school or linking with other school priorities.

Challenges in evaluating school mental health promotion programs were identified (Hazell et al 2002). From an intersectoral perspective assessing the educational evidence about policy, teacher professional development and changed school practices may not be evidence the health sector recognises as legitimate. However, education systems and school staff can be more interested in these educational outcomes than mental health per se. What is required is acceptance of outcomes that match priorities of both sectors.

The evaluation by the Hunter Institute of Mental Health, nearing completion, looks at the nature and the level of success of the training and development. Additionally there is a focus on school change through in-depth case studies of 16 schools monitoring how they undertake the whole school approach with MindMatters. This evaluation is a time series design with data collected on three occasions over a 3 year time frame. Student level outcomes have been collected using in-school controls. Data on two measures, resilience and help seeking, have been collected from all grades in the secondary school at baseline and then on two additional occasions. Changes in scores are compared with baseline data for comparable unexposed students (Hazell et al 2002). The MindMatters evaluation reveals at this early stage the complexity of the school site in determining how interventions are actually occurring at school, year level or cohort and classroom levels. The idiosyncratic nature of each school is created by the school history and context, school system, the nature of the teaching group, leadership stability and whether champions for the project with power within the school exist within that staff. The MindMatters evaluation will also examine the issue of fidelity and sustainability. These appear to be helped by strong training and development commitment and/or strong curriculum review procedures.

National Dissemination

The governance of the national dissemination is a central part of the national implementation due to the Australian federal system, where state sectors and systems have responsibility for education and health and Federal or Commonwealth departments act as funding agents for national perspectives. MindMatters is a Commonwealth funded approach that uses major contractors to undertake the implementation of the MindMatters concept and resources. In this case, MindMatters uses The Australian Principals Association Professional Development Council (APAPDC) and the Curriculum Corporation as the major contractors to provide training and development to schools across Australia. Maximising the level of acceptance of MindMatters in systems and sectors was critical to increase any needed reinforcement or coordination. Other governance issues include:

- each state has a working party or reference group representing a range of stakeholders
- a project officer linked to the central training group is located in each state/territory
- a national reference group and working parties provide guidance
- training using generic materials combined with relevant state and sector aspects is undertaken by a national team

- training is free but schools need to provide funding for teacher replacement time and travel expenses.

The training is characterised by being active in terms of working through the local context involving the articulation of school factors, using the same learning and teaching methods as contained in the resource and encouraging flexible application within the classroom and the school within the existing sector or school policy frameworks. Teachers find that the topics and training have personal as well as professional meaning. In part, this reflects the nature of teaching as a potentially stressful occupation and the high demands in some worksites. The addition of Staff Matters in 2005 is intended to support teachers' mental health.

Staff Matters is both a web-based resource and a training and development approach linked in with the whole school concept of MindMatters. There is a general concern in the Australian education sector about the quality of school work life. With its link to better outcomes for students Staff Matters emphasises personal, collegiate, organisational and community approaches to health and well-being. On the website are additional research, resources and activities such as:

- exploring values and beliefs in relation to health
- building collegiality on worksites
- staff need for good relationships with students for work satisfaction
- strategies for making professional development a worthwhile personal experience
- sourcing support and understanding from the community
- website links to major Australian helplines and mental health information sites for staff experiencing distress.

Schools are undertaking Staff Matters as part of MindMatters. Schools new to mental health promotion are coming to see the importance of mental health through this different approach.

By late 2005, 2346 schools with secondary enrolments have been represented in the 56 623 participants representing 84% of all schools in Australia with secondary enrolments. These participant numbers represent only the first involvement with MindMatters – participants often come to a range of follow-up sessions. Capacity-building sessions with individual schools are not included in these figures. An initial evaluation based on three states indicates that:

- 98% of participants indicate they will use the resource back at school
- over 70% will use the resilience booklets and the bullying and harassment materials
- 45% will use the loss and grief materials
- just over 30% are working on a whole school approach
- approval rating for the nature of the training is high – participants rate it on average between 7 and 8 out of 10
- 2 day training sessions are rated as more successful than 1 day.

During 2002 MindMatters was extended, focusing on students with high support needs. Seventeen schools have been involved in the pilot of MindMatters Plus which aims to identify pathways of care in school communities. The purpose of the MindMatters Plus initiative is prevention and early intervention for mental health problems. Within existing whole school action for mental health, MindMatters Plus aims to provide examples of coordinated approaches to mental health and education initiatives, school sites, staff and local communities including doctors in general practice and youth health agencies. Expected outcomes include the development of a range of sustainable school-friendly models that allow schools to respond more effectively to students with additional needs in mental health. From 2005 the MindMatters Plus demonstration school learnings will be integrated with the general MindMatters project to provide insights into working with young people with high needs within a whole school approach.

A programme for parents, Families Matter, has recently been implemented through national parent organisations covering parents in state, independent and catholic schools. The concept of Families Matter is to provide an opportunity for parents, carers and family members to be involved in the discussions on health and well-being.

Key Recommendations for Replication

* The approach to mental health promotion needs to be undertaken using education systems, processes and language in the training and in the dissemination.
* Training needs to reflect and model the actual nature of the material being promoted.
* The teacher emerges as a key to the success of a school mental health promotion initiative.
* Training needs to respect the professionalism of teachers providing development in educational terms as well as acknowledging them as individuals in a worksite.
* Funding bodies need to make investments over time and understand how the dissemination occurs within an individual school and across states and sectors.
* Coordinated multi-level training needs to occur that includes teachers, principals, year level coordinators as well as mental health workers linked to the school.
* Transference to other countries (for example, Germany) has involved an incorporation of that country's relevant cultural context, a similar consultation structure and the use of the training methodology of actively experiencing the MindMatters activities.

The Future

Interim funding has been allocated until May 2006 while discussions continue about directions for 2006 and 2007. The evaluations from the various components of the project will form the basis for those discussions. The direction at this stage appears to be more intensive work with particular schools and a regional emphasis. There is a high level of cooperation between contributing organisations for this model. Plans also exist for a rewrite of the kit that will incorporate learnings from the project but maintain the original look and feel of the MindMatters 2000 kit.

References

Australian Health Ministers 1992 National Mental Health Plan. Australian Government Publishing Service, Canberra

Hazell T, Vincent K, Waring T et al 2002 The challenges of evaluating national mental health promotion programs in schools: a case study using the evaluation of MindMatters. International Journal of Mental Health Promotion 4(4):21–27

Sheehan M, Marshall B, Cahill H et al 2000 SchoolMatters: mapping and managing mental health in schools. Commonwealth Department of Health and Aged Care, Canberra. Online. Available: http://www.curriculum.edu.au/mindmatters

Sheehan M, Cahill H, Rowling L et al 2002 Establishing a role for schools in mental health promotion: the MindMatters project. In: Rowling L, Martin G, Walker L (eds) Mental health promotion and young people: concepts and practice. McGraw-Hill, Sydney

Wynn J, Cahill H, Rowling L et al 1999 MindMatters, a whole-school approach promoting mental health and well-being. Australian and New Zealand Journal of Psychiatry 34(4):594–601

Youth Research Centre and Centre for Social Health 1996 Mental health education in Australian secondary schools. AGPS, Canberra

Tackling School Bullying

The 'Bullying Prevention Programme' was developed in Norway in the early 1980s as a response to the growing body of research pinpointing bullying as a serious social problem in Scandinavian countries (Olweus et al 1998). The principal programme developer, Dan Olweus, defines bullying in the following way: 'a student is being bullied or victimized when he or she is exposed, repeatedly and over time, to negative actions on the part of one or more other students' (Olweus 1993). Bullying is characterised by an imbalance of power or strength, otherwise known as an 'asymmetric power relationship' in which the bully performs aggressive, intentional behaviour repeatedly over time (Olweus 1997, Olweus et al 1998). Bullying can be direct as a physical or verbal assault on a victim, or it can be indirect such as excluding someone from a group or spreading malicious rumours about the victim. Evidence suggests that bully/victim behaviour patterns that develop become established and consistent over time, and are likely to continue throughout the school years unless systematic adult efforts are made to remedy the situation (Olweus 1978). The Olweus' Bullying Prevention Programme (1993) applies a whole school approach in modifying the school environment in order to address the negative impact of bullying among primary and secondary school children. This multi-level programme seeks to bring about change at the level of the individual, the classroom and the school in order to reduce opportunities and rewards for bullying behaviour. A detailed account of the implementation of the programme may be found in Book Nine of the 'Blueprints for violence prevention' series (Olweus et al 1998) and in the text by the originator of the programme, Dan Olweus (1993) titled 'Bullying at school: what we know and what we can do'.

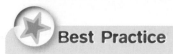

Best Practice

Bullying Prevention Programme

. . . .

(Olweus 1993, Olweus et al 1998)

The Bullying Prevention Programme is a comprehensive and multi-level school-based programme designed to reduce and prevent bullying problems among primary and secondary school children through shifting normative beliefs, improving peer relations and reorienting school systems where necessary. Research suggests that causes of bullying stem from micro-level individual personality characteristics, i.e. aggressiveness, coupled with meso-level classroom factors such as teachers' behaviour as well as macro-level environmental factors such as school organisation and local community attitudes. Therefore, the core components of the programme are multi-level, targeting the individual, the classroom and the school as a whole. The programme actively involves students, parents, teachers and administration in adopting a no-tolerance approach to bullying and providing support and protection to victims of bullying. This type of programme is often referred to as a 'whole-school' approach as it emphasises universal and democratic involvement of all school members in developing and maintaining school policy (Smith et al 2003).

This programme has been implemented in several countries around the world including Canada, Germany, the US, the UK, Belgium, Spain and Switzerland (Smith et al 2003). Interest in the programme has increased due to reports citing school bullying and violence as an international problem, and calling for a integrated and coordinated global response involving national strategies and policies (O'Moore 2004).

Programme Content

The Bullying Prevention Programme involves specific measures for the macro (school), meso (classroom) and micro (individual) levels. The programme does not have a prescribed end date, and should be integrated into the school ethos such that it may be rolled over into subsequent years. Full details of the programme are available in the book 'Bullying at school: what we know and what we can do' (Olweus 1993).

School level:

Establish a Bullying Prevention Coordinating Committee: This committee, comprised of the school principal, a guidance counsellor, a school psychologist, teacher, parent and student representatives, coordinates programme interventions and provides continuity in anti-bullying efforts.

Olweus bully/victim questionnaire: This anonymous student questionnaire or needs assessment can identify the forms of bullying in the school, parent/teacher awareness, characteristics of school bullies and the locations where bullying takes place.

School conference day: A half-day or full-day conference, to be attended by staff, student representatives and parents, can increase awareness of bullying in the school, disseminate questionnaire findings, instigate involvement, commitment and responsibility for the programme and develop aims for a Bullying Prevention Programme at the school.

Improving supervision and outdoor environment: Most bullying activity occurs on the playground (Olweus et al 1998). It is important, therefore, that schools have a coordinated plan to ensure sufficient adult supervision during school breaks and recess, and at locations of previous bullying.

School meetings with parents: Contact between the school and parents, and parent participation in committees and activities, are necessary for programme success (Stevens et al 2001).

Classroom level:

Classroom rules: By involving students in setting up classroom rules against bullying, they feel responsible for their enforcement and empowered to resist bullying.

Positive and negative consequences of rule breaking: Verbal praise and friendly attention are good positive reinforcers of students' positive actions. If a child violates the rules in some way, however, the teacher should pair the negative consequence with a clear statement of what the desired alternative behaviour is and encourage 'change activity' (Olweus et al 1998).

Classroom meetings: While the content will depend on the age and maturity of the students, classroom meetings are a useful way to discuss rules, consequences of rule breaking and role-play situations.

Classroom meetings with parents: Teachers should make parents aware of the anti-bullying discussions going on in the classroom and alert them to any particular incidents. Parents should be encouraged to discuss their child's experience in school and express their worries.

Individual level:

Serious talks with bullies: The principal aim is to get them to stop their bullying behaviour. The teacher should have some proof or reliable information from a number of sources before approaching the bully.

Talk with the victim: The teacher should also speak with the victim in order to determine the nature of the bullying. As victims may be afraid of the repercussions of 'tattling' on a bully, they should be supported and protected against further bullying as much as possible.

Involving the parents: The teacher should arrange a meeting with the bully and his/her parents to discuss the situation and potential solutions. It may be helpful to involve the victim and the victim's parents in the meeting, if the teacher believes both parents will be cooperative.

Evaluation Findings

The first evaluation of the programme was conducted by Olweus (1997) and Olweus et al (1998), which followed four cohorts of 2500 students in total. Questionnaires were administered pre-intervention, 8 months post-intervention, and 20 months post-intervention. The main findings were:

- more than 50% reduction in students reporting incidents of bullying in their schools; this was observed for both genders and across all age groups (Olweus 1997)
- several of the variables produced more significant effects at 20 months post-intervention rather than at 8 months post-intervention
- there was a noticeable reduction in other anti-social behaviours, i.e. vandalism, theft, alcohol use
- the social climate of the classrooms improved significantly, with increased order and discipline, increased school life satisfaction and a more positive attitude towards school work
- girls were generally more receptive to the anti-bullying intervention, and they were more willing to play an active part in challenging school bullying.

A clear dosage–response effect was shown in classroom interventions, such that those classes who exhibited the largest reduction in bully/victim problems had followed the implementation of the complete programme more rigorously than other classrooms.

Subsequent evaluations have produced somewhat mixed findings. Evaluations have been undertaken in Canada, Germany, the US, the UK, Belgium, Spain and Switzerland (Smith et al 2003). Some replications added new components to the original programme, e.g. a peer conflict intervention in Canada and additional support materials in the US. However, these replications had less positive outcomes than the original programme, so there is no evidence that the added components had a positive effect (Smith et al 2003). In Belgium, for example, the programme was replicated in 18 Flemish schools with a total of 1104 children aged 10–16 years participating (Stevens et al 2000). In this study, there were positive effects on school children participating in the programme as compared to a control group. In particular, analysis of the effects on bullying and victimisation found a mixed pattern of positive changes in primary schools and no change in secondary schools. Results, however, were confounded in a number of ways, i.e. participant attrition, whereby bullies tended to drop out of programme participation, as well as differences between the intervention and control groups at baseline. Indeed, the authors of this study noted that further follow up and evaluation is necessary, as several replications of this programme have failed to produce the positive results of the original programme.

Programme Implementation Features

Theoretical framework: Developmental models of aggressive behaviour, research on the development of anti-social behaviours in children and behavioural modification theories all contributed to the development of four key principles for the Bullying Prevention Programme (Olweus 1997, Stevens et al 2001). The principles are as follows:

1. school teachers should demonstrate warmth, positive interest and involvement with students
2. school staff should maintain strict limits to unacceptable behaviour

3. in cases of rule violations, adults should apply fair and non-physical penalties on bullying students
4. adults both at school and at home should act as authorities, though not necessarily authoritarian, e.g. severe and dictatorial.

Needs assessment: A school or community survey, such as the Olweus survey mentioned previously, is useful in determining the extent of a bullying problem in an individual school, district or location so that specific and targeted interventions may be planned.

Increase adult awareness and involvement: In order to implement this programme successfully, teachers and parents must be aware of the extent of bullying problems in the school (Olweus et al 1998) and engage in teacher–parent meetings as well as discussion groups for parents of involved children.

Sequence of intervention activities: The implementation of this programme requires a number of steps including setting up the Bullying Prevention Coordination Committee, administering the Olweus student questionnaire and analysing results, holding staff training in the programme components, arranging a school conference to cover the topic, etc. The questionnaire should be administered in late spring as children then have the opportunity to reflect on experiences during the past year and appropriate interventions can be implemented the following autumn. Analysis of the questionnaire, teacher training and setting up committees should occur during the summer, and the conference and programme implementation be scheduled for early autumn (Olweus et al 1998).

Staffing and training: The coordinating committee with a programme coordinator is responsible for ensuring that the school implements the programme as prescribed and that staff, teachers, parents and students are familiar with the programme and are actively engaged (Olweus et al 1998). All members of the coordinating committee and the classroom teachers must understand the programme and its components and, therefore, should attend 1 or 2 day training sessions as organised by the programme coordinator. Teachers' skills and practices have played a critical role in defining outcomes of the intervention (Stevens et al 2001), with technical assistance available via telephone consultation for the programme coordinator every 3–4 weeks during the first year of implementation (SAMHSA 2004).

Booster training: Annual training booster sessions are important to make staff aware of new methods and procedures in delivering the programme, to train new teachers and to refresh the concept, aims and objectives of the programme in the minds of existing staff.

Multidisciplinary support: In situations where there is more severe bully/victim problems, the Bullying Prevention Coordinating Committee is encouraged to link with social workers, counsellors and school psychologists to lend multidisciplinary support (Stevens et al 2001).

Key Recommendations for Replication

Account for school structure/culture: The implementation of the Bullying Prevention Programme may be more difficult in certain school systems and can be influenced by contextual characteristics such as the role of religion in private religious schools, the socioeconomic demographics of the school population (O'Moore 2004) and even cultural differences in the organisation of the school guidance and psychological services (Stevens et al 2001).

Consultation between programme designers and users: It is important to establish a working connection between programme designers and programme users. Such a linkage helps to improve the intervention's fit with the context in which the programme has to be implemented (Stevens et al 2001).

Staff time/energy: Implementing this programme requires that staff take the time to learn about the programme and constantly work to sustain the initiatives at the different levels. Taking short cuts will only undermine the potential of the programme. The active and enthusiastic involvement of the principal and key staff members may help to keep up the momentum of the programme, particularly through the critical first year.

Family support: Replications of the programme have enjoyed success by adding further interactive components with parents, such as providing them with communication skills training (Stevens et al 2001). None of the previously evaluated programmes provided activities specifically for parents of the children involved, and this may be a programme element that organisers should consider introducing in future replications.

Community level component: Though the original Olweus programme acts on the school, classroom and individual levels, some replications now also include community-level components such as convening meetings with community members and incorporating anti-bullying messages and strategies into youth-related activities in the community, e.g. scouting and sports (Olweus et al 1998).

Integrate teacher training into initial teacher education: To enhance the dissemination and sustainability of this programme, bullying prevention teacher training should be incorporated into teacher education at both pre-service and in-service levels (O'Moore 2004). This would raise teachers' awareness of the issue of bullying, increase their self-efficacy in dealing with bully/victim problems and strengthen teachers' motivation to administer the prevention programme.

Establish a regional/national anti-bullying advisory board: A regional or national anti-bullying advisory board would help to provide guidance for local administrators dealing with both school and workplace bullying. Such a board would also be useful as a repository for evidence-based advice and guidance on how to develop and implement school policies to offset the problem of bullying, and would be in a position to deliver on international recommendations from the World Health Organization (O'Moore 2004).

Targeted Interventions

A number of school-based programmes have been designed for students who are at higher risk by virtue of their life circumstances or increased exposure to stress. Such programmes, which usually involve teacher training and parent involvement, address the enhancement of coping skills and cognitive skills training in preventing the onset of problems such as depression and suicide. The 'Coping with Stress' course for 15–16-year-olds, developed by Clarke et al (1995), is an example of a cognitive mood management programme which aims to prevent the development of depression in students with elevated risk of clinical depression. A fuller description of this programme may be found in Chapter 7. The 'Penn Prevention Programme' (Jaycox et al 1994), which includes cognitive and social problem-solving skills, has also been applied successfully with younger children aged 10–13 years with an elevated risk of depression. The 'Penn Resiliency Programme' (Gillham & Reivich 1999, Gillham et al 1995) also addresses improved coping skills and cognitive thinking in children with symptoms of depression. This programme has been adapted across different sites, including in China (Yu & Seligman 2002), and the positive outcomes have been sustained for up to 2 years post-intervention.

Specific programmes for children of parents with alcohol problems ('Students Together and Resourceful', Emshoff 1990) and the 'Children of Divorce Intervention Project' (Pedro-Carroll et al 1999) have provided support and skill training in developing coping strategies, social skills and improved adjustment. The 'Resourceful Adolescent Programme' (Shochet et al 2001) is a resilience building programme which has been implemented with 14–15-year-olds in Australia. This programme includes both an adolescent version and a combined parents–adolescent version. Adolescents in both groups were found to have significantly lowered levels of depression and hopelessness at 10 months follow up compared to the comparison group.

Suicide Prevention Programmes

With regard to suicide prevention, most school-based programmes address suicide awareness and education for adolescents and may also include general coping skills training. By and large these programmes are delivered by teachers who have received additional training, followed by school counsellors, social workers, school nurses and mental health specialists. Many of these programmes target all students in a particular class with the aim of increasing overall awareness, confidence and skills of peer confidantes in identifying and obtaining help for suicidal peers. Garland and Zigler (1993) describe the main aims of such programmes as being:

- to raise awareness of the problem of adolescent suicide
- to train participants to identify adolescents at risk from suicide
- to educate participants about mental health resources and referral techniques.

While many of these interventions have been successful in increasing students' knowledge and improving attitudes about suicide, few studies have measured behavioural outcomes. A small number of studies have moved beyond awareness raising to include behaviour change and coping skills training, e.g. Israeli studies by Klingman and Hochdorf (1993) and Orbach and Bar-Joseph (1993). A systematic review of school-based curriculum suicide prevention programmes by Ploeg et al (1996, 1999) concluded that, overall, 'there is insufficient evidence to support school-based curriculum suicide prevention programs for adolescents' (1999:15). Guo and Harstall (2002) also concluded that there was insufficient evidence to either support or not support these programmes largely due to poor quality evaluations. Studies by Overholser et al (1989) and Spirito et al (1988) reported a worsening of suicide-related attitudes, with increased levels of hopelessness and maladaptive coping responses among male students. Shaffer et al (1991) also reported negative effects particularly for students who had previously attempted suicide. These findings have led to concern that suicide prevention programmes can in fact be harmful to certain students (Lister-Sharp et al 1999). While these negative findings have been limited to first generation studies, which have been less sophisticated in their design and content and also less rigorous in their evaluation methodology, the potential of negative outcomes, particularly for vulnerable students, cautions against implementing these programmes and points to the need for significant training, back up and support. More comprehensive programmes, which include teacher training, parent education, stress management and life skills, together with the introduction of a crisis team in the school have achieved more positive outcomes, including significant reductions in both suicide and attempted suicide over a 5-year period (Zenere & Lazarus 1997). More detailed evaluation is needed before topic-specific suicide prevention programmes are to be recommended over good quality generic skills programmes in this area.

Link with other Services

In addition to school-based interventions there is a recognised need for complementary interventions which involve family members and local communities as well as a broad range of health and welfare services. The school can be an important link in ensuring awareness of, and access to, appropriate sources of support and professional help for young people when needed. Linkage between schools and outside agencies is an important feature of the health promoting schools initiative and the development of a partnership approach, with better integration of the health services with the everyday life of the school, is encouraged. The active participation of students in developing a school journal, containing youth-friendly information on mental health, is highlighted in the 'School Journal' case study. This is a good example of a process which involved partnership between young people, schools, parents, teachers, mental health service users and mental health professionals in raising awareness of mental health and support services.

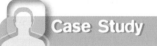

Case Study

The School Journal

Anne Sheridan

Introduction

The School Journal is a mental health promotion initiative targeting young people aged 15–18 years in the north west of Ireland. It aims to engage with young people to support them to produce information on mental health issues and services in a positive and teenage-friendly way. The resulting product is a homework diary with over 50 pages exploring mental health issues such as relationships, depression, anger management, abuse, sexuality, etc. The first edition of the Journal was produced in 2000 with subsequent editions produced in 2002 and 2005. An evaluation of the project took place in 2001 and the second revised edition of the Journal included the recommendations of student users.

Background

A mental health needs assessment with young people undertaken in 1999/2000 indicated a need for information on a range of issues affecting their mental health (Sheridan 1999). Young people recommended that this information be presented in a sophisticated and well-designed format to appeal to their age group and raise the profile and image of mental health in general.

A review of existing information available to young people on mental health confirmed a gap in the provision of youth-friendly information and the School Journal project became an attempt to address this. Three health professionals, a child psychiatrist, mental health social worker and mental health promotion officer agreed to work together on the project. Initially the idea was to produce a high quality and well designed range of leaflets through working in partnership with young people. A group of 13 young people became involved in the project and after initial working sessions the group rejected the idea of leaflets as not being effective or useful for young people. The idea of a school homework journal incorporating information on mental health emerged as a more acceptable and practical resource for young people throughout a whole school year.

The first edition of the School Journal was launched in September 2000 and in 2001 an evaluation was undertaken to assess user satisfaction (Share 2001). Focus groups with student users indicated that the journal had been received very positively by them. There was a high level of satisfaction with the content, design and layout of the Journal. Young people referred to the content being relevant and written in a way they could relate to and understand. The evaluation showed that boys and girls had read the journal and liked the sense of humour and variety it contained. They also noticed the services directory and said things like 'it's good to know they're there if you should ever need help'.

Student participation on the production of the School Journal was validated by the evaluation. Within the Health Service Executive North West (HSENW) (formerly the North Western Health Board (NWHB)) the participation of young people in the planning of services for children and young people has been a stated objective of the Regional Children's Services Planning Structure since 2002. The HSENW area 'Mental Health Promotion Strategy and Action Plan' further recognised that 'increased student participation in decision making and planning results in positive mental health benefits' (NWHB 2004).

Programme Implementation and Recommendations

A number of key factors contributed to the success of this project. They are as follows:

Needs based: The initial project idea came as a direct result of needs assessment and consultation with young people about mental health (Sheridan

1999). This led to a number of recommendations from young people as to how their positive mental health could be promoted. These included the provision of teenage-friendly information on mental health issues, positive tips on coping and information on services. They wanted the information to be presented positively and to include very few 'don't's and 'no's. Their fears and anxieties about help seeking and the need to promote this were also prioritised.

Partnership with young people: Aside from the partnership between the Health Promotion Department and the Child and Family Mental Health Service this project also developed a partnership with young people. To date over 50 young people have been involved in the production of three editions of the School Journal. A broad range of young people have been involved and their involvement has been supported by their parents and school principals. Young people were recruited from schools, out of school Youthreach centres and a community arts project on mental health. From the outset it was agreed that the final say in all aspects of the content, design and layout of the final product should be with the young people. This meant that, aside from the personal commitment to this partnership by the professionals involved, it was important to secure the support and commitment of the organisation of the HSENW. The support of school principals and key teachers was encouraged throughout the project through information sessions and training events. Parents were invited to information sessions on the project so that they understood what their young people were involved in and so that they could meet the professionals involved.

The group-work process: A lot of attention was paid in the early stages to group formation and promoting dynamic working relationships within the groups. Group exercises and team-building strategies ensured that group cohesion was developed. A working agreement was endorsed by all which included issues such as membership, respect, confidentiality, participation, length and frequency of working sessions. As almost all working sessions took place on Saturdays, which meant that young people had to give up their free time, it was agreed that one residential working session would take place during the school week. Transport was provided for the young people to attend the working sessions. A number of group-work methods were used throughout the working sessions including first ideas, small group discussion, inputs from visitors, drama, information inputs, internet research and large group discussion. All comments and suggestions were recorded and final agreement achieved by consensus. The group had several meetings with the graphic designers and advised them on design of the Journal. The content was written and rewritten until the group was satisfied.

Group capacity building: Although young people know instinctively what works with their age group they did require further information, skills and training in mental health promotion. Negative attitudes towards help seeking were common in the groups and it was important to challenge these attitudes and help young people understand that professional services can really make a difference to young people in distress. Involving young people who themselves had experienced mental health difficulties helped achieve this. Other people were also invited to meet the group to talk of their own experiences where members felt a lack of understanding or awareness of particular issues, e.g. what it is like to grow up in a family where a parent has an alcohol dependence problem. This was followed by members of the group writing on the subject and the text being passed back to the presenter for comments. Young people were also involved in the marketing of the Journal and were provided with training in presentation and media skills to enable them do this.

Well established relationship with schools: There is a long history of partnership between the HSENW area and post-primary schools in the area. This relationship provided opportunities to market the Journal, to plan its dissemination and to receive regular feedback on barriers encountered.

Implementation Challenges and Experiences

A number of challenges and experiences in the implementation of the School Journal are worthy of note.

Attitudes and faith: In general, working in partnership involves an openess to attitudes which are different. This is particularly the case when working with young people. Aside from the attitudes of the individuals involved, there are organisational attitudes to be considered. These need to be managed so that the essence of youth involvement is not stifled by organisational inflexibility. This poses a challenging and dynamic question – are we willing to set aside our own beliefs and attitudes and trust the advice from young people as to what works? This takes faith at a number of different levels.

Marketing the Journal: A targeted and strategic marketing plan is an essential part of any project such as the School Journal and should be underway from the start. In developing the second edition of the Journal there were attempts to improve this aspect of the overall project. From the outset, schools were involved. Meetings were held with key teachers at different points to keep them informed of the project. Drafts were circulated to teachers and principals so that they could get a sense of the finished product. Successful dissemination involved forward planning on their part to include the Journal on the student book list for the coming year. Suggestions and comments from teachers and principals were considered by the group and some were taken on board. For example, teachers and principals recommended that the Journal would have a nominal cost so that it would be valued by students. This was initially agreed and later reviewed when it emerged that collecting a fee from students became a barrier to its dissemination. Presentations at conferences nationally and internationally provided opportunities for members of the group, including the young people, to promote the project. The evaluation of the Journal highlighted some disappointment among the initial group of young people as to their role in the overall marketing of the Journal and they felt that they had more to offer in this regard.

It is demanding work: Working on a mental health promotion project such as the School Journal demands a big time commitment from everyone. But so does everything that is worth doing! To access young people most of this work time has to be at weekends. This can be particularly draining after a hard week's work. Working sessions need to be carefully managed so that the work is focused and productive. Like any document, the final editing and proofreading is laborious and coming at a time when everyone is over-familiar with the content. Having at least two outside readers is essential to ensure that typos are kept to a minimum.

It is enjoyable and energising work: Working directly with young people in creating the School Journal continues to be an enjoyable and rewarding experience for everyone involved. The creativity and energy created by the group along with the personal commitment and sense of ownership to the project is remarkable. The encouragement and maintenance of that sense of individual responsibility to the project can only happen through a process of engagement which promotes a partnership which does good work while also having fun.

Key Recommendations for Replication

The overall recommendation is that health professionals, particularly health promotion professionals, should engage young people in partnership to develop programmes aimed at their age group. In attempting to do this the following recommendations will help.

Select a varied group: The more representative the group is the more likely that the end product will be accessible to all young people in the group targeted.

Help the group to form: Allow time at the start to settle everyone in to the group. Having outside facilitators could be helpful here, e.g. a youth drama group.

Contract well with the group: Everyone likes to know how long a project will last, how much time will be involved and what supports are available.

Be prepared for the hard work: It is time consuming and there are a lot of organisational issues to get right, e.g. practical matters such as arranging travel for the group.

Have the budget confirmed: It is morally wrong to start working with young people if the budget to complete the project has not been fully secured.

Ensure that the project 'fits': The investment in terms of time and money is substantial so before embarking on a similar project ensure that the various stakeholders are on board as well as the structures to facilitate dissemination.

Develop a marketing strategy: This needs to be part of the project from the start. The group needs to know that there is a market for the product and have ideas as to how to tap into that market to ensure as broad a dissemination as possible.

Plan sessions well: There is nothing worse than having a group of young people eager to work but the preparation hasn't been done.

Plan an evaluation strategy: Again this should be developed from the outset so that the researcher has a chance to contribute to the aims, objectives and design of the project.

Provide opportunities for the young people to celebrate their work: This is important for all of us but particularly so for young people who have given their free time to a project.

References

NWHB (North West Health Board) 2004 Mental Health Promotion Strategy and Action Plan 2005–2010. Manorhamilton, Ireland

Share 2001 The mental health School Journal: evaluation report. Unpublished report, NWHB, Manorhamilton, Ireland

Sheridan A 1999 Consultation with young people on mental health. Unpublished report, NWHB, Manorhamilton, Ireland

The potential of a school-based programme to link with and influence the broader community is illustrated by a case study from Pakistan. The 'School Mental Health Programme' is a school-based education programme which is designed to increase understanding of common mental health problems and reduce stigma. In this initiative, the school serves as a gateway to the local community and the programme, operating through the school children, positively influences the knowledge and attitudes of the school children, their parents and neighbours.

Case Study

School Mental Health Programme

Malik H Mubbashar, Khalid Saeed, Zainab Farhan

Background

Mental health has been one of the most neglected areas of general health considerations in Pakistan. The subgroup on the National Programme for Mental Health Care in Pakistan (Planning Commission Government of Pakistan 1998) concluded that there were an estimated one million people with severe mental illnesses and 10–15% with mild to moderate mental illnesses in the country which has a total population of 150 million. Furthermore, an estimated 16–22/1000 of children between the ages of 3 and 9 years suffer from severe mental retardation (Durkin et al 1979, Hasan & Hasan 1981) while the prevalence rates of epilepsy are 9–18/1000 (Aziz et al 1994). There is one psychiatrist for every 500 000 people in Pakistan (Planning Commission Government of Pakistan 1998).

In 1986 a community mental health programme was started in the rural areas of Rawalpindi. The objective of this programme was to raise awareness about mental health problems in the community, train doctors in primary health care in diagnosing and treating common mental disorders in the community and to develop a system of supervision and referral with the specialist mental health care service. Earlier in this programme it was realised that schools can be a powerful medium and can play an effective role in stimulating community efforts for mental health care provision. It was believed that the school children can become the main source of information for their family, friends and neighbours, particularly in areas of low literacy. They have an essential role in the rural communities where they function as the eyes and ears (Mubbashar et al 1986).

Implementation

A school mental health programme was started in the rural areas of Rawalpindi in 1988 (Mubbashar 1989). The aim was to encourage better use of the mental health services that were being integrated into primary care. The programme works directly with school children and their teachers, and the children share their knowledge and understanding with their families, friends and neighbours.

The objectives of the school mental health programme were:

- to develop greater awareness of mental health among school children, school teachers and the community
- to provide essential knowledge about mental health principles to the school teachers to enable them to:
    - impart such knowledge to school children
    - recognise common mental health problems in school children
    - provide essential psychological support and counselling when required by school children
    - increase community awareness of mental health needs and services.

The programme was designed in four phases: familiarisation, training, reinforcement and evaluation.

Familiarisation phase:

Before the start of the programme, the district school authorities were contacted; the aims and objectives of the programme were explained and their cooperation was sought. This phase involved collection of background information on the existing educational facilities. In addition, teams visited various schools of the field area to assess current mental health knowledge among the heads of the schools, teachers and students and their willingness to support and own the programme. During this phase, medical camps were organised at various schools once a week to provide them with counselling on various medical and mental health problems. The aim of this initiative was to gain their confidence and establish rapport with the school authorities for the acceptance and success of the programme. During this phase, the knowledge of teachers about mental health and illnesses was also assessed. It was noted that the majority of teachers had very limited knowledge of mental health and many teachers shared the rural community's views about the causation of mental illness being due to the influence of evil spirits. The socioeconomic stress and unhappy, difficult environments were also considered as potent causes of mental ill health.

Training of teachers phase:

The training was mainly directed towards changing the attitudes of the teachers towards mental health. In addition, it was aimed to provide them with knowledge of common mental health problems and the basic aim of psychological counselling when needed. The training of school teachers was conducted either in one of the central high schools of the area or on the premises of the local education authority offices. The training took place mostly during the 3 month long summer vacation when the children were off, but the teachers were only allowed to take either the first or the second half of the vacation. The training used locally developed manuals, case studies and an interactive methodology, besides having a pre- and post-training evaluation.

Reinforcement phase:
During this phase the following activities were carried out:

- visits to schools
- propagation of the programmes through slogans and contests
- organisation of parent/teacher associations.

The slogans were:

- smoking is injurious to health
- mental illnesses are not due to possessions by evil spirits but are like any other bodily disease and are treatable
- people are different and some of them have disabilities. Do not laugh at other people with disabilities but help them.

Numerous posters carrying these slogans were designed by the school children themselves, which are displayed now in most of the class and staff rooms. The teachers, from their own resources, organised the production of the rubber stamps carrying these catchy phrases, which were put on the children's note books as well as on all the letters being sent out by the local post offices.

Evaluation phase:
During this phase, studies were carried out in the following areas to evaluate the impact of the school mental health programme:

- changes in knowledge and attitudes of teachers regarding mental health before and after training (Bhatti 2000)
- impact on the knowledge and attitudes of the community after initiation of the school mental health programme (Rahman et al 1998)
- impact on the knowledge and attitudes of school children after the initiation of the school mental health programme (Saeed & Mubbashar 1999)
- use of the school mental health programme as a tool for the promotion of social capital (Saeed et al 1999)

In light of these studies it was concluded that the school mental health programme improved school children's awareness of and attitudes to mental health problems, and that there was a positive change even in the attitude and knowledge of their friends and neighbours. There is, however, no study demonstrating the translation of this change in knowledge and attitudes into a change in mental health related practices.

Implementation Challenges

Over the last 16 years, the major challenge has been to increase the reach of the programme to a wider population. However, this has been a slow and often difficult process facing resistance from mental health professionals not keen on the public health approach, and teachers often taking it as an additional task. Another problem identified was the lack of intersectoral coordination. Field experience had shown that, until there is a strong political will combined with commitment of adequate resources, it might be difficult to generalise the programme. In light of this experience, a pilot programme has been initiated in consultation with provincial governments and departments of health and education, involving one district of each of the four provinces of Pakistan and Kashmir since 2002. The evaluation of this particular initiative would be instrumental in identifying the mechanisms which need to be put into place for countrywide implementation of the programme.

Recommendations

In light of our experiences in Rawalpindi, we feel that the school mental heath programme is a cost-effective method of combating stigma and raising public awareness about mental health problems. There is a need to carry out longitudinal, system-based studies focusing on the programme's inputs, processes, outputs and impact, which would be helpful in furthering the reach of the programme.

References

Aziz H, Ali S M, Frances P et al 1994 Epilepsy in Pakistan: a population based epidemiological study. Epilepsia 35(5):950–958

Bhatti N 2000 Pre- and post-training evaluation of knowledge and attitudes of school teachers regarding mental health. Unpublished dissertation to the College of Physicians and Surgeons, Pakistan

Durkin M S, Hasan Z M, Hasan K Z 1979 Prevalence and correlates of mental retardation among children in Karachi, Pakistan. American Journal of Epidemiology 147(3):277–294

Hasan Z, Hasan A 1981 Report on a population survey of mental retardation in Pakistan. International Journal of Mental Health 10:23–27

Mubbashar M H 1989 Promotion of mental health through school health programme. Eastern Mediterranean Region Health Services Journal 6:14–9

Mubbashar M H, Malik S J, Zar J R 1986 Community based mental health care programme. Report of an experiment in Pakistan. Eastern Mediterranean Region Health Services Journal 1:14–20

Planning Commission Government of Pakistan 1998 Report of the subcommittee on mental health and substance abuse. Ninth five year plan (1998–2003) Prospective plan 2003–2013. Planning Commission Government of Pakistan, Islamabad

Rahman A, Mubbashar M H, Gater R et al 1998 Randomised trial of impact of school mental health programme in rural Rawalpindi, Pakistan. Lancet 352:1022–1025

Saeed K, Mubbashar M H 1999 Evaluation of the impact of school mental health programme: a study of knowledge and attitudes among girl students at Rawalpindi, Islamabad. Journal of College of Physicians and Surgeons Pakistan 9(7):325–327

Saeed K, Wirz S, Gater R et al 1999 Detection of disabilities by school children: a pilot study in rural Pakistan. Tropical Doctor 9:151–155

Generic Principles of Effective Mental Health Promotion Programmes in Schools

Based on the research evidence and the programmes reviewed in this chapter, the following characteristics of successful school-based interventions have been identified.

Adopting a whole school approach

Programmes adopting a whole-school approach, which embrace changes to the school environment as well as the curriculum and involve parents, families and the local community, are more likely to be effective. The health promoting school initiative provides a useful framework for strengthening the school's capacity as a mental health promoting setting for living, learning and working. This requires a comprehensive approach with the use of coordinated and multiple strategies aiming to bring about change at the levels of the individual, the classroom and the school.

Adopting a social competence approach

Traditional topic-specific approaches are recognised as being of limited value. Reviews of the evidence endorse a social competence approach, which brings a focus on the promotion of resourcefulness and generic coping and competence skills, rather than interventions focusing on the prevention of specific problem behaviours such as suicide (Jané-Llopis et al 2005, Mentality 2003). The social competence approach supports the use of interactive methodologies that embrace a more participatory approach for students. Effective social competence promotion programmes include opportunities to reinforce the application of these skills throughout a range of social contexts beyond the classroom, i.e. in the home, youth centres and other community-based settings. Peer-led approaches and mentoring programmes are recognised as potentially useful approaches.

Theory-based interventions

Programmes need to be grounded on sound theories of child development and learning. Interventions guided by a strong theoretical base have been found to lead to improved outcomes (Harden et al 2001, Jané-Llopis & Barry 2005, Zins et al 2004).

Interventions over multiple years

It is increasingly recognised that once-off or short-term interventions are not likely to produce long-term effects (Greenberg et al 2001a). Therefore, sustained interventions over multiple years are more likely to produce long-lasting positive outcomes (Wells et al 2001).

High-quality implementation

The level and quality of programme planning and delivery are influenced by contextual factors in the school setting and the presence of a supportive implementation system. This includes the level of engagement and cooperation from students, teachers and parents, support from the school organisation and management, teacher training and provision of support resources, quality of materials and the overall readiness of the school to implement the programme. Teacher training in the skills and confidence needed for effective programme delivery is highlighted as being critical to programme success.

Evaluation

The incorporation of systematic evaluation methods contributes to the ongoing improvement and sustainability of school-based mental health promotion programmes. The multifaceted nature of the majority of school programmes calls for research approaches that take into account the contextual and dynamic nature of the school as a setting (Rowling 2002). Parson and Stears (2002) provide a useful discussion of this issue in the context of evaluating health promoting schools. The evaluation of whole school approaches requires careful documentation of actual programme implementation, assessing the role of contextual factors in facilitating effective delivery and measuring multiple programme outcomes using a variety of measures drawn from a variety of sources.

Sustainability

While many programmes can demonstrate their success in the short term, many fail to sustain their impact over a longer period. It is, therefore, important to identify organisational and system-level practices and policies that will ensure the sustainability of high quality programmes. The sustainability of successful programmes is dependent on their successful adaptation to the ecology of the school and community in which they occur (Price & Lorion 1989). Comprehensive programmes that target multiple protective and risk factors have greater potential to endure in school settings than have discrete, short-term interventions that target single, topic-specific issues.

References

Aber L, Jones S, Brown J et al 1998 Resolving conflict creatively: evaluating the developmental effects of a school-based violence prevention program in neighborhood and classroom context. Development and Psychopathology 10(2):187–213

Apter A 2001 Adolescent suicide and attempted suicide. In: Wasserman D (ed) Suicide, an unnecessary death. Martin Dunitz, London:181–195

Battistich V, Schnaps E, Watson M et al 1996 Prevention effects of the Child Development Project: early findings from an ongoing multi-site demonstration trial. Journal of Adolescent Research 11:12–35

Beautrais A L, Joyce P R, Mulder R T 1996 Risk factors from serious suicide attempts among youth aged 13 through 24 years. Journal of the American Academy of Child and Adolescent Psychiatry 35(9):1174–1183

Botvin G J, Tortu S 1988 Preventing adolescent substance abuse through life skills training. In: Price R H, Cowen E L, Lorion R P et al (eds) Fourteen ounces of prevention: a casebook for practitioners. American Psychological Association, Washington DC:98–110

Botvin G J, Eng A, Williams C L 1980 Preventing the onset of cigarette smoking through life skills training. Preventive Medicine 9(1):135–143

Botvin G J, Renick N, Baker E 1983 The effects of scheduling format and booster sessions on a broad-spectrum psychosocial approach to smoking prevention. Journal of Behavioral Medicine 6:359–379

Botvin G J, Baker E, Botvin E M et al 1984a Alcohol abuse prevention through the development of personal and social competence: a pilot study. Journal of Studies on Alcohol 45:550–552

Botvin G J, Baker E, Renick N L et al 1984b A cognitive-behavioural approach to substance abuse prevention. Addictive Behaviors 9:137–147

Botvin G J, Baker E, Dusenbury L D et al 1990a Preventing adolescent drug abuse through a multimodal cognitive-behavioral approach: results of a three-year study. Journal of Consulting and Clinical Psychology 58:437–446

Botvin G J, Baker E, Filazzola A et al 1990b A cognitive-behavioural approach to substance abuse prevention: a one year follow-up. Addictive Behaviors 15:47–63

Botvin G J, Baker E, Dusenbury L D et al 1995 Long-term follow-up results of a randomized drug abuse prevention trial within a white middle-class population. Journal of the American Medical Association 273:1106–1112

Botvin G J, Mihalic S F, Grotpeter J K 1998 Blueprints for violence prevention. Book five: Life Skills Training. Center for the Study and Prevention of Violence, Institute of Behavioural Science, University of Colorado, Boulder, Colorado

Botvin G J, Griffin K W, Diaz T et al 2000 Preventing illicit drug use in adolescents: long-term follow-up data from a randomized control trial of a school population. Addictive Behaviors 25(5):769–774

Botvin G J, Griffin K W, Paul E et al 2003 Preventing tobacco and alcohol use among elementary school students through Life Skills Training. Journal of Child and Adolescent Abuse 12(4):1–17

Browne G, Gafni A, Roberts J et al 2004 Effective/efficient mental health programs for school-age children: a synthesis of reviews. Social Science and Medicine 58:1367–1384

Bruene-Butler L, Hampson J, Elias M J et al 1997 The 'Improving Social Awareness-Social Problem Solving' project. In: Albee G W, Gullotta T P (eds) Primary prevention works, vol 6: issues in children's and families' lives. Sage, California

Caplan M, Weissberg R P, Grober J S et al 1992 Social competence promotion with inner-city and suburban young adolescents: effects on social adjustment and alcohol use. Journal of Consulting and Clinical Psychology 60(1):56–63

CASEL (Collaborative for Academic, Social and Emotional Learning) 2003 Safe and sound: an educational leaders' guide to evidence-based social and emotional learning programs. CASEL, Chicago

Clarke G N, Hawkins W, Murphy M et al 1995 Targeted prevention of unipolar depressive disorder in an at-risk sample of high-school adolescents: a randomized trial of group cognitive intervention. Journal of the American Academy of Child and Adolescent Psychiatry 34(3):312–321

Coleman J 1997 Key data on adolescence, 2nd edn. Routledge, London

Dryfoos J G 1997 The prevalence of problem behaviours: implications for programs. In: Weissberg R P, Gullotta T P, Hampton R L et al (eds) Enhancing children's wellness, vol 8: issues in children's and families' lives. Sage, London.

Dryfoos J G 1998 Safe passage: making it through adolescence in a risky society. Oxford University Press, New York

DuBois D L, Holloway B E, Valentine J C et al 2002 Effectiveness of mentoring programs for youth: a meta-analytic review. American Journal of Community Psychology 30(2):157–197

Durlak J A, Wells A M 1997 Primary prevention mental health programs for children and adolescents: a meta-analytic review. American Journal of Community Psychology 25(2):115–152

Elias M J, Weissberg R P 1989 School-based social-competence promotion as a primary prevention strategy: a tale of two projects. Prevention in Human Services 7:177–200

Elias M J, Gara M, Ubriaco M et al 1986 Impact of a preventive social problem-solving intervention on children's coping with middle-school stressors. American Journal of Community Psychology 14:259–275

Elias M, Zins J, Weissberg R et al 1997 Promoting social and emotional learning. ASCD, Alexandria, Virginia

Emshoff J G 1990 A preventive intervention with children of alcoholics. Prevention in Human Services 7(1):225–253

Fagan A A, Mihalic S 2003 Strategies for enhancing the adoption of school-based prevention programs: lessons learned from the Blueprints for violence prevention replications of the Life Skills Training program. Journal of Community Psychology 31(3):235–253

Felner R D, Adan A M 1988 The school transitional project: an ecological intervention and evaluation. In: Price R H, Cowen E L, Lorion R P et al (eds) Fourteen ounces of prevention: a casebook for practitioners. American Psychological Association, Washington DC:111–122

Felner R D, Brand S, Adan A M et al 1993 Restructuring the ecology of the school as an approach to prevention during school transitions: longitudinal follow-ups and extensions of the School Transitional Environment Project (STEP). Prevention in Human Services 10(2):103–136

Garland A F, Zigler E 1993 Adolescent suicide prevention: current research and social policy implications. Special issue: adolescence. American Psychologist 48(2):169–182

Gillham J E, Reivich K J 1999 Prevention of depressive symptoms in school children: a research update. Psychological Science 10:461–462

Gillham J, Reivich K, Jaycox L et al 1995 Prevention of depressive symptoms in school children: two year follow-up. Psychological Science 6:343–351

Gordon J, Grant G 1977 How we feel. Jessica Kingsley, London

Gorman D M 2005 Does measurement dependence explain the effects of the Life Skills Training program on smoking outcomes? Preventive Medicine 40:479–487

Gottfredson D C 1990 Changing school structures to benefit high-risk youths. Understanding troubled and troubling youth: multidisciplinary perspectives. Sage, California

Green J, Howes F, Waters E et al 2005 Promoting the social and emotional health of primary school-aged children: reviewing the evidence base for schools based interventions. International Journal of Mental Health Promotion 7(3):30–36

Greenberg M, Kusche C, Cook E et al 1995 Promoting emotional competence in school-aged children: the effects of the PATHS curriculum. Development and Psychology 7:117–136

Greenberg M T, Domitrovich C E, Bumbarger B 2001a The prevention of mental disorders in school-aged children: current state of the field. Prevention and Treatment 4(1). Online. Available: http://journals.apa. org/prevention/volume4/pre0040001a.html November 2005

Greenberg M T, Domitrovich C E, Graczyk P et al 2001b A conceptual model for the implementation of school-based preventive interventions: implications for research, practice and policy. Report to the Center for Mental Health Services. Prevention Research Center for the Promotion of Human Development, Pennsylvania State University, Pennsylvania

Griffin K W, Botvin G J, Nichols T R et al 2003 Effectiveness of a universal drug abuse prevention approach for youth at high risk for substance use initiation. Preventive Medicine 36(1):1–7

Griffin K W, Botvin G J, Nichols T R 2004 Long-term follow-up effects of a school-based drug abuse prevention program on adolescent risky driving. Prevention Science 5(3):207–212

Grossman J P, Tierney J P 1998 Does mentoring work? An impact study of the Big Brothers, Big Sisters program. Evaluation Review 22:403–426

Guo B, Harstall C 2002 Efficacy of suicide prevention programs for children and youth. Health Technology Assessment, series A. Alberta Heritage Foundation for Medical Research, Edmonton

Haney P, Durlak J 1998 Changing self-esteem in children and adolescents: a meta-analytic review. Journal of Clinical Child Psychology 27(4):423–433

Harden A, Rees R, Shepherd J et al 2001 Young people and mental health: a systematic review on barriers and facilitators. EPPI-Centre, England. Online. Available: http:// eppi.ioe.ac.uk 13 October 2005

Hawkins J D, Von Cleve E, Catalano R F 1991 Reducing early childhood aggression: results of a primary prevention program. Journal of the American Academy of Child and Adolescent Psychiatry 30:208–217

Hodgson R, Abbasi T 1995 Effective mental health promotion: a literature review. Health Promotion Wales, Technical Report No 13

Hodgson R, Abbasi T, Clarkson J 1996 Effective mental health promotion: a literature review. Health Education Journal 55:55–74

Hurry J, Lloyd C 1997 A follow-up evaluation of Project Charlie: a life skills drug education programme for primary schools. Initiative paper 16. HMSO, London

Jané-Llopis E, Barry M M 2005 What makes mental health promotion effective? Promotion and Education Suppl2:47–55

Jané-Llopis E, Barry M M, Hosman C et al 2005 Mental health promotion works: a review. Promotion and Education Suppl2:9–25

Jaycox L H, Reivich K J, Gillham J et al 1994 Prevention of depressive symptoms in school children. Behaviour Research and Therapy 32:801–816

Jekielek S M, Moore K A, Hair E C 2002 Mentoring: a promising strategy from youth development. Child Trends Research Brief. Online. Available: http://www.childtrends. org/Files/MentoringBrief2002.pdf 17 November 2005

Kellam S G, Rebok G W, Ialongo N et al 1994 The course and malleability of aggressive behavior from early first grade into middle school: results of a developmental epidemiologically based preventive trial.

Journal of Child Psychology and Psychiatry 35:259–281

Klingman A, Hochdorf Z 1993 Coping with distress and self-harm: the impact of a primary prevention program among adolescents. Journal of Adolescence 16:121–140

Lister-Sharp D, Chapman S, Stewart-Brown S et al 1999 Health promoting schools and health promotion in schools: two systematic reviews. Health Technology Assessment 3(22):1–207

Lloyd C, Joyce R, Hurry J et al 2000 The effectiveness of primary drug education. Drugs: Education, Prevention and Policy 7(2):109–126

McGill D 1998 Blueprints for violence prevention. Book two: Big Brothers, Big Sisters of America. Center for the Study and Prevention of Violence, Institute of Behavioural Science, University of Colorado, Boulder, Colorado

Mentality 2003 Making it effective: a guide to evidence based mental health promotion. Radical mentalities – briefing paper 1. Mentality, London

Offord D R, Kraemer H C, Kazdin A D et al 1999 Lowering the burden of suffering: monitoring the benefits of clinical, targeted and universal approaches. In: Keating D P, Hertzman C (eds) Developmental health and the wealth of nations: social, biological and educational dynamics. The Guilford Press, New York

Olweus D 1978 Agression in the schools. Bullies and whipping boys. Hemisphere Press (Wiley), Washington DC

Olweus D 1993 Bullying at school: what we know and what we can do. Blackwell, Cambridge

Olweus D 1997 Bully/victim problems in school: knowledge base and an effective intervention program. The Irish Journal of Psychology 18(2):170–190

Olweus D, Limber S, Mihalic S 1998 Blueprints for violence prevention series. Book nine: bullying prevention program. Center for the Study and Prevention of Violence, Institute of Behavioural Science, University of Colorado, Boulder, Colorado

O'Moore M 2004 Guiding framework for policy approaches to school bullying and violence. Presentation at the OECD international policy conference Taking Fear out of Schools, 5th–8th September 2004, Stavanger, Norway

Orbach I, Bar-Joseph H 1993 The impact of a suicide prevention program for adolescents on suicidal tendencies, hopelessness, ego identity and coping. Suicide and Life Threatening Behaviour 23:120–129

Overholser J C, Hemstreet A H, Spirito A et al 1989 Suicide awareness programs in the schools: effects of gender and personal experience. Journal of the American Academy of Child and Adolescent Psychiatry 28(6):925–930

Parson C, Stears D 2002 Evaluating health-promoting schools: steps to success. Health Education 102:7–15

Pedro-Carroll J L, Sutton S E, Wyman P A 1999 A two year follow-up evaluation of a preventive intervention for young children of divorce. School Psychology Review 28:467–476

Pentz M A, Dwyer J H, MacKenna D P et al 1989 A multi-community trial for primary prevention of adolescent drug abuse: effects on drug use prevalence. Journal of the American Medical Association 261:3259–3266

Perry C L, Klepp K, Sillers C 1989 Community-wide strategies for cardiovascular health: the Minnesota Heart Health Program youth program. Health Education Research 4:87–101

Ploeg J, Ciliska D, Dobbins M et al 1996 A systematic overview of adolescent suicide prevention programs. Canadian Journal of Public Health 87(5):319–324

Ploeg J, Ciliska D, Brunton G et al 1999 The effectiveness of school-based curriculum suicide prevention programs for adolescents. Ontario Ministry of Health, Public Health Branch, Toronto

Price R H, Lorion R P 1989 Prevention programming as organizational reinvention: from research to implementation. In: Shaffer D, Phillips I, Enzer B (eds) Prevention of mental disorders, alcohol and other drug use in chilgren and adolescents. Office for Substance Abuse Prevention, Washington DC:97–124

Prinz R J, Blechman E A, Dumas J E 1994 An evaluation of peer coping-skills training for childhood aggression. Journal of Clinical Child Psychology 23:193–203

Reid J B, Eddy J M, Fetrwo R A et al 1999 Description and immediate impacts of a preventive intervention for conduct problems. American Journal of Community Psychology 27:483–517

Resnicow K, Botvin G J 1993 School-based substance abuse prevention programs: why do effects decay? Preventive Medicine 22(4):484–490

Rhodes J, Englund S 1993 Schools-based interventions for promoting social competence. In: Glenwick D S, Jason L A (eds) Promoting health and mental health in children, youth and families. Springer, New York

Rowling L 2002 Mental health promotion. In: Rowling L, Martin G, Walker L (eds) Mental health promotion and young people: concepts and practice. McGraw-Hill, Sydney, Chapter 2:10–23

Rowling L, Martin G, Walker L 2002 Mental health promotion and young people: concepts and practice. McGraw-Hill, Sydney

Rutter M, Smith D J (eds) 1995 Psychological disorders in young people: time trends and their causes. John Wiley, Chichester

Rutter M, Maughan B, Mortimore P et al 1979 Fifteen thousand hours: secondary schools and their effects on children. Open Books, London

SAMHSA (Substance Abuse and Mental Health Service Administration) 2004 The Olweus Bullying Prevention Program. SAMHSA Model Programs. Online. Available: http://www.modelprograms.samhsa.gov/

Shaffer D, Garland A, Vieland V et al 1991 The impact of curriculum-based suicide prevention programs for teenagers. Journal of the American Academy of Child and Adolescent Psychiatry 30:588–596

Sheehan M, Cahill H, Rowling L et al 2002 Establishing a role for schools in mental health promotion: the Mind Matters project. In: Rowling L, Martin G, Walker L (eds) Mental health promotion and young people: concepts and practice. McGraw-Hill, Sydney

Shochet I M, Dadds M R, Holland D et al 2001 The efficacy of a universal school-based program to prevent adolescent depression. Journal of Clinical Child Psychology 30(3):303–315

Shure M B, Spivack G 1988 Interpersonal cognitive problem solving. In: Price R H, Cowen E L, Lorion R P et al (eds) Fourteen ounces of prevention: a casebook for practitioners. American Psychological Association, Washington DC:69–82

Smith P K, Ananiadou K, Cowie H 2003 Interventions to reduce school bullying. The Canadian Journal of Psychiatry 48(9):591–599

Smith E A, Bechtel L J, Minner D et al 2004 Evaluation of Life Skills Training and Infused-Life Skills Training in a rural setting: outcomes at two years. Journal of Alcohol and Drug Education 48(1):51–70

Spirito A, Overholser J, Ashworth S et al 1988 Evaluation of a suicide awareness curriculum for high school students. Journal of the American Academy of Child and Adolescent Psychiatry 27:705–711

Stephens T, Dulberg C, Joubert N 1999 Mental health of the Canadian population: a comprehensive analysis. Chronic Disease in Canada 20(3):118–126

Stevens V, De Bourdeaudhuij I, Van Oost P 2000 Bullying in Flemish schools: an evaluation of anti-bullying intervention in primary and secondary schools. British Journal of Educational Psychology 70:195–210

Stevens V, De Bourdeaudhuij I, Van Oost P 2001 Anti-bullying interventions at school: aspects of programme adaptation and critical issues for further programme development. Health Promotion International 16(2):155–167

Tilford S, Delaney F, Vogels M 1997 Effectiveness of mental health promotion interventions: a review. Health promotion effectiveness reviews, no 4. Health Education Authority, London

Trudeau L, Spoth R, Lillehoj C et al 2003 Effects of a preventive intervention on adolescent substance use initiation, expectancies, and refusal intentions. Prevention Science 4(2):109–122

Waldron H B, Kaminer Y 2004 On the learning curve: the emerging evidence supporting cognitive-behavioural therapies for adolescent substance abuse, suppl 2. Addiction 99:93–105

Weare K 2000 Promoting mental, emotional and social health: a whole school approach. Routledge, London

Weissberg R P, Caplan M, Harwood R L 1991 Promoting competent young people in competence-enhancing environments: a systems-based perspective on primary prevention. Journal of Consulting and Clinical Psychology 59(6):830–841

Wells J, Barlow J, Stewart-Brown S 2001 A systematic review of universal approaches to mental health promotion in schools. HSRU, University of Oxford, Oxford

Wells J, Barlow J, Stewart-Brown S 2003 A systematic review of universal approaches to mental health promotion in schools. Health Education 103(4):197–220

WHO (World Health Organization) 1997 Life skills education in schools. Programme on Mental Health, WHO, Geneva

WHO 1998 WHO's global school health initiative: health promoting schools. WHO, Geneva

WHO 2001 The world health report 2001. Mental health: new understanding, new hope. WHO, Geneva

Wynn J, Cahill H, Holdsworth R et al 2000 MindMatters, a whole school approach to promoting mental health and well-being. Australia and New Zealand Journal of Psychiatry 34:594–601

Yu D L, Seligman M E 2002 Preventing depressive symptoms in Chinese children. Prevention and Treatment. Online. Available: http://www.journals.apa.org/prevention/volume5/pre0050009a.html 18 November 2005

Zenere F J, Lazarus P J 1997 The decline of youth suicidal behavior in an urban multicultural public school system following the introduction of a suicide prevention and intervention program. Suicide and Life-Threatening Behavior 27(4):387–402

Zins J E, Weissberg R P, Wang M C et al (eds) 2004 Building academic success on social and emotional learning: what does the research say? Teachers College Press, New York

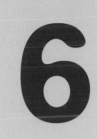

Promoting Mental Health in the Workplace

6

Introduction

The workplace is a key setting for promoting the mental health of the adult population as many people spend a large proportion of their time at work. The importance of work in terms of role fulfilment, self-identify and participation in society is well recognised. Mental health promotion in the workplace has a wide range of social and health benefits and can also contribute to improved productivity. The promotion of employee well-being leads to greater work and life satisfaction, reduced work stress with resultant increases in the productivity and profitability of oraganisations (Pfeffer 1998), while unrecognised mental health problems at work such as job-related stress, depression and anxiety contribute to reduced productivity, low job satisfaction, absence from work and increased health care costs. Transition periods such as entering work, going back to work, unemployment and retirement may lead to mental health problems if people are not given sufficient support. This chapter examines the importance of mental heath in the workplace and considers the role of the workplace in promoting good mental health. Work-related stress is increasingly recognised as being damaging to people's mental health and a range of individual and organisational level strategies for protecting employees' mental health and reducing the negative impact of stress are examined. Given the importance of work to mental health and overall well-being, developing the competencies and skills in securing and successfully maintaining a job deserves special attention. In this chapter we explore a model programme which explicitly sets out to develop job search skills to enable unemployed people to secure employment and thereby prevent the negative mental health impacts of unemployment. We also examine the importance of work for people with mental disorders and the role of employment as a mechanism for promoting mental health, quality of life and the reintegration of people with mental disorders in society.

Rationale for Promoting Mental Health in The Workplace

The workplace is one of the key environments that affects our mental well-being and health and there is a growing awareness of the role of work in promoting mental health. Work is seen as an important source, not only of financial security, but also of personal identity, self-esteem, time structure, social recognition, relationships and participation in a collective effort that contributes to society. The WHO report 'Mental health and work: impact, issues and good practices' (2000) identifies three main issues that employers need to address in promoting the mental health needs of their employees:

1. recognition and awareness of mental health as a legitimate concern of organisations. As disability and absenteeism costs increase in the workplace, employers are faced with the challenge of developing policies and effective strategies to address these issues
2. effective implementation of workplace policies and anti-discrimination provisions. This requires that human resource managers appreciate the full implications of existing legislation and the enforcement of anti-discrimination legislation regarding the employment of people with mental health problems
3. understanding the need for early intervention and assistance programmes to meet employees' mental health needs, as well as reintegrating employees back into the work environment.

Traditionally, however, many workplace health initiatives have placed more emphasis on physical health and safety issues in the workplace than on mental health. The promotion of mental health is relevant to many aspects of employment including health safety, equal opportunities, bullying and harassment and work–life balance initiatives (Mentality 2003). However, few health and safety policies in the workplace have explicitly addressed mental health issues such as the impact of work stress and the prevention of mental health problems such as depression.

The important role of policy and legislation in supporting workplace health promotion initiatives is also recognised. Policy initiatives such as the 1989 EU Framework Directive on Health and Safety (EU Health and Safety at Work Directive 1989) recommend a holistic approach towards health promotion at work, encompassing both the psychological and physical health aspects of occupational health and safety policy. This directive makes it mandatory for organisations within the EU member states to assess the health and safety risks to its workers and employers are obliged to provide protective and preventive services, full information on health and safety issues and consultation and participation rights to workers on matters affecting workplace health and safety. Stress represents an important occupational risk to health; however the assessment of psychosocial factors relating to health has not received the same attention as traditional physical hazards. Cooper and Cartwright (1997) point to the fact that there are skills and training deficiencies in undertaking risk assessments on the psychosocial factors pertaining to health and argue for the provision of more comprehensive and professional training for labour and factory inspectors in this regard. Jané-Llopis et al (2005) report that the 2001 European Council conclusions on combating stress and depression (European Commission 2002) and the Communication on Health and Safety at Work (Commission of the European Communities 2002) emphasise the importance of good working conditions, social relations and the promotion of well-being at work. In addition, regulatory policies in relation to sexual harassment, bullying and discrimination in the workplace, when implemented effectively, can impact positively on mental health. Occupational health services and the provision of employee assistance programmes, have an important role to play in supporting mental health promoting initiatives. Traditionally, employee assistance programmes (EAPs) were established to assist employees with alcohol and drug addiction problems; however, they have broadened their scope to also include personal and work-related difficulties. EAP services may include on-site and telephone counselling or referrals to appropriate agencies for additional support.

The low participation of small and medium-sized enterprises (SMEs) in health promotion and occupational health services has been highlighted as an area of concern. SMEs account for a major proportion of EU businesses, for example, with some 40% of companies employing fewer than 10 people. Clearly, different approaches need to be adopted in meeting the needs of such smaller companies, as access to specific occupational health services or programmes may be more difficult. A number of countries have instituted group practice models where there is shared resourcing of specific services for employees and employers of SMEs. The provision of outreach occupational health and health promotion services to specific employee groups, such as those engaged in the construction industry and agricultural sector, have also been developed to meet these needs.

The impact of mental health problems in the workplace has serious consequences not only for the individual employee and his/her family but also for the productivity of the organisation. The UK Department of Health and the Confederation of British Industry have estimated that 15–30% of workers experience some form of mental health problem in their working lives. One in five workers are estimated to have some type of mental health problem at any given time, with depressive disorders being one of the most common. The WHO (2000) report on mental health and work identified the following consequences of mental health problems at work:

- absenteeism – increase in sickness rates, particularly short periods of absence, depression, stress and burn out, physical health problems such as heart disease, backache, high blood pressure, ulcers, sleeping problems, etc.
- work performance – reduced productivity and output, increased error rates and accidents, poor decision making, planning and control

- staff attitude and motivation such as burn out, loss of motivation and commitment, poor timekeeping, long hours with diminishing returns, labour turnover
- relationships at work – tension and conflict between colleagues, poor relationships with clients and increase in disciplinary problems.

Implementing Mental Health Promotion in The Workplace

Creating Healthy Workplaces

The creation of healthy workplaces entails more than providing a safe working environment. A healthy workplace involves creating an environment that is supportive of the psychosocial aspects of work, recognising the potential of the workplace to promote workers' mental health and reduce the negative impacts of work-related stress. Many of the factors that influence the positive health and well-being of workers relate to the social environment at work, such as the style of management, working culture and levels of social support, as well as job security. A positive social climate, good team work, supportive management structures with clear roles and responsibilities and good opportunities for job development have been found to be supportive of positive health and reduced work-related stress (Michie 2002). A culture of consultation and involving people in decisions is protective of positive mental health especially in dealing with organisational change. On the other hand, an organisational culture of high demand and low job control, together with an unsupportive and bullying management style can have serious negative impact on workers' mental health. The Whitehall II study reported that low job control, high job demand, low social support at work and a combination of high effort and low rewards were all associated with poor physical and mental health (Stansfeld et al 1999). In particular, psychological demands, work overload, low social support and an imbalance in effort and reward were found to be associated with an increased risk of mental disorder in both men and women.

An empirical review of the evidence on work factors associated with negative mental health and absenteeism (Michie & Williams 2003) found the key factors to be:

- long hours worked, work overload and pressure
- the effects of these on personal lives
- lack of control over work and lack of participation in decision making
- poor social support
- unclear management and work role and poor management style.

Promoting employees' well-being and mental health requires change at the individual and organisational levels. Many interventions have focused on individual change without consideration of the broader organisational context. Israel et al

218

(1996) propose a model of occupational stress and health, which can be used as a framework for developing interventions. This model suggests that a comprehensive ecological approach is needed for interventions to be successful and requires multiple interventions aimed at different levels of practice such as the individual, work group, department and the organisation as a whole. Therefore, a comprehensive policy of mental health at work includes addressing the mental health of the organisation itself as well as that of the individual employees (WHO 2000). The gain to both individuals and the organisation is reflected in reduced absenteeism, improved well-being and productivity. The WHO report on Mental Health and Work (2000) showcases examples of good practices in workplace mental health promotion from around the world and the reader is referred to this report for further details.

Reviews of the evidence (Mentality 2003, Williams et al 1998) suggest that an effective workplace health improvement policy should include:

- promoting the mental health and well-being of all staff
- offering support and assistance to workers experiencing mental health problems in the workplace
- adopting a positive approach to employing workers with a history of mental health problems.

Each of these aspects of mental health promotion in the workplace will now be addressed and details of intervention programmes examined.

The Workplace and Stress

Occupational stress is of increasing importance due to structural changes in the working environment. Globalisation of the world economy has impacted on job restructuring, more contract work, greater workload demands and higher job insecurity. Employees are faced with greater demands which contribute to higher stress levels and adverse health outcomes (Tennant 2001). Job stress has been defined as the harmful physical and emotional response that occurs when the requirements of the job do not match the capabilities, resources or needs of the worker (NIOSH 1998). Job stress is one of the most common work-related problems in EU countries (WHO 2000) and can cause poor physical and mental health and lead to increased rates of work-related injuries and accidents. In Europe, 28% of employees report stress at work, while in Japan the figure may be as high as 63% (WHO 2000). There is also concern about increased risk of work-related illness in developing countries that have experienced rapid industrialisation. While many countries have minimum standards for health and safety features related to the physical aspects of the workplace, there is no specific legislation addressing the psychological or mental aspects of the work environment, including the impact of job stress, in many countries.

As Michie (2002) points out, the workplace is an important source of both demands and pressures causing stress, but also structural and social resources to counteract stress. The following factors have been identified as potential causes of work-related stress:

* overwork
* lack of clear instruction/role clarity
* unrealistic deadlines
* lack of decision making
* job insecurity
* isolated working conditions
* surveillance
* inadequate childcare arrangements
* sexual harassment
* bullying
* discrimination.

Stressors at work increase the risk of anxiety, depression and burn out (Jané-Llopis & Anderson 2005). The mental health impacts are significant because mental health problems occur frequently and they often go unrecognised and untreated. In reviewing the occupational stress literature, Tennant (2001) reports that specific acute work-related stressful experiences contribute to depression and that enduring structural occupational factors can also contribute to psychological disorders such as burn out and alcohol abuse.

Cooper and Cartwright (1997) propose a three-pronged strategy for managing stress at work. The three approaches include:

1. primary interventions – concerned with organisational and structural change and actions to modify or eliminate sources of stress inherent in the work environment

Box 6.1

Sources of stress at work

(based on Michie 2002, WHO 2000)

* intrinsic to the job – poor physical working conditions, work overload or underload, time pressures, physical danger, lack of control over pacing, shift working, inflexible work schedule, unpredictable or unsociable working hours
* role in organisation – role ambiguity, role conflict, responsibility for people, conflict relating to organisational boundaries
* career development – over-promotion, under-promotion, lack of job security, thwarted ambition, low social value to work
* relationship at work – poor relations with work colleagues including those in superior and subordinate positions, social or physical isolation, interpersonal conflict and violence, lack of social and practical support
* organisational structure and climate – low levels of participation in decision making, restrictions on behaviours, budgets, office politics, lack of effective consultation, poor communication, financial difficulties, non-supportive culture

2. secondary interventions – concerned with early detection and management of stress by increasing awareness and improving the stress management skills of the individual worker through training and activities. Health promotion programmes such as physical fitness and lifestyle modification programmes are also included in this category

3. tertiary interventions – refers to the treatment, rehabilitation and recovery process for individuals who are stressed or have experienced ill health as a result of stress. These interventions include counselling services and supports provided, for example, through EAPs. Comprehensive systems and procedures to support the rehabilitation and return to work of employees who have experienced stress-related problems is another aspect of tertiary interventions.

Cooper and Cartwright (1997) note that while there is considerable activity on the secondary and tertiary level interventions in the workplace, primary or organisational level strategies are comparatively rare.

Individual Focused Approaches

Strategies to deal with work stress may be directed at the individual employee or may be focused on the organisational characteristics of the workplace. The individual employee-focused interventions tend to be directed at enhancing coping capacity usually through the use of stress management training. These interventions include cognitive-behavioural approaches such as stress inoculation training, relaxation techniques, social skills training, social support, training in time management and encouraging staff to enhance the balance between work and home life. The object of teaching effective coping skills before stress exposure is to prepare the individual to respond more favourably to negative stress events and reduce the psychological impact. The evidence is somewhat mixed on the

---

Box 6.2

A range of possible strategies to reduce workplace stressors

(a summary based on Elkin & Rosch 1990)

- redesign the task
- redesign the work environment
- establish flexible work schedules
- encourage participative management
- include the employee in career development
- analyse work roles and establish goals
- provide social support and feedback
- build cohesive teams
- establish fair employment policies
- share the rewards

effectiveness of these approaches in reducing negative mental health outcomes in the workplace (Murphy 1996, Van der Klink et al 2001). Evidence on individual stress management approaches suggest that while they can temporarily reduce experienced stress, their long-term effects remain unclear. Likewise, lifestyle and health promotion interventions such as physical exercise appear to be effective in reducing anxiety, depression and psychosomatic distress, but do not necessarily alter the link between the stressor and the experience of psychological strain (Cooper & Cartwright 1997). As a result, it is difficult to sustain the benefits of such programmes if the work environment or source of the stress remains unchanged. In general, stress management approaches that focus on changing the individual's capacity to deal with stress without changing the source of the stress are of limited effectiveness. Management tend to have a preference for supporting individual-level interventions rather than addressing issues concerning power and organisational change (Kjell Nytro et al 2000). However, it is now clearly recognised in workplace health promotion practice that there is a need for comprehensive interventions that will target individual and organisational issues in the workplace and recognise the need for organisational and social change to reduce stressors that are beyond the individual's control.

Organisational Approaches

Organisational approaches refer to interventions that change work organisation and environmental features in an effort to reduce work-related stress. Organisational interventions can include many types, ranging from structural changes such as staffing levels, work schedules, job structure and physical environment to psychosocial changes such as social support, increased participation and control over work, management style and culture. Many work reorganisation interventions have focused on promoting well-being by enhancing job control, enhancing choice in one's work and a sense of autonomy. Job control has been found to be a significant mediator of change in work reorganisation interventions for stress reduction (Bond & Bunce 2001). In organisational downsizing, for example, it is suggested that the effects on the worker can be reduced if individual control, clarity and participation in the process is facilitated (Parker et al 1997). Lack of job control is associated with alcohol dependence and poor mental and physical health, while increasing control has been found to reduce sickness absence (Stansfeld et al 2000). Social support at work is protective of the negative impact of job demands and can have a significant effect on workers' health and well-being (Stansfeld et al 2000). For both men and women, high job demands and low social support at work have been found to be predictive of depression (Pattani et al 2001).

The control–demand model of work-related stress (Karasek 1990, Karasek & Theorell 1990) provides a useful framework for interventions at work. This model highlights the important relationship between the level of job demand and degree of control over work in determining work-related strain and risks to health. The model predicts that when job demands are high and levels of control and decision-making latitude are low, work strain is more likely to result. However, high job demands combined with high levels of control are less likely to lead to work strain and are more conducive to positive achievement. Research on the model indicates that level of control is the more important predictor of the two

were held once a week for three weeks and sessions 4–6 were held once every two weeks over a 6-week period. One important feature of the sessions is that the actual strategies for improvement are drawn from the participants, based on their own experiences. Active learning processes, such as modelling and rehearsals of newly learned skills, were incorporated into the training sessions.

Session one: This focuses on understanding the existing helping networks within the workplace and exploring how social support from others can help solve problems and reduce stress at work. Participants map out their own social networks and analyse the strengths and weaknesses of their own network.

Session two: This looks at strengthening these helping networks by refining interpersonal skills, such as clarifying misunderstandings, providing constructive feedback and asking others for help.

Session three: This session deals with teaching the participants training activities to aid in training others on CSP concepts and skills.

Sessions four and five: These deal with increasing worker participation in decision making.

Session six: This session is dedicated to techniques which can be used to maintain new skills in the long term and enhance occupational self-esteem.

Evaluation

The programme was evaluated in a large-scale randomised study in which group homes were randomly assigned to receive the programme or be in the control group (Heaney et al 1995a). Data were collected from group home staff via self-administered questionnaires, 1 month before the programme began and five weeks after the intervention. The results of the study indicated that the CSP intervention resulted in increased perceived social support, interpersonal skills, group problem solving, positive work team functioning, job satisfaction and employee mental health among those employees who attended at least five of the six CSP sessions (Israel et al 1996). For CSP to have been really effective, participants must have been able to use their new skills and knowledge back in the group homes. Results of the programme evaluation showed that participants reported higher levels of supervisory support, they experienced higher levels of praise and feedback, had more contact with co-workers, had a greater ability to handle disagreements and overload at work and a better work team climate compared to the control groups (Heaney et al 1995a). The results also suggest that the CSP increased the coping resources, enhanced the mental health and the job satisfaction of participants, and increased the quality of social interactions for direct-care staff who attended most or all of the projects. As a result of this increased job satisfaction, the high rate of staff turnover that was noted during the programme could be addressed by the CSP.

Direct-care providers reported an improvement in the relationship with their house managers. However, for house managers, the relationship with supervisors and co-workers remained unaffected as they reported no change in received praise or feedback. An explanation for this could be that only direct-care staff and house managers were included in the programme. Other grades, such as supervisors and other co-workers in a home, were not involved. House managers, therefore, had the sole responsibility for enhancing the nature of these types of work relationships. A change in the perception of the relationship between house managers and care providers does not necessarily indicate an actual improvement. As experiences were shared between participants, a deeper understanding of the role of a house manager may have been gained and thus care providers viewed their managers in a more positive light. However, increases in perceived support, whether real or not, have also been shown to enhance health and buffer stress (Heaney 1991).

The findings regarding the train-the-trainer aspect of the programme, however, were less impressive. As part of the evaluation, in the last CSP session of the programme, participants were asked whether up to that time they had conducted training activities in their group home. Approximately one third of the participants reported that they had not conducted any CSP training activities back in their own group homes thus concluding that the train-the-trainer approach was not successful (Heaney et al 1995a). However, 90% of the participants did state that they had used new skills back in the home, suggesting that the indirect transfer of the CSP concepts and skills to non-attendees may have occurred through role modelling.

Process evaluation of the intervention indicated that there was little variation in the delivery of the programme across groups, thus indicating consistency in the programme's implementation. Participants also commented on the importance of hearing the experiences of others in different group homes and this contributed to building rapport and information exchange among the participants.

A possible explanation for the sometimes limited effects of the CSP is that efforts to change work-related attitudes and behaviours have limited success unless the organisation reinforces them. The assumption was made that direct-care providers had an autonomous input into the home as an organisation, thereby neglecting to consider other staff at all organisational levels who also have an input. Provider agencies were encouraged to support the sustainability of the CSP concept in the workplace but no guidelines were given on how to do so.

Programme Implementation

Theoretical input: The programme is based on the principles of social learning theory (Bandura 1977). This theory suggests that modelling and rehearsal of new behaviours are crucial to the learning process. Skills transfer is facilitated by providing the learner with general principles that guide successful performance, the problems and situations used as examples should be similar to those encountered regularly in the workplace and the training should increase the likelihood of participants being able to generate a skill in a wide variety of situations and settings. The participants practise new skills until they have a feeling of mastery and are then encouraged to use the skills in the workplace.

Skilled trainers: The trainers play a key role in facilitating the group process and ensuring the effective transfer of skills. Trainers need to be perceived as being knowledgeable and admirable by the participants and provide unconditional positive regard for participants (Janis 1983).

Active learning approach to skills development: The sessions encouraged participants to analyse their own social networks and develop skills to strengthen them. Similarly, approaches to facilitate participation in decision making were practically implemented through role-play situations. Methods to maintain these skills were also suggested and practised.

Group format and the sharing of experiences: The programme was implemented with participants in a group format. This allowed for a variety of experiences to be shared and discussed. This also facilitated the active learning processes such as skills development and role play, so that these skills could be modelled and transferred to the group home setting.

Inclusion of recipient and provider of support in training sessions: Each of the participants was a provider of support to colleagues and managers, but also a receiver of support from other colleagues and managers. The exploration of experiences from both these roles provides each grade with an insight into and an understanding of each other's work.

Locally based: Each of the programme sessions was provided in a convenient location to participants to allow for ease of access. Some were in community and conference centres, as well as in local hotels. This feature was important in maintaining good attendance rates.

Train-the-trainer approach: Ensuring that every member of a group home participated in the course was not feasible, so the feature of training direct-care providers and home managers to transfer skills to their colleagues was important. This cascade approach to training seeks to ensure a wider dissemination of the programme and its benefits. However, it would appear from the evaluation that this aspect of the programme needs to be developed further in order to ensure that training activities are actually implemented back in the workplace. Further support and evaluation of this aspect of the CSP is recommended.

Key Recommendations for Replication

The CSP demonstrates that an approach emphasising the enhancement of social support and participation in decision making can be effective in promoting employee mental health and well-being and can have a positive effect on existing work relationships. The majority of workplaces share similar sources of stress and, as a result, this model can be adapted to most workplaces where there are a number of persons working together. Little special equipment is required to implement this programme so it is logistically feasible to implement in most worksites. Important lessons have been learned from the evaluation of this programme that should be considered when contemplating replicating this model. The following recommendations are highlighted.

Tailor the intervention to the needs of the employees: Take into account specific sources of stress and the larger organisational context. As this programme is orientated toward maximising social support resources within the workplace, current relationships, sources of conflict and staffing structure within the organisation should be addressed.

Consult with the organisation and stakeholders: Implementation of this programme should be based on an identified need for such an intervention within the organisation. It is important that all stakeholders are consulted and involved in adapting the programme in the workplace setting. The development of a steering committee, comprised of key stakeholders, is recommended for programme planning and implementation.

Terms of reference: Establish the functions of the committee and its role in developing the manual, hiring and training facilitators, finding locations for the sessions and determining grades of staff to attend the sessions. Also evaluation methods, process, impact and outcome will need to be considered at this early stage.

Facilitate participation and attendance: Strategies will need to be employed to facilitate participation rates, as the more sessions that are attended the greater the impact on programme outcomes. To facilitate attendance consider ways of ensuring that workplaces are adequately staffed to allow for others to attend or provide reimbursement for days off which are used to attend the programme. Such conditions should be agreed upon with management early on in planning the programme.

Integration of the CSP concept into the organisation: The original CSP did not encourage provider organisations to make the goals of the CSP an important priority. Ensuring that the organisation buys into the concept and goals of the CSP can contribute to time and resources being set aside to facilitate programme implementation. Such an approach will also make it easier for programme participants to return to the worksite and develop structures to sustain their own skills and those of their colleagues. The intervention should also support the creation of a training context and a work context that explicitly support and encourage the implementation of newly acquired skills and knowledge. For example, organisational rewards could be provided to staff who successfully implement new skills and actively enhance the work relationships in their group homes.

Inclusion of all grades in programme: The inclusion of all grades in the programme is recommended from the evaluation of the original model. This will ensure that all grades of participants are responsible for dissemination of the programme's concept, rather than just one or two who may not have the autonomy to orientate the organisational structure.

Incorporate an ecological approach to behaviour change: Exchanges of social support take place between people but the people exist in a complex social environment. Therefore, the programme should incorporate an ecological approach to behaviour change and actively facilitate the creation of organisational norms and policies that inhibit undermining social interactions and reward the provision of social support (Heaney et al 1995a, b).

Unemployment and Mental Health

The negative impact of unemployment on health is well documented (Dooley et al 1996, Ezzy 1993, Jin et al 1995). The relationship between unemployment and poor health has been found to hold after adjusting for possible confounding variables such as social class, poverty, age and pre-existing health status (Wilson & Walker 1993). Unemployed people have poorer physical and mental health and higher rates of mortality. Dooley et al (1994) report that people who become unemployed have over twice the risk of increased depression and diagnosis of clinical depression than those who remain employed. An association between unemployment and suicide has been found in a number of studies (Johansson & Sundquist 1997). Blakely et al (2003), based on analysis of data from the New Zealand census over a 3-year period, found that being unemployed was associated with a two to threefold increase in relative risk of death by suicide compared with being employed. However, in determining the direction of causality, the role of mental health problems in both suicide and unemployment needs to be taken into account. In relation to mental health, unemployed people report experiencing higher levels of anxiety, depression, uncertainty about the future, anger, shame and loss of self-esteem following job loss (Breslin & Mustard 2003). The duration of unemployment also tends to have a cumulative effect in that those who are unemployed longer report the greatest level of psychological distress. A number of interventions have been developed with the aim of improving the mental health of those who are unemployed and improving their chances of finding a job (Price & Kompier 2005). Re-employment, particularly in good quality jobs, has been shown to be one of the most effective ways of promoting the mental health of the unemployed (Lehtinen et al 1998). An example of a large-scale intervention designed to assist job search through enhancing self-efficacy is the 'JOBS' programme, which has been developed and successfully implemented across a number of different countries. Details of the programme and its adaptation across cultures will now be examined.

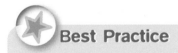 **Best Practice**

The JOBS Programme

(Caplan et al 1989, Vinokur et al 1995, Vinokur et al 2000).

The JOBS Intervention Project, developed by researchers at the University of Michigan (Caplan et al 1989, Vinokur & Schul 1997), was designed as a preventive intervention for unemployed workers. This programme targets job loss as one of the most consistent antecedents of depression and aims at providing job-seeking skills to promote re-employment and to combat feelings of anxiety, helplessness and depression among the unemployed. The intervention goals are to prevent the deterioration in mental health of unemployed workers, which often results from job loss and prolonged unemployment, and to promote high-quality re-employment. While the intervention is aimed specifically at enhancing job-search skills, it also incorporates several mental health promotion elements such as enhancing participants' self-esteem and sense of control, job-search self-efficacy and inoculation against setbacks.

A programme of research at the Institute for Social Research at the University of Michigan produced detailed information on the problems facing unemployed persons and their families, particularly those associated with job search (Caplan et al 1989), economic hardship (Vinokur et al 1991a) and family difficulties (Howe et al 1995, Price et al 1998). After a series of studies documenting these problems and analysing the needs of unemployed workers and their families, the Michigan Prevention Research Centre (MPRC) developed and evaluated the JOBS programme to aid unemployed workers to effectively seek re-employment and cope with the multiple challenges and stresses of unemployment and job search (Caplan et al 1997, Price & Vinokur 1995).

The JOBS programme has been evaluated and replicated in randomised trials involving thousands of unemployed workers and their partners (Caplan et al 1989, Vinokur et al 1995). The programme returns unemployed workers to new jobs more quickly, produces re-employment in jobs that pay more (Vinokur et al 1991b) and reduces mental health problems associated with prolonged unemployment (Vinokur et al 1995), particularly among those most vulnerable to mental health problems (Price et al 1992). In addition, the programme has been shown to inoculate workers against the adverse effects of subsequent job loss (Vinokur & Schul 1997). The JOBS programme also inoculates participants against subsequent job-loss setbacks because they gain an enhanced sense of mastery over the challenges of job search (Vinokur & Schul 1997).

Programme Content

The intervention consists of five intensive and active half-day workshops held over a 1- to 2-week period. The intervention, in the form of training seminars, applies problem-solving and decision-making group processes, inoculation against setbacks and social support together with learning and participatory job-search skills. Pairs of male and female trainers work with groups of 12–22 people. The programme aims to:

- enhance the job-seeking skills of participants
- increase the self-esteem, confidence and motivation of the participants in their job search
- fortify resistance and persistence in the face of setbacks and barriers
- use confidence and skills to achieve re-employment in stable settings
- extend the benefits to the family of the job seeker.

The essential components of the programme model include:

- content that focuses on the enhancement of job-search skills
- delivery format with two trainers conducting a workshop
- delivery process of training that maximises active learning processes, as opposed to didactic passive learning.

The 'JOBS manual for teaching people successful job search strategies' (updated version by Curran et al 1999) is a structured guide that describes the steps necessary for setting up and implementing the programme; the process of hiring trainers, the training period for the trainers and the intervention seminars.

Programme Evaluation

The intervention was originally tested through two large randomised field studies, JOBS I and JOBS II, conducted with recently unemployed people (Caplan et al 1989, Vinokur et al 1995, Vinokur et al 2000). With a follow-up period of 2.5 years post-intervention, the programme has produced impressive results indicating that participants in the intervention group achieved significantly better employment outcomes in terms of better quality and higher paying jobs and also improved their mental health through enhanced role and emotional functioning and reduced depressive symptoms. Using prospective screening, JOBS II also indicated increased benefits to high-risk participants in reducing depression symptoms. In particular, programme participants, in comparison to the control group:

- had higher confidence in job-seeking ability
- showed greater sense of self-efficacy
- had lower levels of depression
- found re-employment sooner (53% intervention versus 29% control)
- had higher quality and better paid jobs at 2.5 years follow up
- showed that the intervention was particularly beneficial to participants at high risk of depression
- showed lower incidence and prevalence of depression at 2.5 years.

Vinokur and Schul (1997) analysed the programme's outcomes to establish the mechanisms though which this intervention produced its significant effects. Enhanced sense of mastery and inoculation against setbacks emerged as significant mediators of the intervention effects on re-employment, financial strain and depression symptoms, particularly so for the high-risk group. The programme has demonstrated that it clearly yields mental health benefits, economic benefits and benefits for those who would be most disadvantaged by job loss. Benefit–cost analyses showed that the JOBS programme brought a three-fold return on investment after 2.5 years, and projected more than a 10-fold return after 5 years, due to increased employment, higher earning outcomes and reduced health service and welfare costs (Caplan et al 1997, Vinokur et al 1991b). The programme, therefore, promotes positive mental health for unemployed workers, prevents the onset of depression among those at highest risk and is cost-effective in terms of increased economic benefits for participants and the state.

Replication of the Programme

The MPRC has worked collaboratively with practitioners in replicating the JOBS programme in many different countries. This takes the form of provision of the programme intervention, training the trainers and data collection instruments for the evaluation. This programme has been disseminated in other countries outside the US including China, Korea and Finland (Vuori et al 2002) and is currently being implemented in the Netherlands and Ireland. The key implementation features together with programme adoption and replication across cultural settings will now be examined in the following case study.

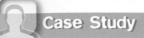
Case Study

Promoting Re-Employment and Mental Health: a Cross-Cultural Case Study

Jukka Vuori, Richard H Price

[Note: Work on this case study was supported by NIMH grant # 5P30MH38330 to the Michigan Prevention Research Centre. Portions of the material for this case have been drawn from Price et al (1998), with permission]

Introduction: The Työhön Program

The Työhön Program is a Finnish adaptation of the Michigan Prevention Research Centre (MPRC) JOBS programme. Both the Työhön Program and the original MPRC JOBS programme are based on the active learning process, social modelling, gradual exposure to acquiring skills, practice through role playing and inoculation against setbacks. The detailed intervention process has only minor alterations to the original MPRC JOBS programme. The programme has been documented in the Finnish Institute of Occupational Health (FIOH) by Mäkitalo et al (1997). Using a randomised field experimental design, the Työhön Program was tested in a difficult labour market situation during 1996–97. The programme was implemented in the context of the European labour market for participants who had been unemployed for a long period of time. At the 6-month follow up, the Työhön Program significantly increased the quality of re-employment in terms of permanence of the attained jobs, especially for those at risk of long-term unemployment. The Työhön intervention also significantly decreased symptoms of distress (Vuori et al 2002). At the 2-year follow up, the Työhön intervention significantly increased active participation in the labour markets, either employed or participating in vocational training. The intervention also significantly decreased symptoms of depression and increased self-esteem (Vuori & Silvonen 2005). In all, the beneficial effects of the group intervention on re-employment and mental health were parallel to those found earlier in the US, but it seems as if the impact of this programme varies depending on the unemployment benefit systems and economic support of the participants.

The later country-wide dissemination of the Työhön Program also had effects on the employment offices, where the group interventions were delivered. The relationship between the labour officials and the unemployed clients had traditionally been an 'over-the-counter' relationship loaded with negative attitudes. The unemployed clients felt that the officials were controlling their life decisions, but on the other hand the unemployed were dependent on the benefits they received. On the other side, the officials often had a pessimistic or negative view of their clients and mutual understanding was poor. The job-search groups based on the Työhön model held by employment office personnel had a positive effect on these attitudes. Labour advisors and counsellors and unemployed clients experienced a different, more open and active way of interacting and this had a positive effect on their relationship and increased positive feedback from the unemployed workers.

The Työhön Program was an adaptation of the original JOBS programme to new cultural and social settings. This new situation also produced new forms of training, delivery and dissemination. Features of adaptation, training, delivery and dissemination of the original JOBS programme and the Työhön Program will now be discussed. For each of these topics, the original features of the JOBS programme will be outlined, followed by a description of how these were modified in the Työhön Program.

Adaptation

JOBS

The JOBS programme was a system for recruitment, delivery and evaluation of a job-search skill enhancement workshop for unemployed job seekers. The JOBS model has the dual goals of promoting re-employment and enhancing coping capacities for the unemployed and their families.

The intervention workshop itself consisted of five intensive half-day workshops held over a 1- to 2-week period that focused on identifying effective job-search strategies, improving participant job-search skills and increasing self-esteem, confidence and the motivation of participants to engage and persist in job-search activities until they became re-employed.

The JOBS programme was delivered by two trainers to groups of job seekers consisting of 12–20 participants. Trainers worked in pairs, explaining principles, modelling and role playing effective job-search techniques, and encouraging active participation from all participants.

Työhön

The most significant modifications were in the appearance and usability of the manuals. The manual of the group intervention was divided into three publications: method manual, trainer manual and participant workbook. The whole method package contained a video showing the main principles and experiences of trainers plus a guide on successful training. The participant workbook was also distributed separately in packages of 10 workbooks. The adaptations in the contents of the method manuals included minor cultural changes and minor changes in scheduling the programme.

Central differences relevant to the implementation of the preventive group intervention were related to differing health systems, social security systems and labour administration systems between Finland and the USA. In Finland, the labour administration, with its extensive network of local labour offices, had a dominating role in services for the unemployed job seekers. Consequently, it was vital for the implementation and wider dissemination of the programme to get the support of labour administration for our efforts. On the other hand, this support enabled the marked success in dissemination of the programme.

Training

JOBS

A training manual and videotapes were available to facilitate training of persons to deliver the JOBS programme (Curran et al 1999). While the manual described each training session in detail, the five basic elements in the programme taught to trainers were as follows:

1. *Job-search skill training*. Participants were invited to acquire and rehearse job-search skills in a safe and supportive learning environment which is critical for effective learning of new skills (Caplan et al 1989).
2. *Active teaching and learning methods*. Trainers used non-didactic active learning methods to engage participants in job-search training. These methods used the knowledge and skills of the participants themselves as part of the learning process, elicited through small and large group discussions, role-playing exercises and other activities (Caplan et al 1997).
3. *Skilled trainers*. Workshop trainers were carefully chosen and rigorously trained to build trust and to work together in pairs as teams to facilitate group processes that promoted learning of skills and coping with job-search tasks.
4. *Supportive learning environment*. In the workshops, trainers modelled and reinforced supportive behaviour and worked to create a positive learning environment through exercises that provided opportunities for participants to learn from and support each other.
5. *Inoculation against setbacks*. Programme participants were provided with a problem-solving process involving identifying or anticipating possible barriers to re-employment and advanced preparation of solutions to overcome them. Inoculation against setbacks is fundamental to effective coping with an inherently stressful job-search process.

Työhön

A trainer supervisor was recruited to the Finnish Institute of Occupational Health (FIOH) to work in a close relationship with the research team. The six trainers for the field experiment were recruited to the labour organisation, but worked under supervision of the trainer supervisor of FIOH. The original trainers were trained for 2 months. Since the trainers were inside the labour organisation, their position strengthened the infrastructure for later scaling up. During the dissemination phase the training typically lasted 1 week, but some offices insisted on having even shorter training. When agency staff attempted to learn the Työhön method on their own, without formal training and just relying on the manual and other materials, fidelity to the original programme was lost and implementation was much less successful.

Delivery

JOBS

As the JOBS programme has become more widely known, foundations, state governments and the governments of other countries have begun to invest in the

JOBS programme and have sought to implement JOBS in their own home settings. One example is the 'Winning New Jobs' project in three communities in California under the sponsorship of the California Wellness Foundation, and the MPRC has collaborated with the Manpower Demonstration Research Corporation.

The programme has been implemented in three sites for 6500 Californians who were recently unemployed. The 5-year project utilised the JOBS intervention programme in three distinctly different communities and service systems. In each case, the programme involved existing community organisations which received funds, staff training and technical assistance from the MPRC and the Manpower Demonstration Research Corporation to implement the JOBS programme. Adoption and implementation of the programme was documented to provide concrete implementation lessons for adoption in other locations.

Työhön

In Finland, the Ministry of Labour and the country-wide national network of employment offices are very dominant regarding services and interventions for the unemployed. Most employment offices have their own facilities and own trainers for their group activities. Many employment offices also use out-sourcing services provided by adult training institutes and by private firms.

The re-invention phase created many of the tools and infrastructure needed later during scaling up and delivery. The manuals and the inclusive video were distributed by FIOH, which also provided training of trainers country-wide. The frequent trainer meetings during the test phase served as models for later trainer support groups. An important asset for delivery was availability of the positive test results. Most of the trained trainers were labour advisors and a smaller number of them were labour counsellors.

Dissemination

JOBS

In addition to the Työhön Program in Finland, in collaboration with colleagues at the Institute of Psychology, National Academy of Sciences, People's Republic of China, MPRC has conducted a new programme of research for implementation of the JOBS programme in seven cities in China. MPRC has actively collaborated with Chinese scientists and service system administrators in the Ministry of Labour to adapt the JOBS programme to the special cultural, social and economic needs and circumstances of the unemployed Chinese workers and their families for whom the programme is being developed.

MPRC has successfully carried out two replications of randomised efficacy trials of JOBS, conducted long-term follow-up studies, conducted several analyses to identify the active ingredients of the JOBS intervention and the psychosocial and motivational processes underlying its success. A new initiative is underway in Ireland serving long-term unemployed workers and the programme has been adapted to the needs of participants of welfare to work programmes in Baltimore, Maryland.

Työhön

The adoption, testing and dissemination of the programme in Finland was sponsored by the Finnish Social Security Agency, the Finnish Ministry of Labour and the Finnish Ministry of Social Affairs and Health. In Finland, employment offices, working under the Ministry of Labour, have a central role in taking care of the interventions for the unemployed job seekers. For job seekers, services of employment offices are free of charge even if they are provided by adult training institutes and private firms as out-sourcing services.

During the test period in Finland, the positive experiences of the offices, trainers and participants spread and other offices became interested. In the early dissemination phase, we had only a vague idea about the extent of later scaling up to the national level. A labour market policy reform was carried out in the beginning of 1998, including, for example, a radical increase in job-search training. This reform boosted our scaling-up efforts. We had the infrastructure, tools and experience for training new trainers for the Työhön job-search method relatively quickly and the potential for larger scale method package delivery. Employment offices started to ask for help in training and our trainer supervisor was assigned full time to speak at information meetings and to train trainers country-wide. Altogether she trained over 300 trainers in employment offices and in firms that worked for employment offices. She also initiated local trainer networks in several areas. Good experiences spread by word of mouth, and at some points the process seemed to advance in all fronts simultaneously. Over 35 000 workbooks were distributed during 1997–2004. This success also facilitated development, publication and dissemination of other related career management programmes in Finland, also applying the MPRC group training principles.

Recommendations

The manuals, videos and other intervention tools related to the delivery of the JOBS programme should be user friendly and comparable in quality to other training material provided to service systems and trainers. We recommend using the available MPRC training manual and videotapes as a starting point in developing and adapting materials for the programme.

The primary vehicle for disseminating the programme is using a thorough training process of new trainers by a skilled and experienced master trainer. The master trainer is a key figure in the implementation and dissemination process of the entire programme. If a wider dissemination is intended, a trainer supervisor would be helpful in many ways. One of the master trainer's main duties, in addition to training, is in planning and designing the adapted training materials. The master trainer could also initiate trainer networks for continuing learning and quality control.

As illustrated in the Finnish national dissemination example above, larger systems mean potential for wider dissemination. Carrying through successful dissemination is often easier if collaboration is done with fewer highly motivated organisational partners from key organisational systems. Partners have to be well motivated to implement the method and it is a substantial advantage if partners have an obvious need for the programme.

Strong leadership support for the implementation of the JOBS programme is crucial for success of dissemination in an organisation. The method should be published in a user-friendly fashion and training support should be readily available. Competing group methods or ideas in the implementing organisation will typically delay or even block the dissemination process. Political or regional pressures to adopt the programme may greatly facilitate the dissemination process.

References

Caplan R D, Vinokur A D, Price R H et al 1989 Job seeking, reemployment, and mental health: a randomized field experiment in coping with job loss. Journal of Applied Psychology 74(5):759–769

Caplan R D, Vinokur A D, Price R H 1997 From job loss to reemployment: field experiments in prevention-focused coping. In: Albee G W, Gullotta T P (eds) Primary prevention works. Sage, Thousand Oaks, California:341–379

Curran J, Wishart P, Gingrich J 1999 JOBS: a manual for teaching people successful job search strategies. Michigan Prevention Research Centre, Institute for Social Research, University of Michigan, Ann Arbor, Michigan (replaces JOBS manual by Curran J 1992)

Mäkitalo M, Tervahartiala T, Saarinen M (eds) 1997 Työhön-ohjelma – Ohjaajan käsikirja [Työhön-program – Trainers manual]. Finnish Institute of Occupational Health, Helsinki

Price R H, Friedland D S, Choi J N et al 1998 Job loss and work transitions in a time of global economic change. In: Arriaga X B, Oskamp S (eds) Addressing community problems: research and intervention. Sage, Thousand Oaks, California:195–222

Vuori J, Silvonen J 2005 The benefits of a preventive job search program on re-employment and mental health at two years follow-up. Journal of Occupational and Organisational Psychology 78:43–52

Vuori J, Silvonen J, Vinokur A et al 2002 The Työhön Job Search Program in Finland: benefits for the unemployed with risk of depression or discouragement. Journal of Occupational Health Psychology 7:5–19

Supported Employment and Mental Health

Work and paid employment play a central role in the lives of all people. Employment is important in maintaining mental health by contributing to one's sense of identity, but it can be especially important in promoting the recovery of those who experience mental health problems (Boardman 2003). Once an employee is absent with mental health problems for more than 3 months, the likelihood is very high that the absence will last more than one year, and if the absence is longer than one year there is a less than 1% chance of the employee returning to work (WHO 2000). Targeted interventions and supports are therefore required to facilitate return to work after treatment for mental health problems. An early return to work can be facilitated by accommodating a gradual return to work in negotiation with the employee, allowing for flexible arrangements such as part-time work, flexitime and temporarily changed duties that involve less job-related stress. As far as possible, keeping people in work will help a return to a normal routine and reduce the likelihood of social exclusion.

According to Schneider (1998) there are numerous arguments for promoting employment for those with mental health problems. To date the majority of mental health service users themselves have stated that they want the opportunity to be involved and be a member of the workforce (Secker et al 2001). This is supported by the United Nations ideology that 'everyone has the right to work' (United Nations 1948). There are also social and health benefits for all stakeholders involved. Employment can provide monetary gains for an employer and employee but also material benefits for society in the form of economic productivity. Similarly, as more people are involved in employment, social security payments are not being paid out and can therefore be channelled into further service and initiative development. It appears that preventing employed people who develop mental health problems from losing their jobs would significantly reduce both the economic costs of increased welfare benefits and the negative psychosocial impact of experiencing social exclusion (Huxley & Thornicroft 2003). It has been found that the combination of having a mental disorder and experiencing discrimination has negative effects on interpersonal relationships. For the worker or employee with a mental health problem or disorder, the benefits of social interaction, activity and a sense of personal achievement that are associated with a workplace environment (Warr 1987) can all contribute to improved health outcomes.

While people with a mental disorder have expressed their desire to work, the existing high rates of unemployment among this population group suggest that the opportunities that do exist may not be appropriate to their needs. Numerous barriers (Box 6.3) can contribute to the low uptake of employment opportunities (Boardman 2003). Discrimination, on the part of employers, seems to be the biggest barrier preventing those with a mental disorder from gaining work (Manning & White 1995). This can be related to society's history of stigma and social exclusion demonstrated to people with a mental disorder (see Chapter 8 for an account of programmes dealing with stigma and discrimination). Many other representatives of society, such as health professionals and GPs, can also underestimate the capabilities of people with a mental disorder in terms of work and employment.

The development of supported employment for people with a mental disorder in the early 1980s indicated an important shift in rehabilitation services. There are numerous types of models which facilitate the development of the concept of supported employment for people with a mental disorder, as discussed in Bond et al (1997), such as the job-coach model, the clubhouse model and transitional employment, the assertive community treatment model and the 'choose–get–keep' model. The features of these initiatives range from priority being placed on building a work history (clubhouse) to that of career planning (choose–get–keep), with others offering a combination of both. The opportunity to participate in work and employment contributes to the rehabilitation and integration of

Box 6.3

Barriers to employment of people with severe mental disorders

(WHO 2000)

- lack of choice in employment services and providers
- inadequate work opportunities
- complexity of the existing work incentive schemes
- financial penalties of working
- stigma and discrimination
- loss of health benefits

individuals with serious mental health problems into mainstream society. To strive for this, the attitudes and structures in mainstream society that exclude people with a mental disorder from participating in everyday life need to be reorientated. This ideology forms the basis for the 'social model of disability'. The conceptual basis of this model can be used to understand the experiences of people with a mental disorder and thus inform dialogue with employers regarding employment opportunities (Oliver 1990).

Work Schemes

The reform of mental health services in many countries has led to the increased emphasis on community mental health services. However, a fragmented development of community mental health services seems to have occurred. The importance of work schemes as part of the range of community services to be provided has not been emphasised and thus has resulted in this population group being neglected with regard to integration into society through the medium of the workplace. However, with improving employment prospects in some countries, new opportunities can be offered to develop and mainstream supported employment work schemes, which to date have been run mainly by non-statutory agencies. The following gives a brief overview of the types of work schemes that can guide different projects.

- Sheltered workshops and employment are beneficial as an introduction to a work situation and for those who find open employment difficult. However, they do not provide employment in the open market and as a result tend to demonstrate low levels of worker movement and may not be commercially viable.
- Pre-vocational training provides people with a period of preparation before competitive employment that includes sheltered workshops, transitional employment and skills training.
- Supported employment places individuals into competitive employment without pre-vocational training. An employee is hired and is entitled to the full company benefits. On-the-job support is given to the employee via trained job coaches (Becker et al 1994) as well as support given to the employer, which ensures programme success. The core principles of supported employment are that the employment services are based on the client's preferences and choices, with continuous assessment and indefinite follow-up support. Rehabilitation is seen as a core component of treatment rather than a separate service, with clients expected to obtain jobs directly and contribute to the community (Boardman 2003).
- Social firms are small to medium sized firms which have been developed, usually with state support, with the main purpose of providing employment to people with a disability such as a mental disorder. In social firms people with disabilities work side by side with non-disabled workers and are paid regular wages and work on the basis of a regular work contract. The required support, however, is provided to workers as needed and an important characteristic of the work environment is the empowering atmosphere for employees with disabilities. A flexible approach is adopted

and there is an emphasis on the potential and abilities of the worker rather than on potential problems and barriers.

- Social cooperatives share the same philosophy of the social firm and provide a protected workplace for persons with disabilities. The social cooperatives function independently from the mental health services but maintain a close working liaison with them.

Numerous studies, mainly from the US, have found that the characteristics of different work schemes can influence the degree of success that people with mental health problems have in relation to obtaining and keeping competitive employment (Schneider 1998). Some work schemes offer a period of preparation before placing clients in competitive work, but more recently clients are placed in competitive work immediately whilst getting 'on-the-job' support. It has been found that a higher number of clients who were placed immediately in supported employment remained employed, earned more money and worked more hours than those who received pre-vocational training. It was concluded that there was no evidence to support the hypothesis that pre-vocational training was more effective in helping clients to obtain competitive employment (Crowther et al 2003). It appears from experimental studies that clients who were involved in individual placement and support (Becker et al 1994) demonstrated superior findings to control groups, with the features of rapid job search and integration of mental and vocational services possibly being the most critical contributors to this difference between groups (Bond et al 1997). Long-term effects of supported employment have also revealed that intervention groups were more likely to be competitively employed in comparison to those who were involved in a pre-vocational programme (Drake et al 1996, McFarlane et al 1995). Another issue to consider in relation to supported employment is the timing of the client's initiation into the programme and empowering the client to decide for themselves the plan for their own rehabilitation programme (Bond et al 1997). It is important to note, however, that there will be clients who may not be suitable to participate in immediate supported employment due to the nature of their disorder and the extent of their present capabilities. Studies to date have not identified the client characteristics that predict who benefits most from the models used in supported employment (Bond et al 1997). In this chapter, specific emphasis will be placed on describing the Clubhouse Model, which has been replicated successfully in many countries around the world and has developed its own set of standards, training processes and fidelity instruments, as well as a programme of research that examines the evidence base for the Clubhouse Model.

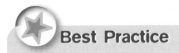 **Best Practice**

The Clubhouse Model

The Clubhouse Model is a facility-based intervention designed to offer people with a serious mental disorder membership in a mutually supportive and empowering community. The programme consists of 'clubhouses' where members receive support and services, with the goal of returning to the workplace as productive employees. The Clubhouse approach is based on the principles of meaningful activity and psychosocial rehabilitation, with work being the central factor in its operation (Boardman 2003). The clubhouse movement arose in the 1950s and proposed that better employment opportunities could be achieved by fostering mental health service users' autonomy in a non-psychiatric setting. The Clubhouse Model originated at Fountain House in New York City in 1948. The Fountain House Clubhouse model represents the original North American application of this rehabilitation approach in which vocational, communal and social services are offered under one roof. The Clubhouse is a building run by clients and staff along egalitarian lines, where clients meet for social activity, mutual support and graded work experience. Membership is voluntary to anyone with a history of mental disorder unless that person poses a significant threat to the general safety of the Clubhouse community. The Clubhouse programmes involve a period of preparation before clients attempt to return to competitive employment. A Clubhouse in a community seeks to remove the social barriers of stigma and isolation, with membership of a clubhouse addressing issues such as low self-esteem, low motivation and social isolation that is often experienced by people living with a mental disorder. Participation in a Clubhouse can promote social inclusion and thus facilitates people to lead a more productive and meaningful life within the community. Clients belong to a Clubhouse of their own free will and membership is lifelong. Currently there are over 317 Clubhouses in 27 countries worldwide (involving 55 000 active members) affiliated to the non-profit corporation, International Center for Clubhouse Development (ICCD) (McKay 2005, McKay et al 2005a). The ICCD maintains a set of Clubhouse standards, a well-documented training process and a certification process. All certified Clubhouses provide comprehensive case management by trained staff and other community support services, including supported education, supported housing, mobile outreach, medication oversight and supported employment, all of which are designed to integrate members into the wider community outside the Clubhouse. Regardless of how or how often a member chooses to use a Clubhouse, all ICCD Clubhouses remain a lifetime source of practical support and companionship.

Evaluation

In the last 20 years, the model has been the subject of an active, international dissemination effort including the development of standards, an international training and certification process. These efforts appear to have standardised the range of programmes that identify themselves as Clubhouses and have informed the development and refinement of standards. The Program for Clubhouse Research was established in 2000 to increase the quality and quantity of research on the clubhouse model. The Program for Clubhouse Research has examined the evidence base for the Clubhouse Model and the outcomes for members participating in Clubhouse programmes (Johnsen et al 2005, McKay 2005a, b). The evidence examined includes findings from multiple and single randomised clinical trials, observational studies, expert consensus and anecdotal evidence. In their review of the evidence, Johnsen et al (2005) have placed more importance on the higher classification of evidence, such as randomised controlled trials (RCT) and observational studies. It is noted, however, in their analysis that adopting this stance may not reflect the qualitative views of all stakeholders involved in this project. Specifically, participation in the Clubhouse components of 'work-ordered day', employment and outreach services were examined. The outcomes evaluated were categorised according to the model's services: employment, education, hospitalisation, housing, social relationships/social inclusion, satisfaction, quality of life and substance abuse/use. The review found that multiple randomised clinical trials consistently show that the Clubhouse Model is effective in reducing the rates of hospitalisation and lengths of stay of participating members. Findings also support the progamme's impact on increased quality of life/satisfaction level for Clubhouse members. Outreach support services are provided to members who are not able to attend the Clubhouse or may have become socially isolated. The findings from the evidence review of outreach indicate that this aspect of Clubhouses seems to delay and reduce hospitalisation rates for Clubhouse members. Some supporting evidence was also found in relation to the impact of Clubhouse on employment outcomes and social relationships and inclusion. Evidence at the RCT level was not found in relation to the other outcomes of the model. However, the lower level evidence did indicate that many of these services and supports are effective and warrant further study. The reviewers raise the question as to whether it is more appropriate to speak of evidence for the model as a whole or evidence for specific programmes or elements within the model. If the latter approach is adopted, then the evidence for the relative effectiveness of specific practices or programmes employed within the Clubhouse Model may be usefully tested and compared.

With regard to employment outcomes, a systematic review by Crowther et al (2003) assessed practices of vocational rehabilitation services for people with severe mental disorder, comparing the effectiveness of pre-vocational training with supported employment in helping participants to obtain competitive employment. The transitional employment programme of the Clubhouse Model was included in this review as pre-vocational training. The review concluded that supported employment is more effective than pre-vocational training in helping people with severe mental health problems to obtain competitive employment. However, a multi-site research study, the Employment Intervention Demonstration Program (Johnsen et al 2004, Macias 2001), conducted an experimental comparison of the Program of Assertive Community Treatment (PACT) and an ICCD Clubhouse programme on employment outcomes. This study concluded that transitional employment jobs, when provided in accordance with the ICCD Standards for Clubhouse Programmes, are either equivalent or superior to non-transitional employment forms of supported employment in every regard (e.g. job tenure, earnings) except hours worked per week. These findings were used to contest the criticisms of transitional employment and the claims that the jobs are inferior in regard to quality, duration or earning potential (Macias 2001). McKay et al (2005b) examined employment outcomes across transitional, supported and independent employment positions in 17 Clubhouses between 1998 and 2001. This study found that individuals with longer Clubhouse memberships tended to work longer and had higher job earnings than those with shorter membership. Masso et al (2001) also examined the effect of attendance rates of one Clubhouse Model, Connections Clubhouse, on 117 randomly selected members on their employment status and their rates of hospitalisation. Results of the study showed that individuals with a high rate of attendance at the Clubhouse had higher rates of employment attainment and more advanced employment status and lower rate of hospitalisation than for members with low rates of attendance.

Other evaluations of Clubhouse include a study conducted by Warner et al (1999) in which a group of Clubhouse users were matched with similar clients but not Clubhouse users, and were then compared in terms of quality of life, service utilisation and treatment costs over a 2-year period. The Clubhouse group achieved a reasonable employment status and good social relationships, and advantages in subjective well-being favoured the Clubhouse group. Over 2 years the pattern of service utilisation and costs also favoured the Clubhouse group. When the two groups were disaggregated for employment status, the Clubhouse group had least treatment utilisation and lower costs.

The Clubhouse costs were analysed using data from a sample of 12 ICCD Clubhouses in 12 countries (McKay 2005). The mean cost per person per Clubhouse visit is reported as $27.12 and the annual cost per member is $3203. These costs need to be considered against the considerable economic benefits arising from the programme in terms of reduced hospitalisation and treatment costs and contributions from taxable income.

Programme Implementation Features

The programme implementation features, which are the unique elements to the success of this programme, are a compilation of the factors that can be found in the ICCD (2005). The principles discussed in the standards are at the heart of the Clubhouse community's success in helping people with mental disorders to stay out of hospital while achieving social, financial and vocational goals (ICCD 2005). Every 2 years these principles as standards are reviewed by the worldwide Clubhouse community and amended as necessary. However the programme's main implementation features remain the same and are as follows:

Membership and active participation: The Clubhouse Model focuses on the strengths and talents of people recovering from a mental disorder. The needs of the client are taken as a starting point in the daily activity. Members are expected to run their Clubhouses by taking on essential tasks and participating in every task (Macias et al 1999). Members participate in planning, decision making and carrying out activities. Staff often act as initiators of the activity but, like the members, participate in every task. Clubhouse members participate in all the tasks of the daily running of the club such as cooking, cleaning, maintenance, administrative duties, guidance of new members, etc. Beard et al (1982) hypothesised that members benefited from participation in the Clubhouse because they felt needed for its successful functioning. When a Clubhouse is doing well, credit must be given to the membership upon whom the Clubhouse is dependent. This reverses the typical provider–recipient role in mental health services and sends a clear message to the members that they are competent and capable.

Work-ordered day: The work-ordered day is at the heart of the Clubhouse practice and functions more as a catalyst for recovery rather than a full-time activity for its members (Johnsen et al 2002). Clubhouse members join work crews to take responsibility for managing, maintaining and contributing to the Clubhouse, with members and staff working side-by-side in a 9-to-5 work setting to perform voluntary work essential to the Clubhouse. The work-ordered day engages members and staff together in the running of the Clubhouse; administration, staff evaluation, training, research and Clubhouse evaluation.

Employment: The Clubhouse enables its members to participate in paid work through the use of three different programmes that assist members in making the transition back into the workplace: transitional employment (TE), supported employment (SE) and independent employment (IE). The desire to work is the most important factor determining placement opportunity.

1. Transitional employment refers to the placement of clients in a series of paid but temporary jobs controlled by the Clubhouse, which is based on agreements made between the Clubhouse and the employers. TE aims to narrow the gap between the daily programme of the club and paid work in the open labour market by helping members develop the skills and confidence required to cope with competitive employment. Clubhouse staff coach members for the work and support them during employment. The Clubhouse guarantees the employer daily staffing for the employment position so in case of illness or other problems another club member or staff employee can act as a substitute. Failure at work is regarded as a natural part of the process and does not hinder a new attempt. Employment is usually part time and lasts between 6 and 9 months. There are no rigid guidelines for length of time on work crews, however, clients are discouraged from seeking competitive employment until they have achieved success in TE, and are free to return to work crews at any time.

2. In the independent employment programme, members with prior work experience and/or job-related education, skills and abilities as well as those who have completed a number of TE placements, are encouraged to seek their own job. Clubhouse independent employment units help members prepare resumes and coach them in job-search and interview techniques. Unlike TE and SE, members go on competitive interviews to get jobs. They can continue to use the services and support of the Clubhouse while they work.

3. Supported employment combines aspects of both TE and IE but the employment positions are not time limited and belong to the members themselves. The main goal is to provide ongoing support to members who have permanent jobs of their own and to ease their integration into long-term employment.

Community participation: The Clubhouse Model, with its focus on the normalising function of community employment and on giving all members a chance to work regardless of psychiatric history, allows the integration and inclusion of members into society and goes some way to challenging some of the myths associated with mental disorders.

Provision of other support services: The Clubhouse can also provide or support members in seeking adult education to develop their own personal skills. Similarly, information and support is given in relation to housing issues, substance misuse and wellness activities.

Key Recommendations for Replication

When considering recommendations for replicating the Clubhouse Model, it is helpful to be aware of the circumstances of expansion for the model programme. In 1977 the founding establishment, Fountain House, was awarded a non-governmental financial grant to establish a national training programme on the Clubhouse Model and thus began the process of replicating the model on a national and international basis. In 1987, the National Clubhouse Expansion Project was founded and developed the International Standard for Clubhouse Programmes (ICCD 2005). The success of the model's replication on a worldwide basis by this time demonstrated that the Clubhouse culture and practice had transcended national, ethnic and cultural boundaries as it is based on universal human values (ICCD 2005). It was then highlighted that the work of the National Clubhouse Expansion Project needed to continue but now at an international level. Funded by dues from member Clubhouses and other sources, the ICCD was developed. This centre provides Clubhouse consultation and certification to Clubhouses nationally and internationally. The centre produces the International Clubhouse Standards, which are a set of best practices and guidelines that define the Clubhouse Model of rehabilitation and ensure the quality of services provided within the clubhouse. The ICCD website (www.iccd.org) provides an in-depth source of information on the centre and the participating Clubhouses and provides links and contact e-mail addresses for all the Clubhouses internationally, with Clubhouses existing in most parts of the world: Albania, Australia, Estonia, Germany, Finland, Japan, Pakistan, Russia, Republic of Ireland, Republic of Korea, South Africa, UK and the US, to name but a few. This ease of access to information and contacts, combined with detailed standards for Clubhouse programmes, has contributed to the success of this model in being replicated. When considering replicating the model it is important to adhere to the core programme implementation features so as to remain faithful to the original model. Two fidelity instruments have been developed to assist in assessing adherence to the Clubhouse Model. It is possible to convert from an existing model of rehabilitation into the Clubhouse approach. The following recommendations for new Clubhouse developments are highlighted:

Establish a Clubhouse community and working group: The Clubhouse Model is based on a community of people and is so before it is a building or a programme. Therefore, it is necessary to bring people together and to develop relationships between members and staff who will be working there each day. This will contribute to the implementation feature of membership and active participation. The Clubhouse working group is comprised of stakeholders representing different interests such as service users, their families, professionals, politicians and community leaders. This group initiates the Clubhouses activity profile and also provides initial education and support, as well as identifying employers for members' employment placements. This group will also be responsible for organising the education of the local community as to what a Clubhouse is all about, possibly via seminars, Clubhouse literature and tours of other Clubhouses. A director for the Clubhouse can then be hired by the working group to continue overseeing the programme.

Clubhouse training: It is important that all involved in the Clubhouse are knowledgeable on this approach to psychiatric rehabilitation. Some existing Clubhouses are certified as training facilities whereby the members and staff of new Clubhouses can spend a period of time in training before they develop their new Clubhouse.

Funding: Funding will need to be secured to assist in the community start up, training and in obtaining an actual location for the Clubhouse building. Funding sources may include local and national government and public or social service agencies. It may be useful to involve representatives from government agencies and organisations that receive funds in the working group.

Clubhouse employment employers: Another important role of the working group is to identify employers for transitional employment placements. The attitude of the work community to people with mental health problems may well be coloured by prejudice and a fear of diversity and unpredictability as well as an element of curiosity. Initiating contact with employers directly rather than random mailing of literature can greatly develop the Clubhouse–employer relationship. Clubhouses that develop such placements early in the programme development experience more success than those that do not. Successful employment programmes can attract new members to the Clubhouse, as well as additional funding from government and private organisations.

Clubhouse members' personal preference: Lavikainen et al (2000) recommend that special attention be paid to the preferences and competencies of Clubhouse members in establishing work arrangements. During the planning stage, resources should be used not only to organise the work tasks but also to prepare each member to meet the tangible circumstances at work and the situational aspects of coping with work. Instead of individualising problems and focusing on assessment, the competencies and capabilities of each member in relation to work situations and the organisation of work tasks should be considered at the planning stage. This will ensure a smoother transition from the work-ordered day to the transitional employment placement.

Generic Principles of Good Practice for Workplace Mental Health Promotion

Effective workplace approaches address the physical, environmental and psychosocial factors influencing mental health, they strengthen modifying factors such as social support, control over decision making and effort–reward balance, and provide skills and competencies for addressing short-term and long-term responses to work-related stress (Israel et al 1996). Based on the research and programmes outlined in this chapter, the following generic principles of good practice for workplace mental health promotion are identified.

Comprehensive Theory-Based Programmes

Using a theoretical model will inform the development of a comprehensive ecological approach combining individual and organisational issues in addressing the complex relationships between work, stress and health.

Supportive Policy

Workplace policy and legislation have an important role in supporting mental health promotion interventions. Integrate the principles of health and safety and policies for handling bullying, harassment and violence at work into the company ethos by establishing company policies.

Supportive Psychosocial Structures

Put in place management and environmental structures that support good communication and social support among staff.

Holistic Focus

Promote good mental well-being by designing work processes and workplaces that promote and protect both the physical and mental health of employees.

Managing Change

Reduce feelings of job insecurity and fear of the future by encouraging transparent organisational processes, which engage employees in decision making and as active partners in the change process.

Tailor Intervention Programmes to the Needs of the Particular Worksite

Assess the needs and resources within the organisation in relation to different types of stressors, modifying factors and responses.

Participatory Approach

Involve participants at each stage of programme planning, implementation and evaluation. It is important to take account of the viewpoints of different stakeholders in the organisation in designing an intervention. Incorporate a joint employee, union and management committee as a key component of interventions with the role of top management and union representatives being crucial in ensuring that all participate (Israel et al 1996).

Establish an Organisational Infrastructure

Comprehensive interventions require a mechanism for integrating the change process at the different systems levels. This may involve setting up a steering group or some other organising structure within the workplace to initiate organisational change. Such a structure needs to foster open communication and shared decision making and clarify key roles and responsibilities for participant members. Different interventions require different roles, with each role requiring different skills, e.g. the role of expert, advocate, enabler and the change facilitator. Clarification of structures, roles and responsibilities is critical to good intervention planning and delivery.

Monitor and Evaluate the Implementation and Effectiveness of Workplace Interventions Particularly with Regard to their Cost–Benefit

Document programme impact in terms of indicators of employee well-being, reduced stress, absenteeism and improved productivity and job satisfaction.

Sustainability

Programmes that are of longer duration and are tailor made for specific employee groups tend to be more effective. Sustaining such programmes in the long term requires the support of senior management so that, ideally, they become an integral part of the organisational culture.

References

Bandura A 1977 Self-efficacy: toward a unifying theory of behavioural change. Psychological Review 84:191–215

Beard J H, Propst R N, Malamud T J 1982 The Fountain House model of rehabilitation. Psychosocial Rehabilitation Journal 5(1):47–53

Becker D R, Drake R E, Concord N H 1994 Individual placement and support: a community mental health center approach to vocational rehabilitation. Community Mental Health Journal 30:193–206

Blakely T, Collings S, Atkinson J 2003 Unemployment and suicide. Evidence for a causal association? Journal of Epidemiology and Community Health 57:594–600

Boardman J 2003 Work, employment and psychiatric disability. Advances in Psychiatric Treatment 9:327–334

Bond F, Bunce D 2001 Job control mediates change in a work reorganisation intervention for stress reduction. Journal of Occupational Health Psychology 6(4):290–302

Bond G R, Drake R E, Mueser K T et al 1997 An update on supported employment for people with severe mental illness. Psychiatric Services 48(3):335–346

Breslin F C, Mustard C A 2003 Unemployment and mental health: examining age as moderator in a population-based survey. Scandinavian Journal of Work, Environment and Health 29(1):5–14

Caplan R D, Vinokur A D, Price R H et al 1989 Job seeking, reemployment and mental health: a randomized field experiment in coping with job loss. Journal of Applied Psychology 74(5):759–769

Caplan R D, Vinokur V, Price R H 1997 From job loss to reemployment: field experiments in prevention-focused coping. In: Albee G W, Gullotta T P (eds) Primary prevention works, vol 6: issues in children's and families' lives. Sage, London:341–379

Commission of the European Communities 2002 Adapting to change in work and society: a new community strategy on health and safety at work 2002–2006. Communication on Health and Safety at Work, COM, 2002, 118 final, 11 March 2002

Cooper L, Cartwright S 1997 An intervention strategy for workplace stress. Journal of Psychosomatic Research 43(1):7–16

Crowther R, Marshall M, Bond G et al 2003 Vocational rehabilitation for people with severe mental illness (Cochrane Review). In: The Cochrane Library issue 4. John Wiley, Chichester

Curran J, Wishart P, Gingrich J 1999 JOBS: A manual for teaching people successful job search strategies. Michigan Prevention Research Center, University of Michigan, Michigan

Dooley D, Catalano R, Wilson G 1994 Depression and unemployment – panel findings from the Epidemiologic Catchment Area Study. American Journal of Community Psychology 22(6): 745–765

Dooley D, Fielding J, Levi L 1996 Health and unemployment. Annual Review of Public Health 17:449–465

Drake R E, McHugo G J, Becker D R et al 1996 The New Hampshire supported employment study. Journal of Consulting and Clinical Psychology 64:391–399

Edwards D, Burnard P 2003 A systematic review of stress and stress management interventions for mental health nurses. Journal of Advanced Nursing 42(2): 169–200

Elkin A J, Rosch P J 1990 Promoting mental health at the workplace: the prevention side of stress management. Occupational Medicine State of the Art Review 5(4):739–754

EU Health and Safety at Work Directive 1989 (89/391/EEC) Official Journal L 183, 29/06/1989:1–8. Online. Available: http://

europa.eu.int/scadplus/leg/en/cha/c11149. htm November 2005

European Commission 2002 Combating stress and depression-related problems. Online. Available: http://europa.eu.int/scadplus/leg/en/cha/c11570a.htm November 2005

Ezzy D 1993 Unemployment and mental health: a critical review. Social Science and Medicine 37:41–52

Grossman R, Scala K 1993 Health promotion and organisational development: developing settings for health. World Health Organization, Regional Office for Europe, Vienna

Heaney C A 1991 Enhancing social support at the workplace: assessing the effects of the Caregiver Support Program. Health Education Quarterly 18(4):477–494

Heaney C A, Price R H, Rafferty J 1995a Increasing coping resources at work: a field experiment to increase social support, improve work team functioning and enhance employee mental health. Journal of Organisational Behavior 16:335–352

Heaney C A, Price R H, Rafferty J 1995b The Caregiver Support Program: an intervention to increase employee coping resources and enhance mental health. In: Murphy L R, Hurrell J J, Sauter S L et al (eds) Job stress interventions. American Psychological Association, Washington DC:93–108

Holloway F, Szmukler G, Carson J 2000 Support systems. 1. Introduction. Advances in Psychiatric Treatment 6:226–235

Howe G W, Caplan R, Foster D et al 1995 When couples cope with job-loss: a research strategy for developing preventive intervention. In: Murphy L R, Hurrell J J, Sauter S L et al (eds) Job stress interventions. American Psychological Association, Washington DC:139–158

Huxley P, Thornicroft G 2003 Social inclusion, social quality and mental illness. British Journal of Psychiatry 182:289–290

ICCD (International Center for Clubhouse Development) 2005. Online. Available: http://www.iccd.org/ November 2005

Israel B A, Baker E A, Goldenhar L M et al 1996 Occupational stress, safety and health: conceptual framework and principles for effective prevention interventions. Journal of Occupational Health Psychology 1(3):261–286

Jané-Llopis E, Anderson P 2005 Mental health promotion and mental disorder prevention. A policy for Europe. Radboud University Nijmegen, Nijmegen

Jané-Llopis E, Barry M M, Hosman C et al 2005 Mental health promotion works: a review. Promotion and Education Suppl2:9–25

Janis IL 1983 Short-term counseling. Yale University Press, New Have, Connecticut

Jin R L, Shah C P, Svoboda T J 1995 The impact of unemployment on health: a review of the evidence. Canadian Medical Association Journal 153(5):529–540

Johansson S E, Sundquist J 1997 Unemployment is an important risk factor for suicide in contemporary Sweden: an 11-year follow-up study of a cross-sectional sample of 37 789 people. Public Health 3:41–45

Johnsen M, McKay C, Corcoran J et al 2002 Characteristics of clubhouses across the world: findings from the international survey of clubhouses 2000. Program for Clubhouse Research, Center for Mental Health Services Research, University of Massachusetts Medical School, Worcester, Massachusetts

Johnsen M, McKay C, Henry A et al 2004 What does competitive employment mean? A secondary analysis of employment approaches in the Massachusetts Employment Intervention Demonstration Project. In Fisher W (ed) Employment for persons with severe illness. Volume 13, Research in community and mental health. Elsevier, Oxford

Johnsen M, McKay C, Campbell R 2005 Examining the evidence base for the Clubhouse Model. Online. Available: http://www.nri-inc.org/Conference/Conf05/Abstracts/Mon1330_FH_McKay.pdf

Johnson J V, Stewart W, Friedlund P et al 1996 Long-term psychosocial work environment and cardiovascular mortality among Swedish men. American Journal of Public Health 86:324–331

Karasek R A 1990 Lower health risk with increased job control among white collar workers. Journal of Organizational Behaviour 11:171–85

Karasek R, Theorell T 1990 Healthy work: stress, productivity, and the reconstruction of working life. Basic Books, New York

Kjell Nytro P O, Mikkelsen A, Bohle P et al 2000 An appraisal of key factors in the implementation of occupational stress interventions. Work and Stress 14(3):213–225

Lavikainen J, Lahtinen E, Lehtinen V 2000 Public health approach on mental health in Europe. STAKES National Research and Development Centre for Welfare and Health. Ministry of Social Affairs and Health, Finland

Lehtinen V, Riikonen E, Lehtinen E 1998 Promotion of mental health on the European agenda. STAKES National Research and Development Centre for Welfare and Health. Ministry of Social Affairs and Health, Finland

McFarlane W R, Stastny P, Deakins S et al 1995 Employment outcomes in family-aided assertive community treatment (FACT). Presented at the Institute on Psychiatric Services, Boston, 6–10 October

Macias C 2001 Massachusetts Employment Intervention Demonstration Project. An experimental comparison of PACT and clubhouse. EIDP, Substance Abuse and Mental Health Service Administration, Massachusetts

Macias C, Jackson R, Schroeder C et al 1999 What is a Clubhouse? Report on the ICCD 1996 survey of USA clubhouses. Community Mental Health Journal 35(2):181–190

McKay C 2005 Recent research findings from the program for Clubhouse research. Issue Brief 2(8). Center for Mental Health Services Research, University of Massachusetts Medical School, Massachusetts. Online. Available: http://www.umassmed.edu/cmhsr/uploads/brief18Clubhouse.pdf November 2005

McKay C, Johnsen M, Campbell R 2005a An examination of the evidence base for the Clubhouse Model. Presentation at the Conference on State Mental Health Agency Services Research, Program Evaluation and Policy. Online. Available: http://www.nri-inc.org/Conference/Conf05/Presentations/Mon1330_FH_McKay.pdf November 2005

McKay C, Johnsen M, Stein R 2005b Employment outcomes in Massachusetts clubhouses. Psychiatric Rehabilitation Journal 29(1):25–33

Manning C, White P D 1995 Attitudes of employers to the mentally ill. Psychiatric Bulletin 19:541–543

Marmot M, Siegrist J, Theorell T et al 1999 Health and the psychosocial environment at work. In: Marmot M, Wilkinson R (eds) Social determinants of health. Oxford University Press, Oxford, Chapter 6:105–131

Masso J D, Avi-Itzhak T, Obler D R 2001 The Clubhouse Model: an outcome study on attendance, work attainment and status, and hospitalisation recidivism. Work 17(1):23–30

Mentality 2003 Making it effective: a guide to evidence based mental health promotion. Radical mentalities – briefing paper 1. Mentality, London

Michie S 2002 Causes and management of stress at work. Occupational and Environmental Medicine 59:67–72

Michie S, Williams S 2003 Reducing work related psychological ill-health and sickness absence: a systematic literature review. Occupational and Environmental Medicine 60(1):3–9

Murphy L R 1996 Stress management in work settings: a critical review of the health effects. American Journal of Health Promotion 11:112–135

NIOSH (US National Institute for Occupational Safety and Health) 1998 Stress at work. NIOSH, Cincinnati

Oliver M 1990 The politics of disablement. Macmillan, Basingstoke

Parker S K, Chimel N, Wall T D 1997 Work characteristics and employee well-being within a context of strategic downsizing. Journal of Occupational Health Psychology 2(4):289–303

Pattani S, Constantinovici N, Williams S 2001 Who retires early from the NHS because of ill-health and what does it cost? British Medical Journal 322:208–209

Pfeffer J 1998 The human equation: building profits by putting people first. Harvard Business School Press, Boston

Price R H, Kompier M 2006 Work, stress and unemployment: risks, mechanisms and prevention. In: Hosman C, Jané-Llopis E, Saxena S (eds) Prevention of mental disorders: effective interventions and policy options. A report of the World Health Organization, Department of Mental Health and Substance Abuse in collaboration with the Prevention Research Centre of the Universities of Nijmegen and Maastricht. Oxford Universitiy Press, Oxford, Chapter 6 (in press)

Price R H, Vinokur V 1995 Supporting career transitions in a time of organisational downsizing: the Michigan JOBS program. In London M (ed) Employees, careers and job creation: developing growth-oriented human resource strategies and programs. Jossey-Bass, San Francisco:191–209

Price R H, van Ryn M, Vinokur A D 1992 Impact of a preventive job search intervention on the likelihood of depression among the unemployed. Journal of Health and Social Behaviour 33:158–167

Price R H, Friedland D S, Choi J N et al 1998 Job loss and work transitions in a time of global economic change. In: Arriaga X B, Oskamp S (eds) Addressing community problems: research and intervention. Sage, Thousand Oaks, California:195–222

Schneider J 1998 Work interventions in mental health care: some arguments and recent evidence. Journal of Mental Health 7:81–94

Secker J, Grove B, Seebohm P 2001 Challenging barriers to employment: training and education for mental health service users. The service users perspective. Institute for Applied Health and Social Policy, Kings College London, London

Shinn M, Rosario M, March H et al 1984 Coping with job stress and burnout in the human services. Journal of Personality and Social Psychology 46:864–876

Siegrist J 1996 Adverse health effects of high-effort/low-reward conditions. Journal of Occupational Health Psychology 1:27–41

Siegrist J, Siegrist K, Weber I 1986 Sociological concepts in the etiology of chronic disease: the case of ischaemic heart disease. Social Science and Medicine 22:247–253

Stansfeld S A, Fuhrer R, Head J et al 1999 Work characteristics predict psychiatric disorder: prospective results from the Whitehall II study. Occupational and Environmental Medicine 56:302–307

Stansfeld S, Head J, Marmot M 2000 Work-related factors and ill-health: the Whitehall II study. Health and Safety Executive, Suffolk

Tennant C 2001 Work-related stress and depressive disorders. Journal of Psychosomatic Research 51:697–704

United Nations 1948 Universal declaration of human rights. Online. Available: http://www.un.org/Overview/rights.html November 2005

Van der Klink J J, Blonk R W, Schene A H et al 2001 The benefits of interventions for work-related stress. American Journal of Public Health 91(2):270–276

Vinokur A D, Schul Y 1997 Mastery and inoculation against setbacks as active ingredients in the JOBS intervention for the unemployed. Journal of Consulting and Clinical Psychology 65(5):867–877

Vinokur A D, Price R H, Caplan R D 1991a From field experiments to program implementation: assessing the potential outcomes of an experimental intervention program for unemployed persons. American Journal of Community Psychology 23(1): 39–74; Journal of Community Psychology 19(4):543–562

Vinokur A D, van Ryn M, Gramlich E et al 1991b Long-term follow-up and benefit-cost analysis of the JOBS program: A preventive intervention for the unemployed. Journal of Applied Psychology 76(2):213–219

Vinokur A D, Price R H, Schul Y 1995 Impact of the JOBS Intervention on unemployed workers varying in risk for depression. American Journal of Community Psychology 23(1):39–74

Vinokur A D, Schul Y, Vuori J et al 2000 Two years after a job loss: long-term impact of the JOBS program on reemployment and mental health. Journal of Occupational Health Psychology 5(1):32–47

Vuori J, Silvonen J, Vinokur A D et al 2002 The Työhön Job Search Program in Finland: benefits for the unemployed with risk of depression or discouragement. Journal of Occupational Health Psychology 7:5–19

Warner R, Huxley P, Berg T 1999 An evaluation of the impact of clubhouse membership on quality of life and treatment utilisation. International Journal of Social Psychiatry 45(4):310–320

Warr P 1987 Work, unemployment and mental health. Oxford University Press, Oxford

WHO (World Health Organization) 2000 Mental health and work: impact, issues and good practices (Harnois G, Gabriel P eds). A joint publication of the WHO and the International Labour Organisation, WHO, Geneva

Williams S, Michie S, Patini S 1998 Improving the health of the NHS workforce. The Nutfield Trust, London

Wilson S H, Walker G M 1993 Unemployment and health: a review. Public Health 107:153–162

Mental Health Promotion in Primary Health Care

7

Introduction

Primary health care is usually understood as the first point of entry to the health services and is ideally based on the principles of a universally accessible service that is comprehensive, integrated, intersectoral and based on community participation. Primary care has an important role to play in strengthening the mental health of individuals, families and communities and in recognising the importance of mental health to overall health and well-being (Jenkins & Üstün 1998). An overview of the relevance of the primary health care setting for promoting mental health is given in this chapter followed by a focus on programmes that are community wide and could form part of a comprehensive and coordinated primary health care service. There is a particular focus on the following interventions: promoting exercise, strengthening access to community and voluntary services, e.g. programmes for families under stress, mood management and depression prevention and training primary health care workers in promoting mental health. A number of programmes and case studies are described that illustrate interventions that are feasible, effective and practical in a primary care setting.

Rationale for Mental Health Promotion in Primary Care

Primary care represents an important setting for mental health promotion. It is the first point of contact with the health services and, therefore, presents an important opportunity for reorienting health services towards the promotion of mental health. The Alma Ata Declaration (WHO 1978) defined primary health care as 'essential health care made universally accessible to individuals and families in the community by means acceptable to them, through their full participation and at a cost that the community and country can afford'. As an approach to care, primary care includes a range of services, accessible through self-referral, including the promotion of health, prevention of disease, diagnosis, treatment, rehabilitation and personal social services. Based on the principles of the Alma Ata Declaration, primary care services are designed to meet the health and social care needs of local communities, providing continuous and comprehensive care from birth to death. Articulated as such, primary care services have a pivotal role to play in promoting mental health, in terms of both its community-wide health focus to service provision and its aim of providing an integrated service which effectively links community health care with specialist services. However, what constitutes primary care services varies considerably across countries and, to date, mental health has been relatively neglected in the delivery of primary care services in many countries. The main focus of primary health care tends to be on physical health and many primary care workers do not have a mental health orientation.

As a setting for mental health promotion, primary health care has the advantage of being an accessible community-based service delivered by health workers who know the local community. Primary care offers a non-stigmatising service with many possibilities for intersectoral collaboration with schools, workplaces, local agencies, voluntary organisations and community groups in the local setting. The primary care system can be expanded into the community by coordinating links with community and self-help groups, local services and supports. Primary care also acts as a gateway to specialist services and, therefore, has a key role to play in terms of ensuring access to community supports and appropriate referral for the sizeable amount of people with mental health problems. Recent research in the UK showed that 15% of people in the community have a diagnosable mental health problem, around 30% who see their general practitioner or primary care physician have a mental heath component to their health problem and some 90% of people with significant mental health problems are cared for entirely in primary care (Sainsbury Centre for Mental Health & NHS Alliance 2002). Therefore, in terms of the pathways to care, primary care services are well placed to ensure early identification of mental health problems, the prevention of subsequent episodes and the general promotion of the physical and mental health well-being of local communities through either direct provision or referral to special services from voluntary and statutory services and agencies.

Primary health care professionals such as doctors, nurses, social workers and other health care staff are well placed to identify the mental health needs of people who are at increased risk due to their specific circumstances, e.g. people living in deprived areas, families under stress, first-time mothers, lone parents and carers. While the primary health care services, due to limited capacity, may not be able to provide direct support themselves, they can nonetheless signpost local services and supports including self-help groups and other statutory and voluntary services. Local primary care staff can play a pro-active role in coordinating services locally, e.g. referral to a home visiting programme, programmes run by the voluntary sector and referral on to specialist mental health and support services. The multidisciplinary nature of the primary care team places them in a good position to coordinate services from across a range of disciplines, agencies and sectors in the local community. Such coordination and cooperation is needed in order to ensure an integrated comprehensive service with joint working between health, social and community services, education, welfare, housing and employment services. As such, the primary care setting offers an opportunity to address both the promotion of mental health and the prevention of mental disorders in a more sustainable way.

While the primary care setting has advantages for mental health promotion there may also, however, be critical organisational and institutional drawbacks. The burden of increasing demands for productivity and efficiency may reduce the likelihood of primary care workers prioritising mental health promotion work. In addition, primary care workers may not be well oriented towards mental health and may not have had an appropriate broad training in this area, i.e. covering not just assessment, treatment and rehabilitation, but also prevention and mental health promotion. The case for promoting mental health as an integral part of overall health care may, therefore, need to be made including making the link between physical and mental health. Likewise, there is a need to organise service delivery so that it is networked and integrated with local community supports and services for promoting mental health. The provision of training and skill development for primary health care workers in developing and implementing mental health promotion programmes is fundamental to mainstreaming and sustaining action in this area.

Mental and physical health are closely interrelated, and mental health impacts on physical health and vice versa. For example, emotional well-being is recognised as a strong predictor of physical health at all ages. Subjective feelings of emotional health are associated with increased general health and greater longevity (Goodwin 2000), while sustained stress and trauma have been found to increase susceptibility to physical illness by damaging the immune system (Stewart-Brown 1998). Mental health problems such as depression and anxiety may significantly influence the onset, course and outcome of physical health problems (Raphael et al 2005). In particular, studies have highlighted the interactions between depression and physical conditions such as heart disease (Hippisley-Cox et al 1998, Kuper et al 2002), stroke (Carson et al 2000, Jonas & Mussolino 2000), diabetes (Anderson et al 2001) and cancer (DeBoer et al 1999). While the complex relationship between physical and mental health states is not yet fully understood, the existing evidence suggests that the impact of physical health on mental health, and of mental health on physical health needs to be much better recognised in primary health care. Primary health care workers need to be more aware of the critical role that the promotion of mental

---

Box 7.1

The importance of primary health care as a setting for mental health promotion

- accessible community-based service
- provision of comprehensive and continuous care from the cradle to the grave
- non-stigmatising service
- multidisciplinary team coordinating service provision between health, social services, community and self-help groups
- gateway for specialist services
- referral to other support agencies and services
- provision of holistic care recognising the links between physical and mental health care
- knowledge of the social milieu of clients and their circumstances
- greater possibilities for intersectoral collaboration in the local community

---

health, and in particular the prevention of depression, has to play in enhancing overall health and the reduction of physical health problems (Box 7.1). There is, therefore, a strong case to be made for ensuring that the promotion of mental health is incorporated in a more holistic manner into the standard delivery of health care for physical conditions.

Implementing Mental Health Promotion in Primary Care

258

There is a growing evidence base for the effectiveness of a range of programmes in primary care including brief intervention programmes to reduce alcohol consumption (Ashenden et al 1997), social prescribing for exercise and creative arts, voluntary sector and self-help programmes (Mentality 2003). Social prescribing refers to mechanisms for linking primary care patients with other non-medical sources of support within the community. Initiatives such as 'Exercise on prescription', 'Prescription for learning' and 'Arts on prescription' have been used with vulnerable populations, including those with mental health problems, and have been found to result in a range of positive outcomes such as enhanced self-esteem, self-efficacy and improved mood and social contact (Mentality 2003). As outlined in this chapter, the interrelationship between physical and mental health is beginning to be more fully recognised. Existing interventions that promote physical health have also been found to have a positive impact on mental health. For example, there is emerging evidence on the benefits of exercise promotion on mental health (Fox 2000) There is great potential for combining mental and physical components in primary health care strategies thereby embedding mental health within more generic health promotion programmes. The specific example of exercise programmes and their impact on mental health will now be examined.

Promoting Mental Health Through Exercise

There is widespread support for a positive and lasting relationship between participation in regular exercise and various indices of mental health, and several consensus documents and reviews have been published in this field. The evidence for psychological benefits, although impressive for mentally healthy individuals, is even stronger for those with mental health problems. For example, Daley (2002) notes that a number of studies have demonstrated a positive relationship between exercise and mental health in people with alcohol misuse problems, people with schizophrenia and those with clinical depression. Some of the improvements in mental health and psychological well-being encompass factors such as coping ability, self-esteem and mood. Fox (2000) notes that the impact of physical activity on the mental health of the public could be viewed from several perspectives:

* exercise may have a substantial indirect effect on mental well-being through reductions in illness and premature death
* exercise may provide a valuable treatment mode for some mental health problems and disorders
* exercise may be useful for the enhancement of life quality of those suffering from mental disorders, even if it is not effective as a cure
* exercise may be effective in the prevention of mental illness and disorders
* exercise may be a powerful medium for improvement in mental well-being among the general population.

Best Practice

The Green Gym Project

The Green Gym project was set up as a result of a joint venture between a local health authority and the British Trust for Conservation Volunteers (BTCV) to encourage the local community to improve their health and environment through participation in conservation activities. The Green Gym offers participants the opportunity to take part in practical conservation activities such as planting hedges, creating wildlife gardens or improving footpaths. Sessions are held once or twice a week within the local community. These sessions are a combination of physical activity, social interaction and team working in order to improve the local environment. A project officer provides training and support so that participants develop the skills and confidence to run the Green Gyms themselves. BTCV continues to support the scheme through its local and national service to community groups. Participants are invited either to attend for a full 3-hour session or to 'drop in' for shorter periods. A warm-up session is encouraged prior to starting work on the task. Leaders are trained in basic exercise physiology including warm-up and cool-down stretches. Leaders are also instructed to encourage participants to work at levels of exertion that are appropriate to their levels of fitness and ability.

Evaluation Findings

Local evaluations of the Green Gym initiative point to a number of physical and mental health benefits for participants (BTCV 1999, 2001). An evaluation of 37 Green Gym participants from the Portslade Green Gym project (BTCV 2001) revealed a significant improvement in mental health, as measured by the mental health component score of the SF-12 health-related quality of life instrument, in the first 3 months of participation. The study used a longitudinal evaluation of the psychological, social and physiological impact of the Green Gym over a period of 6 months. A series of validated questionnaires and physiological measurements were administered at three time points: baseline, 3 months and 6 months. There was also a strong trend in the decrease in depression scores on the Hospital Anxiety and Depression Scale during the same time period. No significant changes were found in the instruments used to measure social support, loneliness and happiness, although the qualitative evidence collected from the interviews suggested that participants valued the opportunity to meet other people which the Green Gym provided. Participants also reported valuing being in the countryside and deriving a lot of satisfaction from the tasks in which they were involved. Case studies of participants also suggest that the Green Gym gave them the confidence to overcome their depression and return to full employment.

Key Recommendations for Replication

The major challenge for any exercise scheme is to find ways to establish long-term maintenance and adherence to exercise. A number of consistent factors have been found to promote exercise adherence and include easy, convenient, accessible and inexpensive exercise settings, frequent professional contact and exercise that is of a moderate intensity (Hillsdon et al 1995). Green Gyms offer an alternative to other exercise prescription programmes and may be a more sustainable and attractive option for members. Evaluation of the motivating factors identified by Oxford Green Gym participants included keeping fit, being out in the countryside, doing something worthwhile, improving the environment and meeting other people. Less important were preparing for the next fitness assessment and weight loss. While these motivating factors may be reflected by the older age profile of the participants, nevertheless it is worthwhile taking these factors into consideration when designing an exercise prescription intervention that can meet the needs of participants.

Strengthening Access to Community and Voluntary Services: Prenatal and Family Support Programmes

Facilitating access to community and voluntary sector support schemes is an important function of primary health care. There are a number of effective community-based programmes that have been developed which have a demonstrated impact on physical and mental health, child neglect, maternal well-being and postnatal depression. As Price (1998) points out, these programmes are of considerable importance as they could be incorporated into standard primary care practice and have both physical and mental health impacts. Chapter 4 has already discussed the 'Prenatal and Infancy Home Visitation' programme and the 'Community Mothers Programme', which are delivered by trained nurses and community mothers respectively. Both these programmes have been shown to produce impressive long-term impacts on both child and maternal health and well-being. In this chapter we will explore the development of programmes for families under stress, which provide support to mothers who are depressed and/ or at risk of further breakdown. The implementation of befriending and day-care support programmes, which are delivered by voluntary organisations and take referrals from primary care health services, are examined.

Access to high-quality social and family support has very positive effects on the mental health and well-being of both parents and young children. The evaluation of home-based social support to pregnant women at higher risk (e.g. those that are socially disadvantaged) provided by midwives (Oakley et al 1996, Olds et al 1997) or lay/community mothers (Hodnett & Roberts 1997, Johnson et al 1993, Marcenko & Spence 1994) strongly suggests that various forms of home support or home visiting during pregnancy improves mental well-being of mothers and their children (NHS Centre for Reviews and Dissemination 1997). Research also indicates that the provision of continuous support from friends or volunteers during labour can reduce postnatal depression and raise self-esteem (Hodnett 1997). However, studies evaluating the outcomes of specifically designed programmes to prevent postnatal depression produce mixed findings. Programmes by Elliott et al (1988) and Zlotnick et al (2001) report that ante-natal education and parenthood support groups for high-risk first-time mothers have lead to reductions in postnatal depression symptoms and mental health related outcomes, such as improved mother–infant engagement (Cooper et al 2002). However, other studies (Brugha et al 2000, Hayes et al 2001, Morrell et al 2000, Stamp et al 1995) found no significant effects on reducing postnatal depression or evidence that the effects are sustained beyond 2 months. Next we will examine the original programme by Elliott et al (1988) as an example of a psychosocial intervention which demonstrated successful outcomes resulting in reduced levels of postnatal depression in first-time mothers.

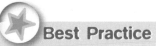 Best Practice

Promoting Mental Health after Childbirth: a Psychosocial Intervention to Prevent Postnatal Depression

(Elliott et al 1988, Elliott et al 2000)

Postnatal depression affects 10–15% of mothers, may lead to chronic mental health problems in a significant proportion of women and can also adversely affect the child (Murray 1995, Murray & Cooper 1997, NHS Centre for Reviews and Dissemination 1997). Elliott et al (1988) conducted a controlled trial of an intervention aimed at reducing the prevalence of postnatal depression in first- and second-time mothers identified as vulnerable to depression. This study was the first attempt to demonstrate that a psychosocial intervention could be effective for postnatal depression. This programme included several components:

* continuity of care up to 6 months after the birth of the child
* an educational component covering at least three aspects: postnatal depression, the common 'realities' of life with a newborn and ways of preparing for the new or changed job of parenting
* the programme acted as a source of information on, or referral to, relevant local and national organisations.

Monthly group sessions were organised for first- and second-time mothers to begin as early as possible in pregnancy and to continue until 6 months post-natal. The programme was advertised as an educational, as opposed to a counselling or psychotherapy, programme with the intention of maximising the uptake of the service. First-time mothers were invited to take part in a programme entitled 'Preparation for parenthood' and second-time mothers to a programme entitled 'Surviving parenthood'.

Group sessions of between 10 and 15 members were chosen rather than individual counselling, thereby providing the opportunity for friendship and emotional support among participants. The group sessions were also used as a second screen to identify those in greater need, for example, for individual counselling. Although the interventions were led by primary care staff, the hospital prenatal clinic was chosen as a venue as this was seen as being more user friendly and accessible. In total, 11 sessions took place from 4 months pregnancy through to 6 months postnatal. Postnatal sessions were included to provide continuity of care during the critical period after giving birth and to avoid women feeling deserted at a time when they most needed support.

Two groups of first-time mothers and two groups of second-time mothers were formed. A psychologist and a health visitor led the groups. In the early group meetings, women were given clearly defined periods each week when leaders in the groups would endeavour to receive telephone calls from the women. Each member was given such times by both her group leader and health visitor. Information on postnatal depression was given in order to prepare mothers for the probability that they would experience some negative emotions after birth and to allow them to experience and express these emotions without feelings of guilt and failure. Both male and female parents were informed about the existence and treatability of postnatal depression and how to recognise it. Early sessions were structured with the group leader providing information personally or using video and audio tapes. Members were then encouraged to raise issues they would like discussed. The proportion of time assigned to 'open discussion' was increased over the course of the first four sessions. The last pregnancy meeting and all the postnatal meetings had no formal agenda. Throughout the programme group leaders aimed to encourage discussion on a variety of issues and to allow the participants to consider a range of both potential problems and solutions using a non-directive style. An outline of the session content is given below:

* Session 1: overview
* Session 2: postnatal depression

- Session 3: new parenthood, caring for two children
- Session 4: abilities of the newborn
- Sessions 5–11: discussion on a variety of issues.

Evaluation

The Leverton Questionnaire was used in early pregnancy to assess vulnerability to postnatal depression (Elliott et al 1988). Eligible and willing first- and second-time mothers were interviewed and were identified as either having vulnerability factors or not. Interviewers were blind as to who was participating in the intervention. Those without identified vulnerability factors were assigned to a control group while those with vulnerability factors were split into an intervention group and a non-intervention group. A total of 32 more vulnerable first-time mothers were invited to the group meetings of whom only three declined and one failed to reply. First-time mothers attended an average of seven out of 11 meetings, whereas second-time mothers attended an average of four meetings. The majority of partners (n = 18) of first-time mothers attended the evening partners' session. However, most second-time mothers felt they could not attend an evening session as a couple because of babysitting requirements. The second session was, therefore, held in the afternoon and only two partners attended. Results from the study revealed that participating first-time mothers reported significantly more positive mood than the group receiving routine care. Significantly fewer women received a diagnosis of depression in the first 2 postnatal months in the intervention group (six out of 48; two cases and four borderlines) than in the control group (17 out of 51; five cases and 12 borderlines). This difference was apparent for both first-time mothers (three out of 22 and nine out of 25 respectively) and second-time mothers (three of 26 and eight out of 26 respectively). Combining these groups, 12% of the intervention group were diagnosed as depressed for 2 or more weeks in the first 2 postnatal months compared to 33% of controls. The differences between the first-time mothers groups persisted to 3 months postnatal, although few first-time mothers were above the threshold for diagnosis of clinical depression. However, for the second-time mothers who had a higher prevalence of depression in the third month than did first-time mothers (four of 26 in the intervention group and six of 26 in the control group), no significant differences between intervention and control groups on the self-report questionnaire data were reported. The outcome data confirmed the impressions gained by the group leaders, that first-time mothers were more successfully engaged in the programme and experienced less depression after childbirth than did the second-time mothers invited to participate in the programme. These results were significant despite a small sample size and an intention to treat analysis (Elliott et al 2000).

Programme Implementation Features

Educational programme: The programme was delivered as an educational antenatal programme as opposed to a counselling or therapeutic intervention, which aided the uptake of the service.

Participant led: The programme was delivered as a self-directed intervention which was guided by the needs of the participants. From the outset, participants were encouraged to influence the course of meetings, and usually did so. The first-time mothers generally welcomed the information provided and sought more information when appropriate. Second-time mothers did not show the same enthusiasm for general information but from the first or second session sought discussion on current issues relevant to them, such as management of the older child, stress in relation to this child or preparation of the older child for the baby. A common theme was the stress imposed on the mother–child relationship by the pregnancy or by the new baby. Participants reported that the meetings were conducted more or less the way they would like.

Continuity of care: This programme catered for the needs of pregnant women in such a way as to provide continuous care up until 6 months postnatal. This continuity of care is especially important at a time when women may be particularly vulnerable and in need of support.

Group process: The programme provided instrumental, emotional and self-esteem support through the group sessions.

Key Recommendations for Replication

The authors, Elliott et al (1988), recommended that for future replication consideration should be given to the provision of facilities closer to members' homes, such as local health centres coupled with more attractive facilities for children. Also, if group meetings were held immediately after antenatal classes, this might encourage more second-time mothers to attend group meetings more regularly. This minimal intervention could be readily offered alongside current antenatal and postnatal provision; however, modifications would be required for women other than first-time mothers as they are less likely to attend group sessions. Liaison and collaboration between health visitors, GPs and midwifery services are essential and the training needs of clients and/or health visitors would need to be examined. Further research would be needed to determine whether the programme would be effective when run within routine services by a health visitor or midwife without a clinical psychologist (Elliott et al 2000).

Family Support Programmes

There are a number of different approaches to delivering social and emotional support to families, such as home visiting and befriending schemes, including involvement of primary health care professionals, volunteers and community mothers. A number of studies have shown that home visiting programmes are beneficial particularly for parents in most need such as those living in disadvantaged areas, ethnic minority groups, refugees, asylum seekers, those in temporary accommodation and teenage and lone parents (Robinson 1999). Chapter 4 has already profiled a number of model programmes in this area and outlined some key aspects of effective implementation. In this chapter we will focus on two specific family support schemes run by the voluntary sector;

Newpin (New Parent Infant Network) and Home-Start. Newpin is a voluntary network based in the UK, where volunteer befrienders work with parents in providing training and therapy to promote personal development and self-esteem. Home-Start is also run by a voluntary sector group which organises volunteers, usually mothers themselves, who visit people's homes and provide emotional support to families under stress. The service is seen as being complementary to statutory services and aims to reduce the needs for professional intervention.

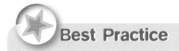 **Best Practice**

The New Parent Infant Network (Newpin)

(Jenkins 1996)

The New Parent Infant Network (Newpin) is a befriending scheme to support families with young children. The original aims of Newpin were to improve the mental health and self-esteem of mothers and thus to reduce child abuse. However, Newpin now also focuses on the minimisation of emotional damage to children and their parents. Newpin provides a safe, stable environment from 9am to 5pm, 5 days a week, for mothers and their children. There is also a 24-hour supportive network encompassing the total centre membership throughout the year. Health visitors, social workers and other local agencies refer suitable families to Newpin. Depending on need, the referred client may then be offered help from a befriender, attendance at the 'Drop-In' (opportunities to attend the centre outside training sessions), a client group or individual counselling or therapy. Many members later go on to train as volunteers. This training consists of 2 half days per week over a 6-month period. One session consists of lectures and workshops on topics such as child development, play, marriage and childbirth, problems in parenting and the befriending relationship. The other session consists of a self-development group run by a group therapist, in which members are encouraged to explore current and past relationships and to come to terms with earlier trauma and loss. At the end of the training, volunteers are assigned to support new clients and continue to receive weekly supervision while befriending.

Evaluation

A case study by Oakley et al (1998) describes the characteristics of clients referred to both the Newpin and Home-Start parent support initiatives and documents key aspects of the referral process. Referral records were examined and qualitative interview data were collected from a sub-sample of families and from staff and referrers involved in Newpin centres based in London. Volunteers and referrers completed questionnaires in the Home-Start study. The kinds of families and problems referred to the two schemes were very similar and mothers' loneliness and low emotional well-being were the main reasons for referral. Children at risk represented a small part of the caseload. Participants in both studies had low levels of social support from family and friends. Most referrals were made by health visitors and there was a significant problem of non-use for both Newpin and Home-Start services. Non-responders in the evaluation were less likely to have used Newpin or Home-Start while responders were less socially disadvantaged, more likely to be white, had fewer children and were more likely to have two parents and older mothers. A quarter of the Newpin and half of the Home-Start sample reported feeling depressed with over half of both samples reporting being referred due to sadness or depression. Nearly twice as many Newpin as Home-Start mothers wanted advice about problems, and the problem most identified by two thirds of the Newpin sample and half of the Home-Start sample was the need for help in coping with depression or stress. This was followed by the need for help with coping with children's behaviour. Most users of Newpin and Home-Start were enthusiastic about the help provided. In their study Oakley et al (1998) highlighted the need for further evaluation of the effectiveness of such schemes in reaching families at greatest risk in order to provide a sound evidence base for policy and service purchasing decisions.

A number of small scale evaluations of the outcomes of the Newpin programme have been conducted which report improvements in self-esteem, depression and social isolation for both volunteers and referred women with young children from highly disadvantaged backgrounds (Cox et al 1991, Pound & Mills 1985). A study by Oakley et al (1995) supported the earlier findings on the benefits for those mothers who were well engaged in improving their self-esteem and sense of connectedness with society. However, the study cautioned that Newpin was unclear about its target group and that dropout rates were an issue. Research on the delivery of Newpin in Australia also reports improved self-esteem and confidence in mothers and reduced problem behaviours in children for families attending for at least 6 months (Mondy 2001).

Programme Implementation Features

Home visits: By delivering a home visiting service, Newpin volunteers are able to visit difficult-to-reach families thereby removing transportation and childcare costs as barriers to service access. This is especially important in reaching and maintaining the participation of geographically, socially or psychologically isolated families and those with heavy work loads or several small children. A home visit also signals a willingness to make accommodations to the family's needs and schedule. This in turn can set the tone for a less formal and more comfortable, friendly and relaxed relationship between the visitor and parent. This may also help the balance of power between parent and professional. The Newpin visitor can also get a more holistic view of the child and family in the home context.

Self-empowerment and support: Anne Jenkins (1996), the founder of Newpin, believes that the absence of hierarchy is crucial in effecting change to help mothers break destructive patterns of behaviour. Instead, there is a strong in-built infrastructure that deals with communications, networking, support systems and responsibility. These are all in play at the same time and it is made clear to each newcomer that they are as vital as the person who may have been a member for over 2 years. Newpin builds a strong supportive structure to help women while they are developing the ability to change themselves. Each woman gets a list of telephone numbers to contact as well as the back up from her own befriender. Mothers can ring people at night and at weekends if they need to talk. For isolated women at home with children this is of obvious help. A strong supportive system is also vital because Newpin's training programme involves extensive therapy. Another core feature of the Newpin programme is that health visitors are encouraged to maintain the mother and child's individual 'uniqueness'. This philosophy means that women aren't coming in as a mother with children to learn how to do things better; rather they are coming in primarily as their own self.

Personal development programme: A therapeutic support group is available to women once they feel ready to participate. An important part of this process is the modular personal development programme which reflects the anticipated stages of growth a mother will experience during her involvement with Newpin. The programme encourages the mother to value herself as a parent and a person, to form a creative and loving relationship with her child, to develop communicating and supportive skills towards others and 'Learning for life', the fourth module, deals with the world of further education or work. The approach which Newpin adopts is the promotion of parental growth and development but without jeopardising the parent–child bond or the child's right to safe autonomy (Jenkins 1996).

Key Recommendations for Replication

The Newpin programme has been implemented in Australia, and Mondy and Mondy (2004a, b) report on their experience of engaging the community in delivering this programme. They highlight the importance of the following features:

- provide parents with a safe and secure base that allows them to modify their early attachment experience
- peer support during the Newpin intervention enables parents and children to grow in confidence, have a greater belief in themselves and their abilities and gain knowledge about child protection issues
- include self-esteem and confidence-building components including, for example, courses on public speaking and computer literacy
- by adopting a strengths-based approach, the Newpin programme works to re-frame attitudes that label women as 'bad mothers' or 'child abusers' to 'parents who are trying to do the best for their kids'
- emphasise the positive aspects of change in the programme rather than the negatives of parenting difficulties
- the centres are places where members can feel safe to explore their own strengths and capacities and receive recognition of their own ability to bring about change
- work with the media in galvanising public opinion and gaining policy support in acceptance of the Newpin message in a non-stigmatising manner, i.e. that parents such as Newpin mothers recognise they have a problem and are working hard to bring about change for a successful future and are deserving of support.

Home-Start is a home visiting programme which offers support to families under stress with at least one child under 5 years of age. In 2003, there were 330 Home-Start schemes in the UK (England, Scotland, Wales and Northern Ireland) and more than 100 schemes internationally. Home-Start schemes have been developed in both rural and urban areas and support both white and ethnic minority families. Each scheme is run by a voluntary group with a multidisciplinary management committee and rooted in its own community. All schemes share the same standards and methods of practice. Evaluations of the Home-Start service have been carried out in the UK, Ireland and the Netherlands. However, significant long-term outcomes for families in receipt of the Home-Start service have not been clearly identified (McAuley et al 2004).

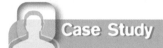 Case Study

Home-Start – a Case Study of a Community-Based Organisation Working with Families with Young Children

Brian Waller

Background

Home-Start is a well-established family support programme aimed at families under stress with at least one pre-school child. The programme is delivered by local Home-Start schemes in which parent volunteers offer regular support, friendship and practical help to families by visiting them in their own home, helping to prevent family crises and breakdown and emphasising the pleasure of family life. Home-based visiting is essential to the Home-Start approach which relies more on a realistic, flexible response and caring attitude than on a clearly structured method of working.

By sharing their time and friendship, volunteers offer families an opportunity to develop new relationships, ideas, skills and confidence. This often leads to renewed interest in the children, an improved response to their needs and greater confidence to avail themselves of other resources within the community. After attending a preparation course, volunteers are matched with a family and visit regularly. The approach varies according to the needs of each family and draws on the flexibility and good humour of the volunteer. Talking with the mother, playing with the children, helping in the home or accompanying the family on outings or appointments may all be offered. Anyone interested or concerned about the welfare of the family with the consent of the family can refer. Referrals usually come from health visitors and social workers. Other referrals come from various workers in the field of health care and from other voluntary organisations. Increasingly, families themselves ask for help from Home-Start. Referrals concern families who may be experiencing stress and difficulties because of a wide range of problems including loneliness, twins/triplets, budgeting problems, depression, marital problems, isolation, illness, disability, single parenting, lack of parenting skills, behavioural problems and mental health problems.

A typical local scheme has between 25 and 30 volunteers who, in the course of a year, support 50–60 families. Each scheme has a paid organiser who recruits, prepares and trains the volunteers and oversees and supports their work with individual families. Home-Start differs from many other family support programmes by focusing on parents' strengths rather than deficiencies and by adopting a holistic approach rather than attempting specific problem resolution. The objectives are to help rebuild parents' confidence and self-esteem and to assist families to widen their network of relationships and support and to use existing community services effectively.

In the UK, there are now over 300 Home-Start schemes. These operate in England, Wales, Northern Ireland and Scotland and cover rural as well as highly urban populations. Schemes are also run in Germany and Cyprus to support the families of service personnel living in British military bases. The Home-Start model has been adopted by other countries and now operates in Israel, Ireland, Norway, Russia, Hungary, Republic of South Africa, Australia, Canada and the Netherlands. In 2001/2, there were a total of 324 schemes operating and in total some 24 000 families and 54 000 children were supported.

Research and Evaluation

A number of studies have been carried out specifically to examine the effectiveness of Home-Start's work. All confirm that, however measured and whether to do with social isolation, mental health, child behaviour or the use of other services, Home-Start interventions work and are acceptable to families facing a range of challenges in their lives. Family support services based on home visiting generally have emerged very positively from the scrutiny of researchers and have demonstrated that over a significant number of variables their impact is substantial, beneficial and of long-lasting duration. Studies carried out to date:

1. Home-Start – a four year evaluation, 2nd edn. Willem van der Eyken, 1982, 1990
2. Crime and the family: improving child rearing and preventing delinquency, David Utting, Jon Bright, Clem Henricson, Family Policy Studies Centre, 1993
3. Family album: snapshots of Home-Start in words and pictures, Sheila Shinman, 1994
4. Negotiated friendship – Home-Start and the delivery of family support, Nick Frost, Liz Johnson, Mike Stein, Lorraine Wallis, School of Continuing Education, University of Leeds, 1996
5. A study of Home-Start, Lyn Rajan, Helen Turner, Ann Oakley, Social Science Research Unit, Institute of Education, University of London, 1996
6. Family health and Home-Start, Sheila Shinman, Brunel University, 1996
7. Needs and outcomes in families supported by Home-Start, Sheila Shinman, Brunel University, 1996
8. The family support outcomes study, Dr Colette McAuley, Queens University, Belfast, 1999

9. Home-Start in Scotland – an evaluation, Alison Kirkaldy, Anthony Crisp, 1999
10. Home-Start Kirklees: Study by Sue Taylor and Nationwide Children's Research Centre, 2001

A further study carried out by Professor Hermanns at the University of Amsterdam, 'Family risks and family support: an analysis of concepts', casts light onto how people cope with stresses and why holistic services such as Home-Start can be helpful.

Key Factors or Conditions that Made the Programme Possible and Ensured its Successful Planning and Delivery

The first Home-Start scheme was established in Leicester, England in 1973 in part as a response to parents of children in public care who felt that their families would not have broken up had early support been available to them. This 'prevention being better than cure' approach, which underpins the work of Home-Start, was seen as attractive by other communities. Over the course of the next few years, a number of similar schemes were set up in other cities and towns. In this initial phase, interested individuals visited the Leicester scheme and were helped and advised how to go about replicating the model.

The social context then and now has been one of rapid change for parents and families. After the stringencies of the post-war period, the growing economy and changing social attitudes placed enormous pressures on family life. Job mobility, patterns of employment in which women were drawn into the workforce and new attitudes to marriage and personal relationships were starting a process, which has continued and accelerated right up until the present time, of seismic change in family life. Traditional patterns of family structure and support were weakening and becoming more complex and diverse.

The expectation that the extended family, including friends and neighbours, could be on hand to help parents no longer held for many. In effect, and not even now fully appreciated, a significant gap has opened up between the needs of families and those who traditionally were able to meet those needs. This is true not only in the UK but in other European and western countries and arguably in other parts of the world. In Southern Africa, for example, it is certainly evident that traditional family structures are crumbling as a result of globalisation, urbanisation, poverty and diseases such as AIDS.

Against a backcloth of changing family structures, Home-Start saw the need to act positively by setting up new schemes. A separate franchising and development organisation, Home-Start Consultancy (later to become Home-Start UK and then just Home-Start), was set up to provide advice and technical assistance to groups and individuals interested in establishing their own schemes. This new organisation was able to concentrate on some of the key issues about core principles, quality standards and training as well as on planning how the Home-Start 'model' could best be replicated elsewhere. One decision taken early on was that the Home-Start approach was essentially a marque – a unique and special way of delivering a particular form of support to families in their own homes – and not a generalised method which might be varied and diluted. In other words, the home visiting pioneered in Home-Start Leicester and the early schemes was seen as not just another way of delivering support to families but a very explicit combination of ethos, values and working rules, based on practical experience as much as on theoretical design. The setting up of Home-Start Consultancy made it possible for these defining characteristics to be strongly embedded into all subsequent schemes.

Throughout Home-Start's development in the UK there has been active interest and support from government. The Department of Health initially, and then the Department for Education and the Home Office, have seen Home-Start as providing an important service to families by providing a range of benefits which complemented government policy and legislation on families and on children. During the last 30 years, successive governments have sought to emphasise the importance of preventive services so that family life can be protected and the costs and damage created by family break up minimised. Home-Start is viewed as a service which offers a coherent and cost-effective response to a wide range of family pressures which could lead to costly problems for individuals, families and the wider community. These include 'mental health' both in the wider sense, i.e., individuals' self-esteem and confidence, and as more specific problems such as anxiety states and depression. Home-Start does not see itself as a treatment service for mental illness as such but the support it offers to parents helps make a difference to people's mental health.

Programme Implementation and Recommendations

The successful growth and development of Home-Start in the UK and in other countries is partly explained by the simple (and therefore replicable) concept which lies behind the service. The notion that parents may need help from other parents at a time when their children are under school age has a universal appeal and potency especially at a time when traditional sources of support are weakening. There have been many challenges, however, which had to be tackled and which could have distracted or damaged the implementation of Home-Start's model service.

Funding is the most obvious issue for any developing voluntary organisation. It has been important for Home-Start to establish, at local and national levels, good links with funders and ensure that schemes are adequately funded from the outset. Schemes and countries that have tried to operate on a practical funding basis have struggled to keep going. The cost-effectiveness of initiatives such as Home-Start should be attractive to funders who might otherwise have to finance more expensive alternatives. Home-Start has worked hard to establish links at an appropriately senior level with officials for ministers to make sure that initial funding is available and that there is a genuine understanding and support for the service's work and potential contribution to local or national government policy.

Some funders or policy makers have sought to influence or change the Home-Start model, e.g. by requesting a change in the age criteria (under school age) or to direct the service towards the resolution of a particular problem such as teenage pregnancy or mental illness. These pressures have been resisted so that the core principles of the service can be protected. Home-Start works best when it is offered to families with young children (when help can be of greatest benefit) and in a holistic way. The service is not about problem resolution as such but about building confidence and support networks.

In most countries where it operates, Home-Start is developed as a non-governmental organisation 'franchise'. This has the advantage of offering local communities real ownership of their scheme and using the strengths of local people and networks. Schemes have generally been started on a bottom up-basis; it is left to local people to decide whether they want to have a Home-Start scheme in their community rather than having one imposed upon them by national or regional planners. This approach, certainly in the UK, has been one of the reasons why so few local schemes have closed. The sustainability record of Home-Start schemes in the UK is remarkable with only six schemes of now over 300 having had to shut down over the last 30 years.

The relationship between local schemes and the national bodies of Home-Start has been generally very positive unlike the traditional tensions and rivalry which often exist elsewhere. This has been achieved partly through the franchise approach – the national bodies do not manage the local schemes – but also through a two-way agreement. The Home-Start Agreement, to which local schemes sign up, requires them to operate within a prescribed and documented framework (the Home-Start Policy and Practice Guide) of principles, working methods and targets. It also requires the national organisation to provide support services to schemes at prescribed levels. There is an agreement review process which allows schemes and the national bodies to review each other's performance.

Written into these documents and systems is a reference to the Home-Start 'ethos'; essentially a statement of values and principles which help to ensure that schemes and the national bodies hold on to a way of working with families and with each other that is respectful, mutual and non-judgemental. Many organisations have explicit principles but Home-Start has worked hard to ensure that these are manifested in day-to-day practice and relationships and are visible and real for the families who use the service. The ethos exists almost as a tangible influence in staff selection, in training and in influencing every aspect of the organisation's work. Perhaps the reason it works is because it is in keeping with the essential design principle of Home-Start; that of parent volunteers working on an equal, respectful basis with other parents.

In recent years, there has been much more demand from funders for hard evidence about impact and outcomes. This did challenge the organisation which had relied heavily on anecdotal and personal evidence of its effectiveness with families. Some resistance was put up to the notions from researchers of 'experimental' and 'control' groups and to terminologies about 'interventions' and 'cases'. Similar objections have been raised about evaluation and monitoring and whether this kind of clinical/quantitative approach can co-exist in an organisation that takes pride in working with individuals on a very personal and confidential basis. Although the process has involved very detailed discussion and thought, it has proved possible to embark upon a series of research projects which do address issues of effectiveness whilst sensitively protecting families from being research guinea pigs or from being denied services.

As the number of Home-Start schemes has grown, there is another challenge presented by the twin threat of bureaucratisation and regulation. It is one thing to operate small scale non-governmental organisations with a human face. It is another to maintain this when the service is provided by many schemes and is moving towards universal coverage. Issues such as health and safety, employment legislation, insurance and management take on a greater significance in a larger organisation and present challenges to Home-Start's ability to retain its ability to work sensitively with people as individuals. The franchise model is of great help here in that it provides for a flat structure rather than a traditional management hierarchy. The model, however, is less easy to 'manage' in terms of achieving consistent levels of quality service and there is a debate as to what limits should be put on the way in which local schemes can diversify their service whilst sticking to Home-Start's core principles and targets.

Key Recommendations for Replication

- In considering the issue of replication, the most obvious point is whether the Home-Start model is relevant and applicable to other countries. It has operated successfully largely in high-income countries such as Norway, the Netherlands, Ireland, the UK, Canada, Hungary, Australia and Israel but is now being established in South Africa and there are plans to set up schemes in Kenya and Uganda. The service is based on local parent volunteers freely helping other families and this may not be a concept that can be assured worldwide. Although Home-Start has been shown to work in relation to problems of relationships, disability, ill health, etc., it is not known whether it can be as successful where there is extensive and primary poverty or where, as in the case of Africa, HIV/AIDS is a major problem for families.
- An international development organisation, Home-Start International, now exists to help interested countries establish Home-Start. Home-Start International has extensive overseas contacts and experience and also performs an important role in coordinating and enabling contact between the eight nations who already have established Home-Start schemes. Home-Start International performs an important function in both these respects and itself offers a model as to how programmes developed in one country can be successfully transferred to other countries.
- A key to the effective development of Home-Start outside the UK has been to ensure that there is high-level government support from the outset for the programme. Countries which have been less successful in trying to use the Home-Start model are those where interested individuals have attempted to set up schemes but without the backing financially and, in terms of policy support, of government.
- There is now at least the beginnings of an international body of literature and research about Home-Start. Some of this has been done in and by individual countries and some with the help of Home-Start International across international boundaries. This work is proving to be helpful in all countries by establishing a credible body of knowledge about effectiveness and about the complex process by which parents can be helped to deal with a wide range of problems.

Future Directions for Application of the Programme

There are three broad directions in which Home-Start looks to develop. The first is about the widening of the service in terms of the number of communities and countries that use the model. In the UK, there are presently 300+ schemes across all four countries – England, Wales, Scotland and Northern Ireland – and operating in rural as well as highly urban areas. There is potential to extend to all communities and this would involve the equivalent of some 500 schemes. The number may not need to be as high as this if some existing schemes extend their boundaries although schemes seem to work best on a local basis where local volunteers know their area and its facilities. Outside the UK, there is scope for Home-Start to be adopted by many more countries faced by similar issues of weakening family links and greater pressures on parents. The Home-Start model is essentially very simple and this makes it potentially very transferable and to some extent adaptable to different social environments. This leads to the second possible direction for the service which is about its adaptability, i.e. the possibility of the basic model being varied somewhat to meet local circumstances. In Israel, for example, Home-Start is used in some communities as the basis for the settlement of new immigrants whose prime problem is essentially one of loneliness and social isolation. In Germany, where the schemes operate with British Forces families, Home-Start works with families who have older children than in the UK simply because there are few other provisions for families experiencing difficulties with children over age for school entry. In the UK itself, many schemes add to the basic home visiting service by offering a range of add-on services such as toy libraries, groupwork sessions and safety equipment services because there is a demand for these services from parents. These variations on the basic service look sensible but it is not known, without research, whether they do add to the effectiveness of the service or whether they might detract from it.

The third possibility for considering a new direction for Home-Start lies in offering the service at the earliest possible stage to families, i.e. before and immediately after the birth of a child. It is known that, at least for some parents, these are particularly stressful times. It is also known that for children the early weeks and months of their lives are of critical importance. Traditionally, Home-Start has been offered to families somewhat later than this and it will be of great interest to know whether a service provided earlier would be of help to families who need support at that time in their lives. As well as these main directions for the service, there are other possible areas for development and consideration. These include a focus on fathers – the service at present tends to concentrate on supporting mothers – and a greater use of male or couple volunteers. Last but not least, it would be interesting to know to what extent any additional training of volunteers in, for example, mental health awareness or even particular skills, would make a difference to the outcomes of Home-Start's work.

. . . .

Voluntary sector programmes, such as those described above, have a critical role to play in building a system of comprehensive coordinated and family-focused promotion and prevention services in the primary care setting. Primary health care staff have an important function in terms of fostering more coordination and joint planning among what often appears as fragmented and family-unfriendly health and social services. These programmes are interdependent with the larger community and their effectiveness rests in part on the availability of other services for families as well as their capacity to connect with them. As Weiss (1993) points out, individual intervention programmes are necessary, but may not be entirely sufficient to reach and support the development of highly stressed or disadvantaged children and families. A major national initiative, Sure Start, was introduced in the UK to improve the emotional development of young children living in disadvantaged communities. Based on comprehensive, community-based projects, adapted to local needs, this initiative provides a range of services such as outreach and home visiting, support for learning and quality play, family health and child development services and support for children with special needs. The National Evaluation of Sure Start (NESS 2004, 2005) provides details on the impact and implementation process of this large-scale initiative.

Mood Management and Depression Prevention in Primary Care

Üstün (1998) argues that the primary care setting is the place where mental health promotion and prevention programmes are most needed. Epidemiological studies indicate the prevalence of mental health problems such as depression and anxiety in community samples and the frequency of their presentation in primary care services (Kessler et al 1994). Üstün et al (1995) report that for every 100 people with a mental health problem in the community, half decide to seek help and attend primary care, where approximately half are recognised. It is estimated that only 5% of those in the community go on to receive specialist services. Depression and anxiety disorders occur in up to 25% of primary care patients and are regarded as more disabling than many chronic physical illnesses (Muñoz 1998). Despite this, there is strong evidence that mental health problems, such as depression, frequently go unrecognised as the diagnosis is missed, and even when recognised a significant number remain untreated (Harris et al 1996, Sartorius et al 1996). Another major barrier to the identification of mental health problems is the stigma attached to mental disorders, which may prevent people who are most in need from disclosing their problems, thus making it extremely difficult for GPs to diagnose and appropriately refer patients. Most people with clinical levels of depression do not seek treatment, either because they do not recognise their problem as a mental health problem or because of stigma. In terms of improving the recognition of depression in primary care, Goldberg (1995) has outlined three approaches:

1. improving the consultation and interview technique of primary carers
2. the use of screening tools
3. bringing mental health services in to primary care.

Educational efforts to reduce stigma and improve awareness of both patients and doctors are described in Chapter 8.

The use of clinical practice guidelines as a tool to support best practice in relation to assessment, diagnosis, management and referral is increasing and, for example, WHO (1996) produced guidelines for primary care of common mental disorders which have been adapted for the UK (WHO Collaborating Centre 2000, Jenkins 2004) and elsewhere in both developed and developing countries. A number of developing countries have integrated mental health promotion and prevention into the routine work of primary care, for example Iran and Pakistan, but systematic research evaluation has not yet been conducted (Mohit 1999). Key features of the Iranian programme, for example, have included use of good practice guidelines, routine data collection on diagnosis, management, referral and outcomes, regular systematic supervision of the front line workers and curriculum consistency between the different cadres and levels of health workers (Institute of Medicine 2001).

Greater recognition of mental health problems such as depression in the primary care setting holds much potential in terms of suicide prevention, as depression is implicated in the majority of suicides (Muñoz 1997). General practitioner training in the recognition and treatment of depression has the potential to bring about reduced suicide risk at the community level. In 1983–1984 the Swedish Committee for the Prevention and Treatment of Depression launched an educational programme on the diagnosis and treatment of depressive disorders for all GPs on the island of Gotland (Rutz et al 1995). The proportion of depressive suicides was found to be significantly lower after the training interventions with estimated savings to society in terms of reduced sick leave and in-patient care from depressive disorders, drug prescriptions and the frequency of suicide (Rihmer et al 1995, Rutz et al 1995). Early recognition and adequate treatment of depression has a critical part to play in suicide prevention.

In addition to the need to recognise depression as a primary disorder, it may also occur as secondary to a range of medical conditions. Depression is more common in people with physical health problems (Peveler et al 2002) and may arise in conjunction with, or as a response to, chronic conditions associated with pain such as endocrine disorders, cerebrovascular disorders and infections such as AIDS/HIV. The prevalence of major depression is one of the highest of all disorders (not just mental disorders) seen in medical settings (Muñoz 1998). The prevalence of depression in the community appears to be increasing worldwide (Murray & Lopez 1996) and is predicted to rise to being second only to heart disease in the global burden of disease worldwide. Depression is related to many other public health concerns including substance abuse, violence, marital disruption and suicide (Muñoz 1998). Epidemiological studies show that major depression affects 17% of adults sometime in their lives and about 10% of them during any 1-year period (Kessler et al 1994). Women have about twice the rate of men. Muñoz (1998) points out that the likelihood of having an additional depressive episode is 50% after the first episode, 70% after two and 90% after three. Therefore, there is a strong argument for an effective identification of depression symptoms and the prevention of depression before it reaches clinical or chronic levels.

The onset of depression and its recurrence are influenced by a range of modifiable risk and protective factors at different stages of the lifespan. The identified risk factors include parental depression, inadequate parenting, child abuse and neglect, stressful life events and bullying (Hosman & Jané-Llopis 2005). Protective factors include sense of control, self-efficacy, stress resistance and social support. It has also been shown that early identification and treatment can effectively reduce recurring episodes (Muñoz 1998). Prevention programmes implemented across the lifespan have provided evidence of the reduction of elevated depressive symptoms thereby reducing the risk for major depressive disorders. Depression is also recognised as a precursor to suicide in both adolescents and older people and, therefore, programmes designed to promote improved emotional functioning and depression prevention have the potential to make a significant impact on suicide prevention (Walker & Townsend 1998).

It is recognised that even in high-income countries there is unlikely to be adequate provision of resources for mental health promotion, prevention and treatment. As depression often goes unrecognised and untreated, an intervention that provides alternative ways to effectively manage mood states and thereby avert the gradual entry into clinical depression has significant implications for population-level programmes delivered through the primary care setting. In order to reach a clinical level of depression, individuals may first go through a spell of gradually worsening depressive symptoms. As the duration, intensity and frequency of these depressive symptoms increases, the individual becomes more likely to develop a full-blown clinical episode of depression. Thus, providing individuals with strategies to manage negative mood should result in improved capacity for self-regulation of emotional health, lower depressive symptoms and reduced risk of developing major depression. As Clarke et al (1995) point out, such interventions hold the promise of reducing human misery and suffering and reducing health care costs by providing an intervention when it might have its most potent effects, i.e. before depression develops and requires more intensive and costly treatment. We will now examine one such programme, the San Francisco Depression Prevention Research project, as an example of a depression prevention programme based on mood management techniques delivered through a primary care setting.

277

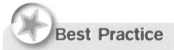

Best Practice

The San Francisco Depression Prevention Research Project

(Muñoz 1997, Muñoz & Ying 1993)

Background

In recognition of the fact that depression is a major public health problem, Muñoz (1998) proposes a framework for a comprehensive approach, which includes the adoption of promotion and prevention perspectives as well as treatment and maintenance strategies. The positive mental health aspect addresses the promotion of healthy emotional functioning and regulation of mood states through interventions designed to teach mood management skills. The prevention aspect addresses the potential of such interventions to reduce the risk of clinical depression, especially for those considered to be at higher risk from depression because of their personal, social, environmental and economic circumstances. One such intervention approach, the San Francisco Depression Prevention Research programme, developed and evaluated strategies for mood management in order to promote healthy emotional functioning and reduce the risk of developing clinical depression for poor ethnic minority patients attending primary care clinics in San Francisco (Muñoz et al 1987, 1995). The intervention, which was in the form of a group-based educational programme adopting a cognitive-behavioural approach, was evaluated by a randomised controlled trial. The evaluation produced impressive results in terms of lowering symptoms of depression for those who participated in the programme and promoting positive and more self-rewarding thoughts and increased pleasant activities. A detailed account of the San Francisco Depression Prevention Research project may be found in Muñoz and Ying's 1993 book titled 'The prevention of depression: research and practice' and in Albee and Gullotta's (1997) book 'Primary prevention works'.

Programme Content

The Depression Prevention Research project focused on low-income primary care patients from ethnic minority groups attending public sector clinics in the San Francisco area. This target group had high-risk markers of poverty and self-perceived health problems. The programme aimed to reduce the risk of clinical depression by teaching participants methods of mood management based on a social learning approach and cognitive-behavioural theory. The programme involved an educational component comprising of mood management skills. The 'Control your depression' book by Lewinsohn et al (1978, 1986) formed the basis for this course. The intervention, labelled the 'Depression prevention course', consists of eight weekly 2-hour sessions with no more than 10 students in the class. The order of group sessions is as follows:

1. Introduction
2. How activities affect mood
3. Increasing pleasant activities
4. How thoughts influence mood
5. Learning to change thoughts
6. How contacts with people affect mood
7. Increasing interpersonal activities
8. Planning for the future.

Participants were taught by trained programme implementers to identify their mood states and to learn to keep track of how specific thoughts, levels of pleasant activities and interpersonal contact either improved or worsened their mood. Course materials included two sections; an outline for participants and lecture notes for the instructors. The outline included homework forms on which the participant could document daily mood levels, frequencies of mood-related thoughts, activities and contacts with people. These forms were reviewed in class to illustrate the relationship between these events. Once these mood states were identified students were then taught to increase those thoughts, activities and interpersonal contact with others that led to positive mood states.

Evaluation

The evaluation study took place in the primary care clinics at San Francisco General Hospital and the University of California, San Francisco (Muñoz et al 1987, Muñoz et al 1995). Patients who had appointments during the recruitment phase of the study were asked if they would like to participate in the study. Two interviews of 2 hours' duration were conducted and a diagnostic screening instrument was used to exclude those who already met the criteria for major depression, dysthymia or other major disorders. These persons were then referred for treatment and screened out of the study. Participants were randomly assigned to an intervention group (n = 72) or control group (n = 78) and were followed up at 6 months and at 1 year. The evaluation aimed to determine depressive symptom levels and the incidence of depression and to determine whether there was an effect on changing the participants' thoughts, activity levels and social activities and whether changes in these variables were related to changes in depressive symptoms. Other factors such as levels of social support and life events were examined to determine if they had an effect on the results. At 1-year follow up the number of new cases of major depression was four in the control group and two in the intervention group; however, the latter two did not attend more than four of the eight sessions. The small number of new cases of major depression did not allow for a good statistical test of differences between the two conditions due to a lack of statistical power. However, the study did indicate reduced pessimism, increased self-rewarding thoughts and less self-punishing thoughts, and engagement in more pleasant and social activities amongst the intervention group. Furthermore, the intervention group reported a significantly greater reduction in depressive levels. The decline in depressive levels was significantly mediated by changes in the frequency of negative thinking and activity levels.

Programme Implementation Features

Adopting a mood-management approach: The programme was designed to provide an educational intervention that would not require individuals to take on the role of a 'patient'. Rather, the participants were involved as students learning about mood management skills. The view of depression as beginning with a problem in emotion regulation, becoming an unhealthy mood state and eventually becoming a major depression disorder forms the framework on which this intervention is based. This leads to a focus on averting problems in emotion regulation and identifying individuals with unhealthy mood states and providing them with methods to strengthen their emotion regulation capacity. Such an approach has widespread applicability in general community, schools and primary health service settings.

A theory-based intervention approach: The social learning and cognitive behavioural framework was utilised in this intervention due to the effectiveness of this approach in exhibiting a major improvement in mood state and reduced levels of depression in comparison with antidepressant medication in clinical populations (Beck et al 1979, Lewinshohn 1975). The theory underlying these treatment approaches was applied to develop an intervention for use in a promotion and prevention context. This theoretical approach posits a

279

reciprocal process in mood management involving mood, thoughts and behaviours. Specific thoughts and behaviours may increase or decrease the likelihood of depressed mood, and depressed mood in turn increases the likelihood that depressive thinking and behaviour will occur. Participants who learn to identify the elements in this process would be able to modify the thoughts and behaviours that lead to depressive mood states, and by reducing the likelihood of these states they would reduce the likelihood of experiencing a clinical episode.

A group-based format: The group-based approach provides individuals with an opportunity to practise and role play new skills and techniques acquired in the sessions. There is also an opportunity to use the dynamics of the group as a support to assist with learning and modelling of skills. A group intervention is also more cost-effective in that one teacher/facilitator can impact on as many as 10 people, thus making it more economically viable than one-to-one approaches and potentially offsetting the higher costs of more expensive treatment methods.

A non-stigmatising model of delivery: The approach used in this study has a number of advantages over other intervention models. For example, due to the stigma associated with mental health problems, participating in a course may be much more acceptable to individuals and health care providers than other interventions to treat depression.

Delivery by trained facilitators: The programme is provided by facilitators who are trained to teach the techniques and methods of the course. As delivery of the course is not limited to mental health professionals alone, the programme can reach a wider population at lower cost. However, it is essential that the facilitators be properly trained to implement the programme effectively and that the intervention provided be carefully evaluated.

Adherence to the programme: While it is recognised that there needs to be some flexibility in how the course is presented in different countries or cultural settings, it is critically important that the basic structure and content of the programme is not modified and that each session should remain the same and be delivered as intended.

Key Recommendations for Replication

The authors recommend that routine and inexpensive methods to identify those at high imminent risk of depression need to be developed. In this way participants who are at higher risk of major depression can be recruited for future intervention trials. Although this study's participants belonged to a group that was at higher risk than the general population as individuals, they had a high lifetime risk rather than a high current risk. The authors also recommend that effective and feasible methods to provide the interventions on a community-wide basis be developed. For example, bibliotherapy has also been shown to be effective in reducing depressive symptoms in older persons with mild to moderate clinical depression. Other adjunctive methods to aid the management of mood and prevention of depression in the primary care and community settings need to be examined.

. . . .

Dowrick et al (2000) investigated the acceptability and efficacy of a problem-solving approach and a group-based 'Coping with depression course' for adults with depression in the community. A multi-centre randomised controlled trial, carried out through the Outcome of Depression International Network (ODIN) group in nine sites across Europe, reported that participants of both interventions were less likely to remain in depression and more likely to report improved subjective mental and social functioning at 6 months post-intervention in comparison to control groups. The problem-solving intervention was found to be more acceptable; however, it was usually delivered in the participants' home whereas participants of the 'Coping with depression course' had to travel to access this group-based programme. Based on the same principles as the Muñoz programme, Clarke et al (1995) developed and implemented a 'Coping with depression course' with adolescents in Oregon, USA. The course consisted of 15 45-minute group sessions in which at-risk adolescents were taught cognitive techniques to identify and challenge negative thoughts that may contribute to future development of depression. Employing cartoons, role play and group discussions, adolescent participants were trained in cognitive restructuring skills to enable them to identify and reduce negative cognitions and thereby reduce the risk of depression. A randomised controlled trial of this cognitive intervention demonstrated a statistically significant reduction in new cases of major depression among the intervention group. At 1 year post-intervention, those students who took the course had incidence rates of 14.5% of affective disorder compared to 25.7% for the control group. The Resourceful Adolescent Program in Australia, which also uses a cognitive approach, reported reduced depressive symptoms in 12–15-year-olds (Shochet et al 2001). These findings suggest that cognitive interventions and problem-solving techniques can be successfully implemented across the lifespan to improve emotional and social functioning and thereby prevent the development of depression among both adults and adolescents at risk. Such programmes can be successfully delivered through the primary care setting as brief interventions that are effective and accessible to community members. A case study of a psycho-educational intervention for low-income women in Mexico will now be examined in order to illustrate the implementation of a depression prevention programme adapted to local needs and circumstances.

Case Study

A Psycho-Educational Intervention for Women with Depressive Symptoms: Programme Implementation in Low-Income Settings

Ma. Asunción Lara

Background

This case study reports on a psycho-educational intervention that was developed and evaluated for low-income women displaying both depressive symptoms and clinical depression (with no suicidal ideation, suicide attempts or psychiatric co-morbidity). This intervention targeted women aged 25 to 45 and was carried out at primary health and mental health settings in Mexico City. The intervention can be considered multi-component. The educational component, which relies on the purposely designed material (Lara et al 1997) written in a comic strip format, seeks to provide information that contributes to the understanding of depression in relation to three aspects; its manifestation, causes and ways of coping with it. The psychological component aims to reduce depressive symptoms using techniques that allow a better understanding of such symptoms and current problems, increasing positive thinking and actions, widening the behavioural repertoire, increasing self-esteem and improving problem solving. The group component involves the creation of an atmosphere of trust and support that facilitates the expression of emotions and change. The approach is gender sensitive in that it considers gender issues associated with the development and maintenance of depression in women. The intervention programme draws from local research findings on women's mental health and clinical practice as much as experience in other countries. Muñoz and Ying's (1993) prevention of depression programme provided a framework to guide the development of the intervention programme. To ensure delivery of the programme according to specifications, a manual was developed (Lara et al 2001). The programme was delivered in two ways: six two-hour weekly sessions or a single 20-minute to 1-hour orientation session. Post-intervention and follow-up assessments showed that both were equally effective in reducing depressive symptoms (Lara et al 2003b) and that the former was slightly better in leading to participants' satisfaction (Lara et al 2003a, Lara et al 2003c).

Key Factors that Made the Programme Possible and Ensured its Successful Planning and Delivery

The following headings (pre-adoption, pilot studies, delivery, efficacy, effectiveness and process evaluation) are related to the implementation that took place as part of the outcome study. Having the research study implemented in a community setting meant that the research itself was complicated since many conditions were difficult to control, although on the other hand it facilitated transference of the programme back to the community. The dissemination aspect addresses issues related to the implementation of the intervention by the community.

Pre-adoption: Creating partnership was crucial to securing support for programme delivery. There are wide cultural differences regarding how to go about locating and motivating suitable partners. We found that there could be agreements at the top levels which did not ensure that the operative level staff would be willing to collaborate, or conversely, staff could be highly motivated because they could more directly perceive the benefits of the programme yet such programmes were not always supported by, nor did they form part of, the organisation's goals. Too many administrative procedures sometimes led to long delays while in some instances too little formality meant starting negotiations all over again every time there was a change in personnel at the decision-making level. Creating partnership entailed showing potential benefits to recipient agencies as well as ensuring that the staff concerned (GPs, psychiatrists, psychologists, nurses and social workers) were involved as much as possible. In this programme, this required providing information on the intervention and asking staff to participate by referring potential candidates. Other benefits of achieving a firm alliance with agencies was the support they provided by appointing their social workers or psychiatric nurses to promote the programme in the community where they are known and trusted, and in conducting follow-up interviews in the participants' homes.

Pilot studies: Investing effort in pilot studies was worthwhile, especially as previous experience was scarce. This was particularly important in a less developed country such as Mexico where there tends to be less local knowledge on many research topics and, since available knowledge comes from the more affluent countries, it applies mostly to the latter's problems and resources. A great deal of adaptation and translation was necessary. In this case study programme, the feasibility study helped determine an appropriate recruitment strategy and obtain knowledge about the target population, the general functioning of the programme, the length of follow up required and suitable partners (Lara et al 1999).

Delivery:

- Programme model: The educational material was the cornerstone in the planning and delivery of the intervention. The appropriateness of the material in terms of culture, gender and social context was a key consideration. Evidence had previously been gathered that the material was easy to read and appealed to women. The structured material helped set out the aims of the programme and structure the sessions around key programme components and activities, thereby increasing programme adherence.

- Implementation support system: The inclusion of a clinical psychologist on the team, together with the high standard of training of the research team and the high morale that prevailed despite the difficulties involved, contributed to the success of the programme. Developing an intervention manual ensured the quality of programme delivery as much as the evaluation of the fidelity of delivery of the intervention by videotaping the sessions. The fact that the manual included guidelines (rules such as keeping what is said in the group confidential, developing an attitude of friendship and support, not judging others, trying not to give advice) for the proper functioning of the group, and that these were explained to the participants, led to respectful exchanges that enabled the intervention to develop within a conflict-free atmosphere. Having well-defined selection criteria for participants was also a crucial issue, since women displaying more severe conditions might not have benefited from the intervention.

Efficacy, effectiveness and process evaluation: Apart from measuring effectiveness in terms of reducing symptoms and increasing self-esteem (Lara et al 2003b), a more qualitative evaluation of participants' subjective perception in terms of the impact of the intervention and reasons for perceiving this impact, useful aspects of the intervention, reasons for attending the intervention, compliance with intervention requirements (Lara et al 2003c) and evaluation of the group process from audiotapes, provided very useful information for further implementation (Lara et al 2004). These results showed which components of the programme participants valued most and allowed the identification of certain group therapeutic factors in the group process and established the basis for further suggestions for the implementation of the programme in the community.

Dissemination

To assure programme sustainability, a training course was designed and delivered on a regular basis. The course is designed to be used by mental health workers who are required to have some experience conducting groups to be familiar with gender issues. As the Institute of Psychiatry has a tradition in continuous education courses in mental health, there were not many obstacles to attracting people interested in replicating the intervention from the beginning. Over the past 5 years, 680 people from both governmental and non-governmental organisations have attended the courses.

At the moment, a study is being conducted to assess dissemination effectiveness and implementation in a sample of 35 of these trained people. Preliminary results show that some institutions have adopted the intervention as one of their permanent programmes for the prevention of depression in women. It has also been found that facilitators consider that the implementation has been facilitated by the educational material for participants, the guide for facilitators and the training course, all of which have led to a high-standard and effective intervention. The fact that the programme is highly structured and provides pre- and post-treatment evaluations has enabled facilitators to structure their work in a more systematic way which in turn has led to recognition from their superiors. Although there have not, so far, been the resources to conduct field observations to assess aspects of fidelity versus adaptation, some of the facilitators mentioned that they try to implement the programme with almost no variation while others have included more sessions to address other aspects such as self-esteem. It would also be important to have outsiders carry on an outcome study to assess the effectiveness of the programme in the community.

The intervention has also been implemented with Latino women in the US. In order to respond to their specific needs, it has proved necessary to gather more information on important issues of depression in this population in order to develop a manual based on a local study which will help local implementation.

New challenges related to implementation are beginning to emerge now that a training course for facilitators is being developed on-line, but at the same time new opportunities are arising since closer contact with trainees (via e-mail) is possible regarding the everyday problems they face in the process of implementing the programme.

Key Recommendations for Replication

The following factors have been identified as contributing to the successful implementation and dissemination of the programme:

- developing and adapting the programme materials for the local setting
- developing an intervention manual to ensure quality of programme delivery
- obtaining additional resources for developing a training programme for facilitators, offering training on a regular basis for participating agencies and following up institutions that have adopted the intervention
- making the educational materials available in bookshops has meant that many people seek more information or advice on how to use it. Having a special contract with the editor to provide books at a reasonable price, so that the material can reach the target population of low-income women, has also proved useful.

Intervention projects, like the one reported here, are long-term multi-stage programmes that therefore require large amounts of human and material resources for their implementation and evaluation, which is a challenge in less developed countries where fewer resources are allocated to research and health care. However, it is clear that evaluation findings, especially those that are sensitive to the importance of implementation, play a critical role in demonstrating the potential of a programme and may, therefore, be vital in securing funding for sustaining an initiative in the longer term.

References

Lara M A, Acevedo M, Luna S et al 1997 ¿Es difícil ser mujer? Una guía sobre depresión [Is it difficult to be a woman? A guide to depression]. Editorial Pax, México

Lara M A, Mondragón L, Rubí N A 1999 Un estudio de factibilidad sobre la prevención de la depresión en las mujeres [A feasibility study on the prevention of depression in women]. Salud Mental 22(4):41–48

Lara M A, Acevedo M, Luna S 2001 ¿Es difícil ser mujer? Guía didáctica para el trabajo de grupo [Is it difficult to be a woman? Manual for group work]. Editorial Pax, Mexico

Lara M A, Navarro C, Navarrete L et al 2003a Seguimiento a dos años de una intervención psicoeducativa para mujeres con síntomas de depresión [Two-year follow-up of psycho-educational intervention for women with symptoms of depression]. Salud Mental 26(3):23–36

Lara M A, Navarro C, Rubí N A et al 2003b Outcome of two levels of intervention in low-income women with depressive symptoms. American Journal of Orthopsychiatry 73(1):35–43

Lara M A, Navarro C, Rubí N A et al 2003c Two levels of intervention in low-income women with depressive symptoms. Compliance and programme assessment. International Journal of Social Psychiatry 49(1):43–57

Lara M A, Navarro C, Acevedo M et al 2004 A psycho-educational intervention for depressed women: a qualitative analysis of the process. Psychology and Psychotherapy: Theory Research and Practice 77(4):429–447

Muñoz R F, Ying Y 1993 The prevention of depression: research and practice. John Hopkins University Press, Baltimore

Mental Health Promotion Training for Primary Care Workers

Primary health care workers include general practitioners or family physicians, nurses, social workers, midwives, psychologists, occupational therapists, counsellors and social care workers among others. Primary health care workers are in a position to support and participate in the delivery of a range of mental health promotion and prevention programmes that are community wide and available to all community members without stigma. They are also in a position to provide mental health advice, to play a role in identifying potential mental health problems and to help community residents access specialist services and expertise in voluntary and statutory services. However, many primary health care staff may not have a focus on mental health and may not have appropriate training to engage in the implementation of mental health promotion initiatives. There is a need for training and skill development in developing and implementing mental health promotion programmes. A training programme for primary health care workers in the promotion of children's psychosocial development will now be illustrated through a case study based on its implementation across seven European countries, namely Cyprus, Greece, Portugal, Serbia, Slovenia, Turkey and the UK.

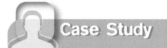 **Case Study**

Promotion of Children's Early Psychosocial Development: the Implementation of a Programme through Primary Health Care Services in the General Population

John Tsiantis, Kalliroi Papadopoulou

Background

This case study reports on a multicultural and interdisciplinary project which focused on the promotion of psychosocial development of infants and young children in the general population (Papadopoulou et al 2002, Tsiantis et al 1996, Tsiantis et al 2000, WHO 1992). The developed approach was applied in Cyprus, Greece, Portugal, Serbia, Slovenia, Turkey and the UK. Of the reported countries, the UK maintained a consultancy role; Slovenia and Turkey did not complete the study. The programme was financially supported by the EU for the member states (BIOMED 1-CT94 1161) and it was partly financed by the World Health Organization, Regional Office for Europe, Division of Mental Health, for the other participating countries. It comprised a three year intervention (pregnancy to 2 years) model, employing public health networks for its implementation. Its aim was to develop a training programme for primary health care professionals (PHCPs) as well as a specific intervention technique in the form of semi-structured interviews, so as to enable PHCPs to sensitise and mobilise parents in their parenting role and to encourage problem-solving strategies within the family. In order to evaluate the effectiveness of the programme an experimental design was followed in the study whereby PHCPs and, consequently, the participating families (recruited through the PHCPs), were assigned to an intervention and a comparison group.

More specifically, the developed training aimed to produce a direct, specific and measurable effect on the attitudes, beliefs and activities of PHCPs regarding their everyday practices. It was designed to sensitise PHCPs to psychological issues and social factors relevant to parenthood, general indicators of good parenting and aspects of children's early psychosocial development and needs. It also aimed to teach PHCPs to use the semi-structured interviews in a fashion that alerts caregivers to their children's needs and encourages them to adopt problem-solving approaches using the parents' own resources where appropriate. Training was based on the principles of empathy, modelling and the development of a parent–child relationship characterised by mutual pleasure and trust, axes that also formed the basis for effective intervention. As a result of training, PHCPs were expected to be more effective in their intervention with families, to be able to define their professional boundaries in relation to mental health personnel and to identify cases for referral to mental health services. Training was organised around three phases of development, namely pregnancy, the first and the second year of the child's life. It comprised 23 3-hour long sessions, with a theoretical and an experiential component (Tsiantis et al 1996). The training programme was attended by the PHCPs of the intervention group.

The intervention was based on the same principles as training and was implemented through five semi-structured interviews, developed for the purposes of the programme (see sample in Appendix 7.1), which served as the main instrument to guide and facilitate PHCPs' contacts with the families. The developed interviews were intricately related to the contents of training and followed the principles of semi-structured interviewing (Cox 1984). They were applied on five pre-scheduled contacts (i.e. during pregnancy and at 6 weeks, 6 months, 12 months and 24 months after birth), by PHCPs of both groups. Throughout the study, PHCPs of the intervention group received group supervision by a mental health professional once a month.

The programme was evaluated both nationally and across the different countries in terms of:

- the impact of training on both the PHCPs' knowledge and attitudes with regard to infant behaviour and development, as well as on practice as assessed by the delivery of the semi-structured interview
- the effect of intervention on maternal emotional well-being, infant language development and behaviour, home environment and mother–infant interaction.

Multi-centre results have provided indications that PHCPs can be trained effectively in methods appropriate to mental health promotion and primary prevention focused on the psychosocial aspects of child development. Training produced changes in the knowledge, attitudes and practice of PHCPs and the intervention produced some effects in relation to supporting mothers in their role and making them feel and cope better (Tsiantis et al 2000). Regarding the effect on participating families, results were not always as expected; positive outcomes were confined to individual countries (Papadopoulou et al 2002) and the total impact of the programme was not as strong as expected.

Key Factors that Made the Programme Possible and Ensured its Successful Planning and Delivery

- The programme was designed so that its content, structure and application would be feasible within existing primary health care resources, working in collaboration with specialist mental health services. Furthermore, it addressed a 'normal' population with interesting implications for children and families in need. In that respect, the developed methods constitute a contribution in the field of mental health promotion and primary prevention.
- The programme addressed a need of PHCPs for better training in issues of parenting and children's psychosocial development, thus improving and expanding their professional opportunities to some extent at least, as well as the need of families for better services regarding issues of mental and not just physical health.
- The inclusion of a theoretical and an experiential component in the training structure ensured both the establishment of theoretical knowledge in PHCPs and the opportunity to discuss and to work out experiences connected with the content of the lectures and their professional practice.
- Supervision was an important component for consolidating the gains of training as well as for maintaining the coherence of the intervention group.
- The application of the semi-structured interviews at specific time intervals facilitated the contacts of PHCPs with the families and maintained some degree of consistency in the way they carried out the intervention.
- Workshops on training and evaluation procedures amongst the participating centres were important for the development of the approach as well as for ensuring the best possible uniformity in its application across the different countries.
- Effective coordination with frequent communication and meetings assisted in resolving administrative problems as well as difficulties in the programme's implementation.

Implementation Challenges and Experiences that Arose in the Course of Programme Delivery

Problems related to the longitudinal nature of the study: Maintaining the motivation of participating PHCPs, especially those of the comparison group, as well as of drop-outs (which is inherent in longitudinal research), presented difficulties in the delivery of the programme. Efforts to maintain motivation and to sustain the comparison group of PHCPs included group meetings with a supervisor once every 3 months in order to discuss implementation problems, regular communication with PHCPs on a personal basis, organisation of social events, lectures on mental health issues which differed from the core issues of the delivered training, facilitation of attendance of conferences, meetings, etc.

Challenges and problems related to the multicultural nature of the study:

• Sample problems: mainly related to the selection of comparable PHCP samples across participating countries due to differences in the public health networks involved in primary care (for example, PHCPs were student health visitors in Cyprus, health visitors in Greece, family doctors in Portugal, pediatricians in Serbia). At the same time, this diversity proved that cooperation across countries is possible and resulted in a community promotion and prevention programme with potential to be applied across different countries and within different primary health care systems.

• Implementation challenges and difficulties: the study took great care in ensuring uniformity in training and the delivery of semi-structured interviews. However, such a multicultural study cannot disregard cultural differences, variations in health care practices as well as the differences in the theoretical orientation of trainers in the different countries. The training workshops, the close cooperation and the existence of concrete training guidelines proved significant assistants in facing this challenge.

• Evaluation issues: problems involved the identification, creation or adaptation of appropriate as well as easy to apply instruments which were not always standardised and the failure to establish inter-rater reliabilities between participating countries.

Key Recommendations for Replication

The developed procedures must:

• be easy to apply within existing health care systems and practices
• be accessible to large portions of the population
• be usable with minimal training
• make effective use of existing primary health care and mental health services.

Future Directions for Application of the Programme

The future regarding the programme's applications may take two directions, deriving from both its strengths and weaknesses:

1. The evidence stemming from the project's evaluation provides indications of the usefulness of community programmes for mental health promotion in the general population. The obtained results suggest that training and interventions, which are not targeted specifically at a particular condition and which address normal populations, may improve the skills of involved PHCPs and may produce some effect on critical issues of parenting. The programme is thus expected to be useful to public health policy makers and consultants as well as to specialists and students in the area of primary health care. It is also recommended to be incorporated in the initial training of PHCPs as well as in programmes for lifelong learning and continuous development within the workplace.

2. The second direction for the programme's future applications stems from its limitations in producing larger scale measurable effects on children and

families. This may suggest that the effects of training 'washed out' into the largely normal population of mothers and young children who were not expected to have significant problems in their psychosocial development. The lack of the expected effect on mothers and children may also be due to the fact that training was more broad based and less focused to the parameters assessed, such as language and infant development. It is possible that if the research had been conducted with mothers who were more disadvantaged or in a situation where the whole population could be considered needy, the impact of training might have been more evident in the outcomes for children and their mothers (Tsiantis et al 2000). This direction has been taken up in a new study (Puura et al 2002, 2005a), with aims and design similar to the presented programme. The difference is that this new approach aimed at early detection of conditions that put a child's development at risk, so that the intervention is focused on children and families according to need. The results of this study confirmed its effectiveness in training PHCPs to apply promotional and preventive methods (Papadopoulou et al 2005), indicated the formation of a partnership in the form of a working alliance between the PHCP and the parent as essential for the provision of help to participating families (Davis & Tsiantis 2005, Tsiantis et al 2005) and had some positive effects on mother–child interaction (Puura et al 2005b) as well as on child and family outcomes (Davis et al 2005), especially in cases where need had been identified.

References

Cox A D 1984 Interviews with parents. In: Rutter M, Taylor E, Hersov R (eds) Child and adolescent psychiatry: modern approaches. Blackwell, Oxford

Davis H, Tsiantis J 2005 Promoting children's mental health: the European Early Promotion Project (EEPP). International Journal of Mental Health Promotion, Special Issue 7(1):4–16

Davis H, Dusoir T, Papadopoulou K et al 2005 Child and family outcomes of the EEPP. The International Journal of Mental Health Promotion, Special Issue 7(1):63–81

Papadopoulou K, Tsiantis J, Dragonas T et al 2002 Maternal postnatal emotional well-being and perceived parenting hassles: does community intervention with normal populations make a difference? International Journal of Mental Health Promotion 4(3):13–24

Papadopoulou K, Dimitrakaki C, Davis H et al 2005 The effects of the EEPP training on primary health care professionals. International Journal of Mental Health Promotion, Special Issue 7(1):54–62

Puura K, Davis H, Papadopoulou K et al 2002 The European Early Promotion Project: a new service for promotion of children's mental health in primary health care. Infant Mental Health Journal 23:606–624

Puura K, Davis H, Cox A et al 2005a The EEPP description of the service and evaluation study. International Journal of Mental Health Promotion, Special Issue 7(1):17–31

Puura K, Davis H, Mantymaa M et al 2005b The outcome of the EEPP: mother–child interaction. International Journal of Mental Health Promotion, Special Issue 7(1):82–94

Tsiantis J, Dragonas T, Cox A D et al 1996 Promotion of children's early psychosocial development. Paediatric and Perinatal Epidemiology 10:339–354

Tsiantis J, Smith M, Dragonas T et al 2000 Early mental health promotion in children through primary health care services: a multi-center implementation. International Journal of Mental Health Promotion 2(3):5–17

Tsiantis J, Papadopoulou K, Davis H et al 2005 EEPP: conclusions, implications and future directions. International Journal of Mental Health Promotion, Special Issue 7(1):103–110

WHO (World Health Organization) 1992 Promoting the psychosocial development of children through Primary Health Care Services. Report on a WHO meeting. Sofia, 13–15 December

Generic Principles of Effective Programmes in the Primary Care Setting

Primary care offers both opportunities and challenges for promoting mental health and preventing mental health problems. The primary health care setting serves as an entry point into the health system and has the potential to serve as a sustained support for maintaining health and well-being. Further research is needed to determine the most effective way of using this opportunity. Based on the research evidence and the programmes examined in this chapter, the following characteristics of successful mental health promotion programmes in the primary health care setting are highlighted in order to guide effective practice:

- programmes adopting a competence enhancement and empowering approach, working in partnership with families and the local community
- programmes and initiatives that adopt an ecological approach, i.e. see the child or adult as a member of a family and the family as a member of the community, engendering a better appreciation of how circumstances affect both the parents' and child's development capacities
- home visiting programmes that seek to address a broad spectrum of family needs are more effective than single focus programmes
- programmes that focus on families with a high level of need such as unsupported and young families, families living in poverty and those having children with a high level of need
- comprehensive programmes that employ multiple methods, are broad spectrum and tailored to meet local needs
- sustained high quality of input and continuity of input so that a relationship of trust and mutual respect is established
- interventions accompanied by interagency and cross-sectoral community working, facilitating access to integrated health, education and social services
- programmes which critically monitor their implementation in context and assess how programme delivery is affected by, and how it can positively influence, formal and informal family services and supports
- programmes delivered in a non-stigmatising and accessible manner, reaching those most in need
- programmes integrating mental and physical health goals, such as exercise programmes
- skilled and trained staff orientated to recognise and respond to the mental health needs of the local community.

291

References

Albee G W, Gullotta T P 1997 (eds) Primary prevention works, vol 6: issues in children's and families lives. Sage, London

Anderson R J, Freeland K E, Clouse R E et al 2001 The prevalence of co-morbid depression in adults with diabetes: a meta-analysis. Diabetes Care 24:1069–1078

Ashenden R, Silagy C, Weller D 1997 A systematric review of effectiveness of promoting lifestyle change in general practice. Family Practice 14:160–175

Beck A T, Rush A J, Shaw B F et al 1979 Cognitive therapy of depression. Guilford Press, New York

Brugha T S, Wheatley S, Taub N A et al 2000 Pragmatic randomised trial of antenatal intervention to prevent post-natal depression by reducing psychosocial risk factors. Psychological Medicine 30:1273–1281

BTCV (British Trust for Conservation Volunteers) 1999 Green Gym: an evaluation of a pilot project in Sonning Common. Oxford Brookes University, Oxfordshire

BTCV 2001 Well-being comes naturally: evaluation of the Portslade Green Gym. Oxford Brookes University, Oxfordshire

Carson A J, MacHale S, Allen K et al 2000 Depression after stroke and lesion location: a systematic review. Lancet 356:122–126

Clarke G N, Hawkins W, Murphy M et al 1995 Targeted prevention of unipolar depressive disorder in an at-risk sample of high school adolescents: a randomised trial of a group cognitive intervention. Journal of the American Academy of Child and Adolescent Psychiatry 34(3):312–321

Cooper P J, Landman M, Tomlinson M et al 2002 Impact of a mother-infant intervention in an indigent peri-urban South African context: pilot study. British Journal of Psychiatry 180:76–81

Cox A, Pound A, Mills M et al 1991 Evaluation of a home visiting and befriending scheme for young mothers: Newpin. Journal of the Royal Society of Medicine 84(4):217–220

Daley A J 2002 Exercise therapy and mental health in clinical populations: is exercise therapy a worthwhile intervention? Advances in Psychiatric Treatment 8:262–270

DeBoer M F, McCormick L K, Pruyn J F et al 1999 Physical and psychosocial correlates of head and neck cancer: a review of the literature. Otolaryngology – Head and Neck Surgery 120(3):427–436

Dowrick C, Dunn G, Ayuso-Mateos J L et al 2000 Problem solving treatment and group psychoeducation for depression: multicentre randomised trail. British Medical Journal 321:1–6

Elliott S A, Sanjack M, Leverton T J 1988 Parents groups in pregnancy: a preventive intervention for postnatal depression. In: Gottlieb B J (ed) Marshalling social support: formats, processes and effects. Sage, California

Elliott S A, Leverton T J, Sanjack M et al 2000 Promoting mental health after childbirth: a controlled trial of primary prevention of postnatal depression. British Journal of Clinical Psychology 39:223–241

Fox K R 2000 Physical activity and mental health promotion: the natural partnership. International Journal of Mental Health Promotion 2(1):4–12

Goldberg D 1995 Epidemiology of mental disorders in primary care settings. Epidemiologic Reviews 17:182–190

Goodwin J S 2000 Glass half full attitude promotes health in old age. Journal of American Geriatrics Society 48:473–478

Harris M F, Silove D, Kehog E et al 1996 Anxiety and depression in general practice patients: prevalence and management. The Medical Journal of Australia 164:526–529

Hayes B A, Muller R, Bradley B S 2001 Perinatal depression: a randomised controlled trial of an antenatal education intervention for primiparas. Birth 28(1):28–35

Hillsdon M, Thoroughgood M, Antiss T et al 1995 Randomised controlled trials of physical activity promotion in free living populations: a review. Journal of Epidemiology and Community Health 49:448–453

Hippisley-Cox J, Fielding K, Pringle M 1998 Depression as a risk factor for ischaemic heart disease in men: population based case control study. British Medical Journal 316:1714–1719

Hodnett E D 1997 Support from caregivers during childbirth. In: Neilson J P, Crowther C A, Hodnett E D et al (eds) Pregnancy and childbirth module of the Cochrane database of systematic reviews, issue 2. Cochrane Library, Oxford

Hodnett E D, Roberts I 1997 Home-based social support for socially disadvantaged mothers. In: Neilson J P, Crowther C A, Hodnett E D et al (eds) Pregnancy and childbirth module of the Cochrane database of systematic reviews, issue 2. Cochrane Library, Oxford

Hosman C, Jané-Llopis E 2005 The evidence of effective interventions for mental health promotion. In: Herrman H, Saxena S, Moodie R (eds) Promoting mental health: concepts, emerging evidence, practice. A report of the World Health Organization, Department of Mental Health and Substance Abuse in collaboration with the Victorian Health Promotion Foundation and University of Melbourne,WHO, Geneva:169–184

Institute of Medicine 2001 Neurological, psychiatric and developmental disorders – meeting the challenge in the developing world. Institute of Medicine, National Academy Press, Washington

Jenkins A 1996 Newpin: a creative mental health service for parents and children. In: Gopfer M, Webster J, Seeman M V (eds) Parental psychiatric disorder. Cambridge University Press, Cambridge

Jenkins R (ed) 2004 WHO guide to mental and neurological health in primary care, 2nd edn. Royal Society of Medicine, London

Jenkins R, Üstün T B (eds) 1998 Preventing mental illness: mental health promotion in primary care. John Wiley, Chicester

Johnson Z, Howell F, Molloy B 1993 Community Mothers Programme: randomised controlled trial of non-professional intervention in parenting. British Medical Journal 306:1449–1452

Jonas B S, Mussolino M E 2000 Symptoms of depression as a prospective risk factor for stroke. Psychosomatic Medicine 62(4):463–472

Kessler R C, McGonagle K A, Shanyang Z et al 1994 Lifetime and 12-month prevalence of DSM-III-R psychiatric disorders in the United States: results from the National Comorbidity Survey. Archives of General Psychiatry 51(1):8–19

Kuper H, Singh-Manoux A, Siegrist J et al 2002 When reciprocity fails: effort-reward imbalance in relation to coronary heart disease and health functioning within the Whitehall II study. Occupational Environmental Medicine 59:777–784

Lewinsohn P M 1975 The behavioural study and treatment of depression. In: Herson M, Eisler M, Miller P M (eds) Progress in behaviour modification, vol 1. Academic Press, New York:19–64

Lewinshohn P M, Muñoz R F, Youngren M A et al 1978 Control your depression. Prentice Hall, New York

Lewinshohn P M, Muñoz R F, Youngren M A et al 1986 Control your depression (revised edition). Prentice Hall, New York

McAuley C, Knapp M, Beecham J et al 2004 Evaluating the outcomes and costs of Home-Start support to young families experiencing stress: a comparative cross nation study. Joseph Rowntree Foundation, York

Marcenko M O, Spence M 1994 Home visitation services for at-risk pregnant and postpartum women: a randomized trial. American Journal of Orthopsychiatry 64:468–478

Mentality 2003 Making it effective: a guide to evidence based mental health promotion. Radical mentalities – briefing paper 1. Mentality, London

Mohit A 1999 Mental health in the eastern Mediterannean region of the World Health Organisation with a view of the future trends. East Mediterranean Health Journal 5:231–240

Mondy L 2001 A study of a child protection program – NEWPIN. What are the experiences of the participants: children, mothers and staff? Unpublished Masters dissertation, University of Newcastle, Australia

Mondy L P, Mondy S 2004a Engaging the community in child protection programmes: the experience of NEWPIN. Australia Child Abuse Review 13(6):433–440

Mondy L P, Mondy S 2004b Situating NEWPIN in the context of parent education and support models. Children Australia 29(1):19–25

Morrell C J, Spiby H, Stewart P et al 2000 Costs and benefits of community postnatal support workers: a randomized controlled trial. Health Technology Assessment 4(6):1–100

Muñoz R F 1997 The prevention of depression: toward the healthy management of reality. Keynote address presented at the Seventh Annual European Conference on the Promotion of Mental Health, Maastricht, The Netherlands, October 9

Muñoz R F 1998 Preventing major depression by promoting emotion regulation: a conceptual framework and some practical tools. International Journal of Mental Health Promotion, Inaugural Issue:23–40

Muñoz R F, Ying Y 1993 The prevention of depression: research and practice. John Hopkins University Press, Baltimore

Muñoz R F, Ying Y, Armas R et al 1987 The San Francisco depression prevention project: a randomized trial with medical outpatients. In: Muñoz R F (ed) Depression prevention: research directions. Hemisphere, Washington DC:199–215

Muñoz R F, Ying Y W, Bernal G et al 1995 Prevention of depression with primary care patients: a randomized controlled trial. American Journal of Community Psychology 23(2):199–222

Murray J 1995 Prevention of anxiety and depression in vulnerable groups. The Royal College of Psychiatrists, London

Murray C J, Lopez A D 1996 The global burden of disease. Harvard University Press, Harvard

Murray L, Cooper P J 1997 (eds) Postpartum depression and child development. Guilford, London

NESS (The National Evaluation of Sure Start) 2004 The impact of Sure Start local programmes on child development and family functioning: a report on preliminary findings. Institute for the Study of Children, Families and Social Issues, Birbeck, University of London, London

NESS 2005 The national evaluation of Sure Start, implementing Sure Start programmes: an in-depth study. Institute for the Study of Children, Families and Social Issues, Birbeck, University of London, London

NHS Centre for Reviews and Dissemination 1997 Effective health care: mental health promotion in high risk groups. Bulletin on the Effectiveness of Health Service Interventions for Decision Makers 3(3):1–12

Oakley A, Mauthner M, Rajan L et al 1995 Supporting vulnerable families: an evaluation of NEWPIN. Health Visitor 68(5):188–191

Oakley A, Hickey D, Rajan L et al 1996 Social support in pregnancy: does it have long term effects. Journal of Reproductive and Infant Psychology 14:7–22

Oakley A, Rajan L, Turner H 1998 Evaluating parent support initiatives: lessons from two case studies. Health and Social Care in the Community 6(5):318–330

Olds D L, Eckenrode J, Henderson C R et al 1997 Long term effects of home visitation on maternal life course and child abuse and neglect: fifteen year follow up of a randomised trial. Journal of the American Medical Association 278(8):637–643

Peveler R, Carson A, Rodin G 2002 ABC of psychological medicine: depression in medical patients. British Medical Journal 325:149–152

Pound A, Mills M 1985 A pilot evaluation of NEWPIN, a home visiting and befriending scheme in South London. Association of Child Psychology and Psychiatry Newsletter 7:13–15

Price R H 1998 Theoretical frameworks for mental health risk reduction in primary care. In: Jenkins R, Üstün T B (eds) Preventing mental illness: mental health promotion in primary care. John Wiley, Chichester:19–34

Raphael B, Schmolke M, Wooding S 2005 Links between mental and physical health and illness. In Herrman H, Saxena S, Moodie R (eds) Promoting mental health: concepts, emerging evidence, practice. A report of the World Health Organization, Department of Mental Health and Substance Abuse in collaboration with the Victorian Health Promotion Foundation and University of Melbourne,WHO, Geneva:132–145

Rihmer Z, Rutz W, Pihlgren H 1995 Depression and suicide on Gotland. An intensive study of all suicides before and after a depression-training programme for general practitioners. Journal of Affective Disorders 35:147-152

Robinson J 1999 Domiciliary health visiting: a systematic review. Community Practitioner 72:15–18

Rutz W, von Knorring L, Pihlgren H et al 1995 Prevention of male suicides: lessons from the Gotland study. Lancet 345:524–526

Sainsbury Centre for Mental Health and NHS Alliance 2002 An executive briefing on primary care mental health services. Sainsbury Centre for Mental Health, London

Sartorius N, Üstün T B, Lecrubier Y et al 1996 Depression co-morbid with anxiety: results from the WHO study on psychological disorders in primary health care. British Journal of Psychiatry 168(30):S38–S43

Shochet I M, Dadds M R, Holland D et al 2001 The efficacy of a universal school based program to prevent adolescent depression. Journal of Clinical Child Psychology 30:303–315

Stamp G E, Williams A S, Crowther C A 1995 Evaluation of antenatal and postnatal support to overcome postnatal depression: a randomized, controlled trial. Birth 22:138–143

Stewart-Brown S 1998 Emotional wellbeing and its relation to health. British Medical Journal 317:1608–1609

Üstün T B 1998 The primary care setting – relevance, advantages, challenges. In: Jenkins R, Üstün T B (eds) Preventing mental illness: mental health promotion in primary care. John Wiley, Chichester:71–80

Üstün T B, Goldberg D, Cooper J et al 1995 A new classification for mental health disorders with management guidelines for use in primary care: the ICD-10 PHC. British Journal of General Practice 45(393):211–215

Walker Z, Townsend J 1998 Promoting adolescent mental health in primary care: a review of the literature. Journal of Adolescence 21:621–634

Weiss H B 1993 Home visits: necessary but not sufficient. The Future of Children 3(3):113–128

WHO (World Health Organization) 1978 Declaration of Alma Ata. International conference on Primary Health Care, USSR, 6–12 September

WHO 1996 Diagnostic and management guidelines for mental disorders in primary care: ICD 10, Chapter V, Primary Care Version, published on behalf of the WHO by Hogrefe and Huber, Goettingen

WHO Collaborating Centre 2000 WHO guide to mental health in primary care. UK version. Royal Society of Medicine, London.

Zlotnick C, Johnson S B L, Miller I W et al 2001 Postpartum depression in women receiving public assistance: pilot study of an interpersonal-therapy-orientated group intervention. American Journal of Psychiatry 158(4):638–640

Promotion of Children's Early Psychosocial Development

7.1

Sample Semi-Structured Interview

Interview with the Mother During the First 3 Months of the Child's Life

Mother's Psychological Health

How do you feel in the new situation, now that the baby is born?

- Positive feelings: reinforce them and encourage the mother to share such feelings with her husband and other members of the family.
- Negative or vague feelings: encourage the mother to talk about her feelings with the child's father, e.g. 'Have you ever talked about your feelings to your husband?'
- If there are communication problems between the couple, the primary health care professional (PHCP) should provide the mother with a model of communication by suggesting that she talks more about her feelings, e.g. 'Could you tell me more about your feelings?'
- The PHCP should be prepared to receive the mother's negative feelings without appraisal or judgement – only to contain them.
- The PHCP should also be prepared to handle the most often encountered negative or vague feelings reported by mothers, such as:
  - fears or feelings of guilt concerning the child's mental and/or physical health and its future development
  - feeling incompetent for the maternal role; doubts over being a 'good mother'
  - feeling neglected or 'abandoned' by others
  - feeling extremely tense, irritable or hopeless, desperate or empty.
- It is important that the PHCP gets insight into the content but also the direction of the mother's negative feelings. These feelings could be:
  - directed toward herself (incompetent for the maternal role, insecure, confused, etc.)

– directed toward the child (s/he is a difficult baby, hard to manage, etc.)
– directed toward the outside world (e.g. the family, the social or medical institutions).

- The PHCP could use the following interventions to handle the above-mentioned difficulties:
  – provide the mother with some crucial information regarding the child's development and child-rearing practices and thus encourage her in her role
  – encourage the mother to share her feelings with her husband and other members of her family and thus look for the necessary support
  – help her to get the necessary specialised psychological or social help when needed. Special attention should be paid to depressed or highly anxious mothers. In such cases PHCPs should arrange consultation with a psychologist or psychiatrist.

Response and Support of the Family

How did the baby's arrival affect the relationships in your family? What about the reaction of your husband (child's father)?

- Positive reactions/changes: reinforce them.
- Negative reactions/changes: encourage the mother to share the baby's care and the household chores with her husband, e.g. 'How about giving your husband an opportunity to take care of the baby? He will feel more competent and you will get some rest and feel more relaxed'.
- Ask about reactions (positive or negative) of other members of the family, e.g. 'What about the reactions of other children? Of grandparents?'
- Encourage the involvement of other family members with the new member of the family.

Mother's Concern for the Child

How do you see your baby's development/well-being?

- Positive views: reinforce them.
- Negative views: express your willingness to share the mother's concern by asking, e.g. 'Could you tell me more about your concern?'
- The PHCP should give the mother relevant information on child development to try and reduce her anxiety.
- The mother should be encouraged to talk about her concern with her husband or the baby's father, e.g. 'Have you already discussed this matter with the baby's father? How does he feel about it?'
- The PHCP should also invite the mother to look for possible solutions together with her husband, e.g. 'What do you both think could be done to improve your child's well-being?'
- If the couple foresees some solution: reinforce it.

- If there are more serious difficulties between the couple: the mother should be encouraged to attend the primary health care service and the paediatrician regularly for support, e.g. 'How about discussing this matter with your paediatrician during your next visit to the service?'
- The mother should be offered the possibility to get specialised psychological help, if she feels like it, e.g. 'How about discussing this matter with a psychologist?'
- The PHCP should be very careful when proposing consultation with a psychologist because some mothers may perceive this as confirmation of their suspicions about the child's health and development.

Mother's Perception of the Child

How do you see your child? Is s/he an easy baby? Or is s/he a difficult one?

- Positive perception: reinforce it.
- Negative perception: try to identify the area of difficulties by asking, e.g. 'In which area do you find your child most difficult: feeding, sleeping, temperament, communication?'
- During this period (0–3 months), mothers often feel the child is a difficult one because of troubles in establishing basic rhythms (feeding, sleep/waking pattern) or because of troubles in communicating with the child. All this should be further explored, but first explore what is pointed out by the mother.

Mother–Child Interaction

Feeding

How do you feed your baby?

- Breast-feeding.
- Bottle-feeding: why?
- Explain to the mother that breast-feeding is desirable in the first 3 months of life although the baby can also progress very well if bottle fed. In both cases encourage close contact between the mother and the baby during feeding (holding close, eye-to-eye contact).

What about the intervals at which you feed your baby?

- Flexible intervals.
- Very strict intervals.
- Encourage the mother to accept that each child has its own rhythm and that some children have difficulties adapting to very strict intervals.

Sleeping

What about your baby's sleeping habits? (How much time does the baby sleep? What is her/his sleep like? How often does s/he cry during the night?)

- Well-established rhythm.
- Difficulties in establishing the rhythm.
- If the mother reports difficulties in the child's sleeping habits, encourage her to think about possible solutions, e.g. 'What do you think could be done to help your child with sleeping? Have you already tried something?'
- The mother should be encouraged to look for solutions together with her husband and other members of the family.

Mother's Emotional Resources for the Child

How do you react when your baby is crying disconsolately in spite of your efforts to stop her/him crying?

- Containment of distress/facilitation.
- Non-containment of distress.
- The aim is to estimate whether the mother is able to contain the child's distress and to facilitate the child or if she has difficulties in containment and reacts with confusion, panic or by ignoring the child.
- If the mother's ability to contain distress is estimated to be low, she should be encouraged to look for support from other members of the family, primarily from her husband, e.g. 'What would you think if your husband takes over the care of the child in such situations?'
- The PHCP could demonstrate in a non-intrusive way some of the activities which might have a soothing or facilitating effect.
- Special attention should be paid if the mother expresses indifference or overt rejection of the child when s/he is in distress (e.g. 'I hate him/her').
- If necessary, consultation with a psychologist should be arranged.

Mother–Child Communication

Can you tell when the baby is crying because s/he is hungry, feels discomfort, is wet or ill?

- The PHCP should encourage the mother to pay more attention to different meanings of the child's signals (e.g. crying at night) and to show by her response that she understood the meaning of the child's message, e.g. 'You will probably have noticed that your baby's crying has different meanings. Your baby will like it if you show, with your response, that you understood her/his message'.

Observation of Mother–Infant Communication

The PHCP should carefully observe the interaction between the mother and the infant, while handling or feeding the baby, during the interview. For this purpose, the mother could be asked to demonstrate the baby's feeding. Special attention should be paid to the following aspects of interaction:

HOLDING	close	distant
HANDLING	tender	rough
EYE-TO-EYE CONTACT	yes	no
TALKING TO THE CHILD	yes	no
ENJOYMENT OF THE CHILD	yes	no
CONTAINING DISTRESS	yes	no
RESPONSIVE TO CHILD'S SIGNALS	yes	no

The PHCP could demonstrate holding and handling the baby, as well as communicating with her/him (talking, smiling, paying attention to child's signals). The period after feeding when the baby is relaxed but still awake is the most suitable time for this purpose.

Mental Health Promotion within Mental Health Services

8

Chapter contents

Introduction

Significant structural changes have taken place in many countries within mental health services over the last decades. There has been a shift in service delivery away from institutional care towards more local comprehensive, community-based mental health care. This move provides increasing opportunities for mental health promotion by ensuring that both the way services are provided and the environment in which they are delivered contribute to improving the health of the 'whole' individual rather than just treating the illness. Mental health promotion within the mental health services adopts a holistic approach towards mental health, taking into account people's mental, physical, spiritual, social and emotional needs in order to promote improved quality of life. Adopting a mental health promotion perspective highlights the need for a more comprehensive approach to service delivery addressing the full range of needs of service users and their families within an integrated and positive model of care. As pointed out by Mentality; 'people with mental health problems will benefit from the same range of mental health promotion programmes as everyone else (2003:43). Therefore, mental health service users will benefit from many of the programmes and approaches discussed in previous chapters, e.g. empowerment and competence enhancement approaches, exercise programmes, social support and employment programmes. In addition, there are specific quality of life issues for mental health service users and their families, in terms of living and coping with long-term mental disorders, that will require targeted interventions in order to meet people's needs. Programmes that promote recovery and strengthen opportunities for user empowerment, together with initiatives to reduce the stigma and discrimination associated with mental disorder, have a key role in promoting the mental health of service users. The integration of the promotion of mental health within the mental health services carries with it the promise of dramatic changes in the culture of service provision and in attitudes towards mental disorders and mental health service users (McGorry 2000).

This chapter provides an overview of the rationale for mental health promotion within mental health services, and then describes key features of mental health promotion programmes which have been pioneered, implemented and evaluated within the context of mental health services. These include programmes to reduce stigma and raise community awareness about mental health, initiatives to enhance recovery of people with mental disorders by empowerment and consumer involvement, early intervention programmes and psychosis prevention, enhancement of social support for carers and finally a consideration of the concept of health promoting mental health services.

Rationale for Mental Health Promotion within Mental Health Services

The rationale for mental health promotion within mental health services derives from the heavy burden of mental disorders, the immense exclusion suffered by people with mental disorders, the impact of mental disorders on physical health and the fact that mental health promotion measures have an effective role to play in improving the social functioning and quality of life of people with mental disorders. Eight of the 10 leading causes of the global burden of disease are related to mental disorders and it is estimated that depression alone will constitute one of the greatest health problems worldwide by 2020 (Murray & Lopez 1996).

People with mental disorders consistently identify stigma, discrimination and social exclusion as major barriers to their health, well-being and quality of life (Mental Health Foundation 2000). Exclusion from employment opportunities, good quality housing, social participation and lack of control and influence in how services are designed and delivered have been identified as contributing to the sense of isolation experienced by people with mental health problems (Bates 2002). Employment is important both in maintaining mental health and in promoting the recovery of those who have experienced mental health problems. As already outlined in Chapter 6, work is crucial for people with mental health problems in that it provides structure, a sense of purpose and identity and a sense of achievement. Unemployment aggravates the social exclusion already experienced by those with mental health problems.

People with severe mental disorders have been identified as being one of the most excluded and vulnerable population groups, with poorer physical health and significantly raised standardised mortality ratios (SMRs) than the general population (Harris & Barraclough 1998, Mentality 2003, Phelan et al 2001). Some of these increased health risks include cardiovascular disease, respiratory infections, diabetes, hepatitis C, obesity, malignancy and trauma. Medications used to treat mental disorders often affect appetite and gastrointestinal function, as well as altering the absorption and metabolism of nutrients. Excessive weight gain occurs in up to half of all patients prescribed anti-psychotic drugs and in some cases is associated with the development of type II diabetes (INDI 2000). Research has also shown that the prevalence of smoking is significantly higher among people with mental disorders than the general population; 70% of those with psychotic disorders living in institutions smoke.

Some of the symptoms associated with mental disorders, such as schizophrenia, may exacerbate or contribute to physical health problems. For example, people with schizophrenia are less likely than healthy controls to report physical symptoms spontaneously. This may be due to cognitive impairment, social isolation and suspicion which may contribute to patients not seeking care or adhering to treatment. However, it would also appear that people with mental disorders are less likely to be offered annual health checks and health promotion interventions, despite their frequent attendance at primary care services (Mentality 2003). Clearly, there is a need to ensure the provision of routine health promotion and prevention services to mental health service users as this could make a significant contribution to their general health.

With the move to community-based care, there has been increasing emphasis on the impact of service provision on the quality of life of mental health service users (see Katschnig et al 2006 for an overview of this area). The quality of life literature has drawn attention to the need for services to ensure the adequate provision of resources for living, i.e. housing, financial and social support, leisure and employment opportunities. The focus on quality of life has also highlighted the importance of the client's perspective including their sense of efficacy and control over their lives, and their ability to fulfil their roles and identities as community members (Zissi & Barry 2006). The focus of services, therefore, extends beyond clinical treatment to consider the needs of the whole person in their social context. This has brought a shift to psychosocial models of intervention designed to build clients' capacities and their personal and social resources for living. Together with supports for economic independence and empowerment (Rosenfield 1992) psychosocial programmes have been shown to have a positive effect on clients' sense of control and quality of life. Therefore, mental health promotion interventions which build on the strengths and capacities of service users and their families, and encourage greater participation and expectations of positive outcomes and recovery, are also likely to contribute to overall subjective well-being and improved mental health.

The remainder of this chapter is devoted to several key projects which exemplify mental health promotion for mental health service users:

1. examples of national campaigns to tackle stigma about mental disorders
2. a mental health community development project developed in collaboration with the mental health services
3. a programme of early intervention and prevention of psychosis which has rapidly disseminated across the world

4. a programme for caregivers
5. an example of a health promoting mental health service.

Stigma Reduction: Community Attitudes and Awareness Raising

The World Health Report (WHO 2001) highlights that the single most important barrier to overcome in the community is the stigma and discrimination associated with mental disorder and people who experience mental health difficulties. People with mental health problems and disorders consistently identify stigma, discrimination and exclusion as major barriers to their health and quality of life (Dunn 1999). Tackling stigma and raising greater public awareness require public education and focused intervention approaches. There are a number of different strategies to tackle stigma that may be used, ranging from sophisticated mass media campaigns to more local initiatives involving information distribution, workshops, community drama and community models of participation. Challenging stigma and promoting increased awareness of, and positive attitudes towards, mental health issues have been addressed through international campaigns such as World Mental Health Day and the World Psychiatric Association's campaign 'Open the doors' (Sartorius 1997, www.openthedoors. com), national campaigns like 'Changing minds – every family in the land' by the Royal College of Psychiatrists in the UK, the 'You in mind' campaign (Barker et al 1993, Hersey et al 1984), the Norwegian Mental Health Campaign (Sogaard & Fonnebo 1995) and the 'Mind out for mental health' campaigns in England (www.nimhe.org.uk/stigmaanddisc), the Scottish 'See me' campaign (www. seemescotland.org), the 'Stamp out stigma' in the USA (www.stampoutstigma. org) and the 'Like minds, like mine' campaign in New Zealand (www.likeminds. govt.nz). Campaigns or mass media interventions, particularly if they are supported by local community action, can have a significant impact on knowledge, attitudes and behavioural intentions. Such interventions can be used to increase understanding, reduce stigma and increase knowledge of coping and sources of support. In other words, they have the potential to impact positively on mental health literacy at the wider community level.

There is a large body of research on the nature and extent of stigma and discrimination (Bhugra 1989, Byrne 2001, Corrigan & Watson 2002, Hayward & Bright 1997, Sayce 2000) and public perceptions and attitudes to mental disorder (Brockman et al 1979, Link et al 1999, Priest et al 1996, Rabkin 1974) to which the reader is referred for further information. This research has largely focused on attitudes to mental disorder and highlights the role of cultural, social, gender and age factors in influencing how people come to understand and explain mental health problems and their origins. Studies that have explored perceptions as part of mental health campaigns suggest that both mental health and mental disorder are still associated with stigma in the mind of the public and that there may be a certain ambivalence to consulting professional sources of help (Barry et al 2000, McKeon & Carrick 1991, Priest et al 1996).

A number of key principles for effective and sustained stigma reduction have been identified (Link & Phelan 2001, Pinfold et al 2003). The approach used needs to address various levels such as the individual, community, organisational and national levels. It is recognised that education approaches alone will not be effective (Byrne 2000) and that contact between the public and service users has been found to have a more direct effect on improved attitudes (Corrigan & Ralph 2004, Pinfold et al 2003). Stigma reduction training programmes for health service staff, which involve users in the delivery of the programme, hold promise as an effective means of addressing stigma among front-line health and welfare staff who interact with mental health service users. Gale et al (2004), in a scoping review on mental health anti-stigma and discrimination, provide an overview of a range of effective approaches to challenging the stigma and discrimination that are associated with mental health problems in England. Based on the existing evidence, this report identifies six key principles that should underpin effective programmes:

1. users and carers are involved throughout the design, delivery, monitoring and evaluation of programmes
2. programmes should be appropriately monitored and evaluated
3. national programmes supported by local activity demonstrate the most potent combination for efficacy
4. programmes should address behaviour change with a range of approaches
5. clear, consistent messages are delivered in targeted ways to specific audiences
6. long-term planning and funding underpins programme sustainability.

Awareness raising and de-stigmatisation have a significant role to play in mental health promotion programmes. Socially shared beliefs and perceptions influence how mental health is interpreted and dealt with in the context of community life. We will now examine public education campaigns aimed at overcoming stigma and promoting greater community awareness. Two different approaches are showcased: an agency-led campaign – the 'Defeat Depression Campaign' (Paykel 2001, Priest et al 1996), and a community development model of raising awareness in Australia – the 'Depression Awareness Research Project' (Sundram et al 2004).

Case Study

The Defeat Depression Campaign

E S Paykel

The Defeat Depression Campaign, undertaken from 1992 to 1996 in the United Kingdom, has been described previously (Paykel 2001, Paykel et al 1997, 1998, Priest et al 1995, Rix et al 1999). It was jointly organised by the Royal College of Psychiatrists (RCPsych) and the Royal College of General Practitioners (RCGP) in order to improve recognition and treatment of depression. There were three specific aims:

1. to educate health professionals, particularly general practitioners, about recognition and management of depression
2. to educate the general public about depression and the availability of treatment, in order to encourage people to seek help earlier
3. to reduce the stigma associated with depression.

The campaign involved many people. Most of the administrative organisation was by Deborah Hart, Public Education Officer at the RCPsych. There were two organising committees: the Management Committee chaired by Robert Priest, particularly responsible for public education activities, with broad membership including other professions and patient groups, and the Scientific Advisory Committee chaired by Eugene Paykel, responsible for scientific advice, consensus conferences and evaluation. Membership and functions of the two committees overlapped a good deal.

Public Education

The campaign had a high media profile, organising press briefings to launch most new initiatives and proactively encouraging coverage in medical and related journals, in newspapers, on television and on the radio at both regional and national levels. These aimed to develop awareness among people experiencing depression, their families and the general public and to de-stigmatise depression by the powerful effects of familiarity. The campaign also devised and used its own logo.

Activities started with a press conference early in 1992, to which a wide range of media were invited, where much material was available. There was a major impact that pleased us all, and for about a week there seemed to be no national newspaper, radio network or television channel that did not feature an item on depression.

Subsequent events included influential personal accounts of depression by a number of public and media figures. One of the heartening aspects of the campaign was the generally sympathetic reception by the press and other media. There was also a considerable increase in media coverage of depression in ways not directly emanating from the campaign, but as a sort of groundswell in response to it.

There were other kinds of public activities. In March 1994, Defeat Depression Action Week took place. During the week, in addition to the now familiar media briefing, there were activities as diverse as a fun run in Hyde Park, a large conference on depression in Leeds and an abseil down the front of Manchester Town Hall. Defeat Depression Action Days on specific themes took place in 1995 and 1996.

To further public education, a pre-existing RCPsych leaflet series was expanded to include titles on depression, depression in the elderly, depression in the workplace and postnatal depression. More than two million copies were distributed to GPs' waiting rooms, hospitals, pharmacies, health promotion services, schools and other sites. Two books were published, on depression in general (Pitt & Calman 1994) and depression in adolescents (Graham & Hughes 1995), both illustrated with cartoons. Factsheets on depression in five ethnic minority languages were distributed, as well as further leaflets on depression in people with learning disabilities, depression in men, manic depression and alcohol and depression. Two audio cassettes and a videotape on self-help were also produced, the last jointly with two mental health user organisations.

Professional Education and Scientific Activities

Professional activities commenced with two consensus conferences in late 1991, dealing respectively with diagnosis and recognition, and with management of depression in general practice. The resultant consensus statement was published in the British Medical Journal (BMJ) (Paykel & Priest 1992). Two more consensus conferences, on depression in the elderly, were also published (Katona et al 1995). Subsequently a number of scientific conferences and workshops on specific aspects of depression were held, with wider participation.

Professional education focused particularly on GPs, who care for the majority of people with depression. In a national campaign with limited resources, much of the direct activity was through printed materials. After publication of the first consensus statement in a high profile medical journal, it was rewritten by a professional writer into easier-to-read guidelines which were distributed by the relevant government Departments responsible for health in England, Wales and Scotland to all GPs and psychiatrists. Subsequently an aide-memoire suitable for a consulting room desk was distributed to GPs. A book (Wright 1993) was written by the editor of the British Journal of General Practice, himself a practising GP member of both campaign committees, and was distributed to all members of the RCGP. The British Journal of General Practice also, through editorials, brought aspects of depression to the attention of its members (Tylee & Katona 1996, Wright 1996).

Two videotaped educational packages led by Dr L Gask, a psychiatrist, covering respectively depression recognition and management and counselling for depression, were prepared and distributed to those involved in GP training. Two videotapes were also produced with the Royal College of Nursing.

Supplementing these activities the RCGP and the Department of Health appointed an RCGP Mental Health Fellow, Dr A Tylee, a GP member of both campaign committees. He established and organised a new national cascade network involving regional educational fellows to train local district GP tutors, who trained GPs directly in mental health and provided local teaching sessions. Considerable emphasis on teaching sessions in depression for local GPs was generated.

As with public education, the GP education activities generated a knock-on effect of much further activity for GPs not directly initiated by the campaign, which was also aimed to improve recognition and management of depression.

Termination of the Campaign

The campaign was conceived as a time-limited 5-year activity. Except for evaluation it was closed, as planned, at the end of 1996. The last few months saw vigorous activity including a conference to summarise the work of the campaign, the launch of the last few leaflets and a book for carers.

The campaign left a legacy. A voluntary association continued public education activities for some years. Joint psychiatric–GP educational activities in other areas, some of which had antedated the campaign, continued. Dr Tylee established an RCGP unit for Mental Health Education at the Institute of Psychiatry, London, where he has since become a Professor. The RCGP subsequently established a new public education campaign, the 'Changing Minds Campaign', directed more generally towards stigma in mental health (Crisp et al 2004).

Evaluation

A key aspect, built in from the beginning, was evaluation. Since the campaign was a national one there could be no external control group, and evaluation depended on before–during–after comparisons of a number of aspects.

The most central evaluation concerned public attitudes. General population surveys were commissioned at baseline, part way through the campaign, and shortly after its close (Paykel et al 1998). Baseline attitudes towards people with depression were generally favourable, but towards treatment with antidepressants they were unfavourable and towards receiving care from GPs they were mixed. There was a progressive and significant change towards more favourable attitudes during the campaign and at its end, particularly in those aspects initially rated unfavourably.

The impact of GP education was studied at the end of the campaign, in a sampled questionnaire survey (Rix et al 1999). Impact was moderate. The campaign was seen as useful but only a minority of GPs had changed practice as a result. Impact of educational materials was highest for the published BMJ consensus statement and guidelines deriving from it, with other materials making comparatively little impact. An impressive 50% had attended a teaching session on depression in the previous 3 years. Campaign materials ranked behind journal articles, postgraduate education and the pharmaceutical industry as useful information sources.

Two other aspects were also monitored (Paykel 2001). The national suicide rate fell progressively over the campaign. Prescribing of antidepressants increased, due to the use of selective serotonin reuptake inhibitors (SSRIs), while tricyclic prescribing remained steady. Both suicide reduction and increased appropriate prescribing were campaign targets, but in both cases there were other potentially influential factors at work.

Some Further Lessons of the Campaign

Some further issues arise in retrospect. First, a considerable asset for the campaign was its origin in the two Royal Colleges. The medical Royal Colleges in the UK are the official bodies responsible for training and examination in the specialties and for representing members of the specialties. They provide an important voice to government in specialty aspects. Because of the two Royal Colleges the campaign acquired standing, so its press briefings and statements were taken seriously by the quality press and media and it could, at times, obtain limited financial help from government.

Second, the RCGP, aware of the increasing importance of public education and attitudes, had a few years earlier appointed a part-time public relations advisor. Her experience, expertise and contacts were invaluable in bringing about press conferences, briefing and media-related activities, and it would have been difficult to start effectively without them.

Third, evaluation was planned from the start. A campaign like this harnesses the energies of many willing people. It is all too easy to forget to consider whether its effects are worthwhile. Until effects and limitation of such campaigns are well established, evaluation is essential.

Fourth, the explicit time limitation was a considerable advantage. By the fifth year the key activities had been accomplished, the participants realised this, and the media became aware that less of what was being said was new. Nevertheless, enthusiasm is not easily relinquished and, without a clear expectation for ending, it would have been much more difficult to bring it to a close.

A limitation was the modest availability of resources. Some funding was provided by the two Royal Colleges, as was infrastructure support. Governmental sources provided support for a few specific aspects. Funding from both these sources was quite limited. Support for many of the activities had to be raised from other sources; often drug companies. It was important to keep this at arm's length. The campaign rigorously avoided any endorsement of specific products or classes of antidepressant, rather presenting evidence for the place and appropriate use of antidepressants in general. Even so there were occasional criticisms attributing marketing aims to the campaign.

An important limitation is the need to be realistic about what can be achieved by a national campaign. Public education was successful because its natural arena is national: in the UK the main newspapers, radio programmes and television channels are national. Local education would have achieved much less. However, professional education largely comprises direct teaching and supervision activities which are in essence local. A national effort can provide materials and a considerable influence from the centre, but in the end it needs to be taken up, reinforced and continued at local level. Some of the activity should be used to influence the teachers at that level.

Within the limits of its aims and its setting, the Defeat Depression Campaign was a clear success. An enduring legacy is apparent in changed attitudes to depression. In the press, depression is a problem which people can be reported as having and which they can acknowledge for themselves. In everyday life, people talk more to their friends about their depressions, present or past.

References

Crisp H, Cowan L, Hart D 2004 The College's anti-stigma campaign, 1998–2003: a shortened version of the concluding report. Psychiatric Bulletin 28:133–136

Graham P, Hughes C 1995 So young, so sad, so listen. Gaskell, London

Katona C, Freeling P, Hinchcliffe K et al (on behalf of the Consensus Group) 1995 Recognition and management of depression in late life in general practice: consensus statement. Primary Care Psychiatry 1:107–113

Paykel E S 2001 Impact of public and general practice education in depression: evaluation of the Defeat Depression Campaign. Psychiatrica Fennica 32:51–61

Paykel E S, Priest R G 1992 Recognition and management of depression in general practice: consensus statement. British Medical Journal 305:1198–1202

Paykel E S, Tylee A, Wright A et al 1997 The Defeat Depression Campaign: psychiatry in the public arena. American Journal of Psychiatry 154:6, Festschrift Supplement:59–65

Paykel E S, Hart D, Priest R G 1998 Changes in public attitudes to depression during the Defeat Depression Campaign. British Journal of Psychiatry 173:519–522

Pitt B, Calman M 1994 Down with gloom! Gaskell, London

Priest R G, Paykel E S, Hart D et al 1995 Progress in defeating depression. Psychiatric Bulletin 19:491–495

Rix S, Paykel E S, Lelliott P et al 1999 Impact of a national campaign on GP education: an evaluation of the Defeat Depression Campaign. British Journal of General Practice 49:99–102

Tylee A, Katona C L E 1996 Detecting and managing depression in older people. British Journal of General Practice 46:207–208

Wright A 1993 Depression – recognition and management in general practice. RCGP Clinical Series. RCGP, London

Wright A F 1996 Unrecognised psychiatric illness in general practice. British Journal of General Practice 46:327–328

Case Study

The Depression Awareness Research Project

Suresh Sundram, Kylee Bellingham

The Depression Awareness Research Project (DARP) was a programme developed, implemented and evaluated by the Mental Health Research Institute of Victoria (www.mhri.edu.au) to determine the effectiveness of using a community development model to promote mental health literacy about major depression in Victoria, Australia.

Background

In response to international (Murray & Lopez 1996) and national (ABS 1998, Mathers et al 1999) identification of major depression as a key contributor to personal, social and economic health costs, a number of national initiatives to tackle major depression were developed in Australia. From a 'National Action Plan for Depression' (Commonwealth Department of Health and Aged Care 2000) formulated under the second National Mental Health Strategy, five target areas were identified including improving mental health literacy about depression. To progress this action plan the federal government established the National Depression Initiative, 'beyondblue' (www.beyondblue.org.au). beyondblue is a not-for-profit company funded by state and federal governments and non-government sources (excluding the pharmaceutical industry) for the purpose of reducing the impact of depression on the Australian community using a public health approach (Hickie 2001). It has three major areas of activity including increasing community awareness of depression in an effort to reduce stigma. Further, a key aspect of its functioning is the active involvement of consumers, carers and the broader community both in its programme development and as the focus of its initiatives. Therefore, the Mental Health Research Institute (MHRI) of Victoria, through its consumer representative Mr Neil Cole, a prominent former state parliamentarian and playwright, received funding from beyondblue for a research programme to develop and evaluate the effectiveness of a community development model to promote mental health literacy about major depression.

As set out in the National Action Plan for Depression, considerations for improving broader depression literacy must take into account barriers to accessing information, appropriate messages and media, and developing supportive social environments that facilitate community-wide change. Large-scale advertising and media have been used by beyondblue as a means to access the broader community. However, for ongoing application it is expensive, time limited and often oriented to the dominant culture. Within Australia, mental health promotion is also often undertaken by community workers who have skills to work with specific target groups such as youth, culturally and linguistically diverse and socially isolated groups. Time and workload often limit the capacity and success of these workers getting information into the community. A model capitalising on the local understanding of community networks and allowing health information to be shared beyond working hours has the potential to build upon the work that so many community workers and agencies are undertaking. DARP sought to develop and evaluate a community development model that had the potential to be economically viable, time efficient, sustainable, capable of responding to community needs and to engender a community sense of learning and support.

The Depression Awareness Research Project

The proposed model incorporated the use of local community members to develop their own community's awareness of major depression. In this approach, 218 voluntary participants from five regions in Victoria, Australia participated in a training programme and then disseminated basic messages about major depression within their community networks. These messages were that depression is common, serious, treatable and is an illness not a character flaw. In three separate rounds of training conducted in each target region, mental health professionals and those who have experienced depression presented information about these core messages. Volunteers also undertook training exercises and discussions about how best these messages could be taken to their local communities. Each volunteer was supported by a local project coordinator in their efforts to share this information with as many members as possible within their established community networks. The evaluation component of the project measured knowledge levels of depression pre- and post-training in the volunteers, and in a sample of those they spoke to on average 17 weeks after education.

The key tenets of this project were that it improves mental health literacy about major depression in the general community, that it is able to be undertaken by local community organisations with minimal specialist mental health input and that whilst maintaining a core evidence-based format it is sufficiently flexible and sensitive to accommodate local community resources, characteristics and baseline knowledge levels. These tenets allow local communities to be active participants in gaining and sharing health knowledge. The programme was conceptualised as a staged model: first, addressing mainstream adult populations across a range of socioeconomic strata; second, developing programmes to address special needs populations such as adolescents, children, indigenous groups and culturally and linguistically diverse communities; third, the widespread dissemination of the programme. The first stage of this project has been completed.

In planning this, it was important to engage community organisations that were able to provide local knowledge of health resources and community networks and basic infrastructure support (office space, telephone, photocopying, computer/internet access, etc.). Collaborative partnerships were formed between MHRI and five community organisations, namely a local municipal council, three non-government psychiatric disability support services and a multi-sectored charitable organisation in a variety of socioeconomic regions (two inner urban, one suburban, one regional centre, one rural/regional). It is anticipated that for stage three it will be these types of organisations that will undertake the programme. However, for stages one and two it is necessary to superimpose over this a research structure to evaluate the effectiveness of this model in achieving its aim of increasing levels of community knowledge about depression. This was done by forming a steering committee comprised of senior management from MHRI, beyondblue and each of the collaborating organisations. This committee oversaw implementation of the programme and its evaluation. It is anticipated that stage three will be initiated and executed by interested community organisations with only advisory and training support from a central organisation, thereby obviating the need for any additional organisational structures. A local area project coordinator was appointed to each area either seconded from the collaborating organisation or employed directly by MHRI, but all based locally with the collaborating organisation. This structure was necessary to ensure both successful implementation and evaluation of the project but direct employment by the community organisation is the preferred model for stage three.

As can be seen from the original impetus to establish a national depression initiative, considerable governmental effort has been expended in targeting depression. Beyondblue has increased community awareness of depression through the general media and the use of popular figures such as sporting stars (Jorm et al 2005). Although it is not possible to quantify the impact of this upon DARP, the DARP programme has operated in an environment where other methods of de-stigmatising and raising community awareness of depression and mental illness have been active. This may have facilitated both community organisation involvement and recruitment of volunteers for DARP.

Programme Implementation: Challenges and Experiences

Role of coordinators: Project coordinators worked with community networks, recruiting volunteer participants then supporting and coordinating them as they developed and initiated community dissemination activities, as well as overseeing the collection of data from these activities to the central research office. These dual roles created tensions for coordinators between maintaining standardised evaluation procedures whilst accommodating local community needs. It was important to instigate a rigorous reporting and supervisory structure back to the coordinating centre to ensure consistent implementation and evaluation across all regions. In stage three, with the reduced need for comprehensive evaluation, this dual role will diminish allowing coordinators to focus on the successful implementation of the model for their local community.

Recruitment of volunteer participants: An important determinant for the success of DARP was the recruitment of adequate numbers of volunteers. A variety of recruitment strategies were used across the regions such as local media coverage, approaching organisations for interested people and 'word of mouth'. With these strategies there was minimal difficulty in recruiting adequate numbers of volunteers and most had a personal or close-hand experience of depression. However, the coordinators reported a number of shortcomings with this relatively non-selective process. These included participants unwilling to initiate dissemination activities, feeling overwhelmed by the task, struggling with depression personally and finding the task confronting, or having high expectations regarding the expertise with which they were to deliver information, hence avoiding presentations. In response to this, the subsequent recruitment and selection of participants was more rigorous and expectations were clarified from the outset. A comprehensive information kit was sent out to individuals and agencies expressing interest in the DARP. Selection criteria were tightened to include only those who were linked to established community networks, were willing and had time to share the DARP information within these networks. Project coordinators discussed with participants concrete strategies and timeframes for accessing networks at the selection interview. All participants were encouraged to discuss with family and/or treating clinicians their suitability for, and obtain adequate support during, their participation in the DARP.

The training programme and package: The training programme and package were a collaborative development by mental health professionals, professional trainers and individual sufferers and carers. It was specifically tailored to the DARP aims to accommodate different learning styles and allow flexibility in the way information about depression could be delivered. Separate information and communication modules equipped volunteers with basic knowledge about depression and skills to assist them in disseminating information within their local communities. The emphasis was on publicising the four fundamental messages about major depression. These simple and straightforward messages resulted from an extensive review of evidence-based treatments and literature and were written for a lay adult audience. Given the difficulties in presenting potentially complex information about a psychiatric disorder to widely heterogeneous audiences, focusing on four simple messages served to establish a 'common denominator' between all participants and regions, ensured some consistency in the information being disseminated and helped lessen volunteers' expectations and anxieties that they be 'experts' on major depression. All information presented in both the training programme and the package of written materials centred on these key messages.

The DARP training was a 2-day group programme with information and training sessions. Information sessions presented by mental health professionals, consumers and carers incorporated background information for the key messages: the prevalence and impact of major depression, signs and symptoms of major depression, potential causes and associated factors, treatment options shown to be effective, outcomes and complications of treatment and personal experiences of major depression. Group exercises, role play, small and large group discussions were facilitated by a professional trainer in conjunction with the local project coordinator throughout the 2 days. This aimed to strengthen communication and interpersonal skills that would assist in the dissemination of information about depression within local communities, reflect on community attitudes about mental illness, particularly depression, and identify local factors (for example cultural, geographical) that would influence their capacity to disseminate the key messages. Each volunteer also received the DARP package of written materials containing an information handbook, supplementary information (booklets, resource lists for local areas), presentation materials (specifically designed fact cards for distribution, overhead transparencies, checklists for presentations) and evaluation materials. These materials were particularly relevant post-training to reinforce information and assist dissemination. They were especially well received when participants required more structure as a base to developing their own style of presentation.

Dissemination of information and evaluation of the programme: To maximise information dissemination by volunteers the project coordinators discussed timeframes and strategies for accessing community networks prior to training, allowed time for alternative strategies to be developed if initial ones were not successful and ensured regular, structured contact to allow volunteers to feel supported. Further, it was found that accessing additional community networks was facilitated by the active involvement of the coordinator in this process and also that in regions of high activity frequent face-to-face contact between coordinator and participants occurred.

The 218 trained volunteers gave 449 presentations to an estimated audience of 7540 people within their communities. Of this estimated audience it was possible to measure knowledge levels about major depression from 5443 people immediately before the presentation and from 2412 people on average 17 weeks after they heard the presentation. In evaluating the DARP a composite score derived from the survey questions was developed to measure knowledge about major depression. The maximum score was 8 indicating very high knowledge levels. A general community survey of levels of major depression knowledge in a representative sample of involved regions prior to DARP revealed a knowledge score of 3.30 ± 1.56 (mean ± standard deviation). The audience who listened to the presentations had a knowledge score of 3.75 ± 1.91 immediately before hearing the presentations. However, on average 17 weeks after hearing the presentation audience members scored 5.24 ± 1.50 on the composite knowledge score. Therefore, hearing a presentation about major depression delivered by a local community member resulted in a 59% higher score in knowledge about major depression than the general community. In a before-and-after measure a 25% increase in knowledge on average 4 months later ($t_{(2412)} = -29.49$, $p < 0.001$) was recorded. Interestingly and importantly there was no apparent effect of length of follow up on knowledge levels suggesting that knowledge gained in this way was not quickly forgotten. It seems, therefore, that the DARP is a successful community development model to improve literacy about major depression that is suitable for use in a wide range of sociodemographic settings.

Key Recommendations for Replication

For subsequent replication (stage three) of this project there will not be the need to comprehensively evaluate its effectiveness thereby simplifying its organisational structure and implementation. It is anticipated that stage three will be undertaken by interested local community organisations with training and advisory support from a central organisation. This training is likely to involve the area coordinator becoming familiar with the training programme for participants, having a good grasp of the knowledge about major depression, understanding the underlying principles of community development and, importantly, understanding how the package may be adapted to more easily integrate with local community values and knowledge. The coordinator is then expected to recruit participants, train them and support participants as they disseminate the information. They will also be required to complete quality improvement and routine evaluation tasks. From this it can be seen that the selection of the individual to the coordinator role is crucial for the success of the project and requires someone well linked to the community with a high level of self-motivation and drive and excellent interpersonal skills. To undertake this task successfully the individual will need to be employed in a full-time or substantial part-time (≥ 0.75 equivalent full-time) capacity. Following this training the coordinator within their local community will require the active support and resources of the community organisation. It is imperative that the agency perceives the programme as a core activity and, thereby, avoids marginalising the coordinator and overly restricting resources.

A key element to the success of the project is the use of a strict timeline. Six months from the time of training of participants to the end of their dissemination activities has been effective. This aims to ensure adequate throughput of volunteers, better budgetary constraints, maintains a quality check and provides a structure for coordinators to work within.

The reduction in the research component of the project with stage three will see a smaller role for any central organising body. The role for a central organisation in stage three is to provide training and expert advice to coordinators and organisations, monitor and oversee the quality of the implementation of each local project and promote and quality-improve the programme.

The success of the programme is ultimately dependent upon the volunteers recruited to the training and a rigorous selection as outlined above is recommended. To facilitate recruitment, the use of local identities or celebrities who can popularise the programme or generally raise community awareness about depression may be very helpful especially in communities with high levels of stigma about mental illness. Further, communities with extensive levels of engagement and cooperation are more likely to be accepting of such a programme. Therefore, disrupted, alienated or traumatised communities will require more intensive effort by the community organisation in recruiting and motivating participation. It equally may be perceived that this model of community development could foster and encourage community interaction.

Future Directions for Application of the Programme

The future of the programme lies in its capacity to attract, train and motivate volunteers from as diverse a population as exists within any targeted community.

Further, it is imperative that coordinators are familiar with modes of communication within their community and are able to work with volunteers in adapting the material to suit specific target groups. If such an approach is adopted it should be feasible to engage with any social or community group. It is anticipated to develop programmes in stage two suitable for schools, young people, indigenous, ethnic/cultural and religious communities. Further, captive groups provide ideal targets and include workplaces, residential facilities, prisons and the armed forces. The model, however, is not limited to major depression and if proven effective could be adapted to other mental and general health issues and, potentially, to other socially important topics.

References

ABS (Australian Bureau of Statistics) 1998 Mental health and wellbeing: profile of adults. Australia, 1997. ABS Cat No 4326.0. ABS, Canberra

Commonwealth Department of Health and Aged Care 2000 National Action Plan for Depression. Mental Health and Special Programmes Branch, Canberra

Hickie I 2001 beyondblue: the national depression initiative. Australasian Psychiatry 9(2):147–150

Jorm A F, Christensen H, Griffiths K M 2005 The impact of beyondblue: the national depression initiative on the Australian public's recognition of depression and beliefs about treatments. Australian and New Zealand Journal of Psychiatry 39(4):248–254

Mathers C, Vos T, Stevenson C 1999 The burden of disease and injury in Australia. Australian Institute of Health and Welfare (AIHW) Cat No PHE 17. AIHW, Canberra

Murray C J L, Lopez A D 1996 Global burden of disease: a comprehensive assessment of mortality and disability from diseases, injuries and risk factors in 1990 and projected to 2020. Harvard University Press, Cambridge, Massachusetts

Recovery and Mental Health Promotion

The move towards community care and the delivery of community-based services has highlighted the importance of meeting the broader needs of mental health service users in the context of their social environments. In discussing the implementation of evidence-based practices in routine mental health service settings, Drake et al (2001) outline a core set of interventions that lead to better outcomes and quality of life for people with severe mental disorders. These include the prescription of medications within specific parameters, training in self-management of illness, assertive community treatment, family psychoeducation, supported employment and integrated treatment for co-occurring substance use disorders. However, Drake et al also stress that mental health services, as well as being evidence based, should reflect the goal of consumers or service users. Drake et al highlighted that 'mental health services therefore should not focus exclusively on traditional outcomes such as compliance with treatment and relapse or rehospitalization prevention', but should be broadened to include helping people to 'attain outcomes such as independence, employment, satisfying relationships and quality of life' (2001:179). There is some evidence of a shift in emphasis from treatment compliance to strategies for promoting recovery and engaging users in a therapeutic relationship with the service. For example, in recent years there has been a growing interest in models of service delivery based on holistic recovery models, i.e. those which address the physical, mental, emotional and spiritual aspects of people within their social setting which can influence personal growth and recovery (Reeves 2002). This includes recognising the importance of social needs such as appropriate housing, employment, leisure opportunities, freedom from discrimination and the need for social networks and support. The recovery model stresses the importance of empowerment and self-directedness and emphasises that the person who has the condition must be given in large part responsibility for, and control of, the recovery process (Frese et al 2001). Anthony (1993) describes recovery as involving the development of new meanings and purpose in one's life as the person grows beyond the effects of the mental disorder. Mental health services embracing this approach are designed to be empowering for service users and stress values such as healing, hope, social connectedness, human rights and recovery-oriented services (Jacobson & Greenley 2001).

In many countries, the user and survivor movements play an important role in service planning and delivery and bring a focus on empowering service users to engage in recovery through increased participation in self-help groups and in their own care plans. There is increasing recognition of the role of self-help groups, through providing natural support networks and mutual help between people experiencing the same problems, in facilitating the recovery process. Research carried out in Canada by Trainor et al (1997) reported that service users found the consumer/survivor organisations to be the most helpful component of the mental health services and that after coming in contact with self-help groups they used fewer mental health services and increased their contact with the wider community. The self-help model recognises and values the experiences of service users in living with and understanding their mental disorder and how this can contribute to helping others in the process of recovery. For example, groups for people who hear voices and self-help organisations such as the International Voices Network show how people are able to help each other and advocate on each other's behalf. Self-help groups and organisations have a key part to play in advocating for users' rights and the provision of user-focused services which promote the recovery, quality of life and mental health of service users.

The active involvement of service users in planning and delivering mental health services is also beginning to be recognised. The ability to make choices about services and how best they should be delivered, together with taking control of their own lives, has been highlighted by service users as being critical to their recovery (Frese et al 2001). Service users value more influence and autonomy in relation to service delivery. There is an emerging body of research on recovery and mental health promotion through special programmes engaging mental health service users as peer counsellors and recruiting users and family members in programme delivery (Felton et al 1995, Frese et al 2001, Peter 2003, Simpson & House 2002). Research by Felton et al 1995 reported that the integration of mental health service users as peer specialists in an intensive case management programme leads to improved outcomes and enhanced quality of life for clients with serious mental disorders and more effective case management. A systematic review of research on involving users in the delivery and evaluation of mental health services found that there were no negative effects on services and that it was generally seen as being worthwhile but that further evaluation is needed (Simpson & House 2002). Such programmes have an important role to play in empowering service users and maximising systems of social support and community networks for both users and their families. We will now examine an initiative from Australia which describes a community development approach to involving service users and carers in improving the quality of mental health services.

Best Practice

Queensland Mental Health Community Development Projects, Australia

The Queensland Mental Health Community Development Strategy was funded and implemented in response to the 1992 Australian National Mental Health Policy (Australian Health Ministers 1992), which highlighted the importance of mental health as an important issue for the Australian public. The strategy is based on a community development approach, which is defined as the 'development and utilisation of a set of ongoing structures which eventually allow a community to meet its own needs' (Bush et al 1998:1). The key priorities of the strategy are 'to involve consumers and carers in the planning, operation and evaluation of services, and to improve intersectoral links between mental health services and other services so as a wide range of support services can be accessed, particularly housing and disability services' (Bush et al 1998:1). The strategy argues that a community development approach is important because 'consumers' and carers become more empowered when they have the opportunity to participate in the planning, implementation, delivery and evaluation of mental health services.

Furthermore, a consumer-focused approach improves the potential for mental health services to address the needs of consumers and carers. As a result of the strategy, a number of mental health community development projects have been funded and implemented. Each of the projects, while funded under a set of overall state-wide objectives, is unique to the setting and community in which each currently operates. The overall framework of the mental health community development projects is based on community empowerment and participation. As part of this initiative, the Sunshine Coast Mental Health Project began in October 1994. The project has a well-articulated model of community development that links the state-wide objectives with well-recognised processes of capacity building. The model embraces the need for change within the relevant agencies and organisations as well as the personal growth of people with mental health problems.

Sunshine Coast Mental Health Project

In the mid 1990s, the Sunshine Coast of Queensland, Australia was a densely populated area, with an increasing demand on a poorly resourced mental health service. A needs assessment was carried out in 1995 by independent researchers which looked at the community history, demographics, non-government and health services, and the basic mental health epidemiology of the area. A total of 30 participants from community organisations and groups were identified and consulted for the needs assessment. The aim of the assessment was to provide direction for the programme and to guide the nature of activities in the community. Among the issues identified were strong discontent with service provision and an absence of consumer involvement in service planning, development and delivery. The need for collaboration between government, non-government and community organisations was also identified. This provided a direction for the project and was used to guide the types of activities to be implemented. The Sunshine Coast project sought to establish a model of practice based on consumer involvement and sustainable partnerships with a wide range of organisations and groups. The implementation features of the Sunshine Coast project include:

- establishment of a pathway of care that is non-invasive and maintains people with mental disorders in contact with their communities
- consumer involvement in the project development and implementation
- appointment of a health promotion officer to liaise between minority groups and mental health services in the area
- a community initiatives team that delivers out-patient vocational and skills training
- inclusion of local mental health services in the community development project
- establishment of a Sunshine Coast Mental Health Committee in 1998.

A comprehensive needs assessment was a vital part of the community development process with feedback from service users being used to stimulate the establishment of consumer reference groups. Consumer 'focus groups' were thus established as a key initiative of the project in order to facilitate greater user participation in service development. Consumers were encouraged to be more self reliant and empowered in developing service initiatives and this led to the development of advocacy skills for clients and their families. Initiatives established through this process included, for example, the 'Self Help Advocacy Resource Place' (SHARP), a mental health information and resource centre which aims to reorientate community attitudes towards mental disorders through education and support. Other consumer-driven initiatives include a 'Mardi Gras' during National Mental Health Week, comic and information booklets, radio programmes and a community service directory. These latter projects promote public awareness of mental health and have contributed to the fostering of positive attitudes towards mental health. As with a lot of these projects, the community development worker acted as the catalyst to initiate these projects but full control of the initiatives was subsequently with the consumers themselves. Consumers were responsible for the direction of the project and had 50% voting rights on the management committee.

Evaluation

Each of the projects has been evaluated in order to determine its effectiveness within its own setting and district. The purpose of the evaluation was to determine (Bush et al 1998:3):

- the extent to which each project has met the original state-wide objectives
- the extent to which each project has met local needs as defined by needs analysis and population based mental health data
- the extent of sustainability of the responses developed by each project
- the cost of the project (directly and indirectly funded) against the utility of a coordinated community response
- the extent to which each project has demonstrated innovations.

The evaluation was based on qualitative information collected during short-term visits to each of the project sites. However, no baseline information was available. A process of triangulation was used to develop consensus concerning the information collected. The method used was post-intervention semi-structured interviews with a sample of key stakeholders. Interviewees included the community development workers, management committee or workers from the supporting organisation, consumers, carers, director of the district mental health services or nominee and other key service providers. Each of the projects was visited and a rapid appraisal process was used to collect information. The appraisal comprised the collection of any reports or profiles of each of the projects and interviews with a selection of stakeholders. In addition, an evaluation project review team was established in order to provide comments at critical stages during the process.

A set of universal questions was posed to the projects which covered topics such as approach of the project, extent of consumer participation, impact of consumer participation and activities undertaken. Specific questions were developed to obtain information from each of the stakeholders. At the end of each site visit, an open feedback session was held at which initial findings of the site visit were fed back to the participants for verification and further discussion.

Key Findings from the Evaluation of the Sunshine Coast Project

From the early stages, the Sunshine Coast project was successful in building consumer and carer involvement. In the first year, an ongoing focus group was established which advocated for and acted on behalf of the community leading to considerable opportunities to empower and increase the skills of consumers and carers. The feelings of discontent, associated with the lack of user involvement in service provision, also significantly improved as a result of the work of the project. Within the project, consumers were responsible for the direction of the work and had 50% voting rights on the management committee. An increase in consumer involvement in service planning, development and delivery through engagement in the various groups was also found. For example, the focus group was developed by consumers into an independent consumer action group. There was also evidence of a net-widening effect in consumer advocacy and self-help beyond the local area and, as a result, various other consumer groups were established.

The mental health needs of the community were promoted in partnership with a wide range of organisations and groups. This resulted in an expanded community-based mental health network, resourced by a directory of services, which was widely disseminated (Bush et al 1998). The network helped in building links between government and non-government services. This led to a more coordinated response to mental health issues on the Sunshine Coast. The project was successful in working with a variety of community organisations to promote public awareness of mental health, promoting access to and utilisation of local media, public facilities and educational institutions. This contributed to fostering positive attitudes about mental health. The collaboration between organisations, groups and services in addressing the needs of those with mental disorders in diverse communities resulted in an expanded community-based mental health network dealing with issues such as life skills training, employment, housing, volunteer support and support for consumers. Human and social capital between partners was seen as a strength of this project. The evaluation reported that there was a strong willingness among key stakeholders to work together as a result of the trust and respect that was developed between consumers, carers and others involved in the project. This positive ethos seems to have spilled over into the activities of the project and contributed to the success of the approach adopted (Bush et al 1998).

The project was found to have had its greatest success in stimulating the establishment and maintenance of consumer self-help and support groups and in contributing to change in existing organisations and the mental health service. The groups that were established appear to have had a great deal of sustainability due to the fact that they had limited reliance on the project's resources and a great deal of consumer participation. The project also linked into other groups and organisations which helped to improve access to services. Consumers were involved in training the Division of General Practice in the Sunshine Coast area. The project reported some initial resistance but that gradually over time the training increased the potential for service providers to become more aware of their attitudes towards mental health consumers. The community development workers provided training to various projects and groups in the area. One of the main strengths of the projects was identified as being the significant increase in consumer and carer empowerment through gaining experience in the running of local projects. 'This substantial investment would appear to provide benefits to the restructure of the mental health services' (Bush et al 1998:92).

Based on the evaluation, it was concluded that the community development approach resulted in the participation of consumers and carers in the planning and delivery of services in the area. The project successfully utilised the formal links between the mental health services and non-government services in order to effectively meet the needs of a diverse group of consumers (Bush et al 1998). The networking approach adopted was seen as an effective way of increasing access to resources for consumers and carers. The project demonstrated how a community development approach could be used in mental health to advance the rights of consumers through individual participation and system brokerage. The Sunshine Coast project was identified as a potential role model for similar projects in the future. However, it is also important to acknowledge the barriers that were found to exist in this project. External issues, such as short-term and uncertain funding cycles, were identified as one of the main barriers to the project. Other potential barriers included local features of distinct and different communities in the area and consumer involvement being made difficult by distance and travel. Consideration of these issues will guide further initiatives in replicating this model elsewhere.

This project signals a clear shift in focus from a clinical to a social model of mental health. The readiness of local mental health services and other community organisations to embrace the objectives of the projects and the community development approach is seen as a key factor in influencing the reform of the mental health services and partnership building in the community. Variation in readiness across the projects was also identified as affecting the time it takes to reach desirable outcomes.

In terms of the overall mental health community development strategy, this initiative is unique in the Australian context. Community development is a relatively unexplored approach to mental health among those with chronic and long-term mental health problems, who often experience marginalisation in the communities in which they live and have difficulties in asserting their rights in mental health services. These innovative projects demonstrate the value of a community development approach and its potential in the reform of mental health services and asserting the rights of service users.

Early Intervention and Mental Health Promotion

The reorientation of mental health services to include the value of early intervention is proposed by McGorry (2005) as one of the key priorities in international mental health. McGorry (2000) makes the case for the integration of efforts to improve positive mental health within preventive interventions in mental health services and points to the benefits in terms of nurturing a more positive approach to service provision. The development of early intervention programmes within the mental health services is relatively recent; however there are a number of models of early intervention being applied in various countries around the world. Chapter 7 outlines the development of effective early intervention programmes in relation to depression within the context of primary care and community services. In particular, there is increasing confidence that early intervention in psychotic disorders may be incorporated into mental health services (Birchwood et al 1997, McGorry 2000). Early intervention strategies in first-episode psychosis seek to reduce the duration of untreated psychosis, provide comprehensive early treatment of the first episode of psychosis, reduce the duration of active psychosis and promote recovery, community involvement and quality of life (McGorry et al 1999).

Edwards et al (2000) provide an interesting account of the development of a range of approaches to early psychosis service initiatives in Australasia, Europe and North America. They point to the fact that the essence of the early intervention approach is that a restructuring of services around the onset phase and early course of psychotic disorders will prove to be more cost-effective. This is particularly the case in relation to young people in the early phase of the disorder as they consume the greatest amount of resources. Schizophrenia and other forms of psychosis that affect young people rank as the third most disabling condition (following quadriplegia and dementia) and pose an enormous burden in terms of human suffering and economic costs. The availability of early detection and intervention programmes to reduce first-onset duration and relapse is therefore of high priority. Bertolote and McGorry (2005) argue that the provision of prompt and effective interventions for young people with early psychosis, for their families and carers, will promote recovery, equity and self-sufficiency and will facilitate the uptake of social, educational and employment opportunities, thereby promoting the individual's rights to citizenship and social inclusion. The early intervention paradigm builds on the strengths and qualities of young people with a psychosis and their families, and encourages greater optimism and expectations of positive outcomes and recovery. McGorry (2000) stresses that recovery rather than reha-bilitation is the goal of early intervention approaches and that quality of life in a positive sense, not merely the abolition of symptoms in the shortest possible time, should be constantly focused upon.

There is emerging evidence that early intervention approaches are more effective than standard clinical care (McGorry 2000) and a number of interven-tions have demonstrated efficacy in the management of early psychosis leading to improved outcomes. Macmillan and Shiers (2000) describe the development of the IRIS initiative in the West Midlands in the UK to promote early interven-tion for young people with psychosis and improved partnership between primary and secondary care. They report using the following core principles for early intervention services, which were identified by IRIS in collaboration with the UK's National Schizophrenia Fellowship:

- youth and user focus
- the importance of early and assertive engagement
- the embracing of diagnostic uncertainty
- treatment to be provided in the least restrictive and stigmatising setting
- an emphasis on social roles
- a family-oriented approach.

We will now examine the Early Psychosis Prevention and Intervention Centre (EPPIC) programme developed by Patrick McGorry and colleagues in Australia. Readers are advised to consult the original publications of the authors for fuller details of this early intervention programme, its development, implementation and evaluation.

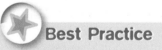 **Best Practice**

Early Psychosis Prevention and Intervention Centre (EPPIC) Programme

(Edwards & McGorry 2002, McGorry et al 2002, Phillips et al 2005)

Introduction and Background

There is growing evidence that both health and social outcomes for people with first episode psychosis are improved if the illness is detected and treated as early as possible (Falloon 1992, Falloon & Fadden 1995, McGorry 2000). The EPPIC

325

model, developed in Melbourne, Australia, is a complex system of interventions which aims to reduce delays in access to treatment and any resulting disruption in psychosocial functioning for young people with early psychosis. EPPIC, which is a component programme of ORYGEN Youth Health, is an integrated service which sees 250 to 300 new clients with first-episode psychosis each year. The EPPIC model includes strategies for early detection of young people at risk of developing psychoses and the provision of intensive phase-specific interventions for up to 18 months after the onset of the disorder. The rationale for early intervention in first-episode psychosis such as schizophrenia includes the early detection of new cases, shortening the delays to effective treatment and the provision of optimal and sustained treatment in the early 'critical period' of the first few years of illness. By delaying the onset of the disorder, reducing the time spent living with disability and accelerating recovery it may be possible to reduce the prevalence of psychotic disorders. The aims and objectives of EPPIC (www.eppic.org.au/contentPage.asp?pageCode=ABOUT) are:

- early identification and treatment of primary symptoms of psychotic illness with correspondingly improved access and reduced delays in initial treatment
- reduction of frequency and severity of relapse and increase in time to first relapse
- reduction of burden for carers and promotion of well-being among family members
- reduction of secondary morbidity in the post-psychotic phase of illness
- reduced disruption in social and vocational functioning and in psychosocial development in the critical period of the early years following onset of illness when most disability tends to accrue.

Early intervention may help prevent the often significant biological, social and psychological deterioration that can occur in the early years following onset of a psychotic disorder. Edwards and McGorry (2002) highlight some of the potential benefits of early intervention as being reduced morbidity, more rapid recovery, better prognosis, preservation of psychosocial skills, preservation of family and social supports and the decreased need for hospitalisation. The following briefly outlines some of the different programmes and services offered by the Australian EPPIC programme.

Youth Access Team (YAT): This is a multidisciplinary mobile assessment and community treatment which provides the first point of contact with EPPIC by visiting new clients to assess their need for treatment. YAT operates a 24-hour service 7 days a week to provide assessment for young people aged 15–29 years presenting with a first episode of psychosis and, if required, intensive home-based treatment. YAT uses networking and community education activities to raise awareness of psychosis in young people and to promote recognition and early referral. A major focus for the team is promoting the client's engagement with treatment. In cases where a young person is likely to take some time to recognise the need for treatment and to be motivated to attend regular appointments, home-based treatment and support can be provided. YAT also attempts to minimise the potential trauma involved in in-patient admissions and facilitates early discharge planning from in-patient care. Triage, which is a sub-component of YAT, is the first point of contact for those seeking EPPIC services. The triage role involves talking to the referrer, the young person, their family and other services to identify current difficulties and to determine whether specialist mental health assessment is required. The urgency of the young person's situation is assessed according to crisis, urgent or non-urgent classification and an appropriate response is arranged (www.eppic.org.au). The philosophy of EPPIC entails treating people in their own environment where possible.

In-patient unit: While most people are treated at home, some individuals with mental health disorders may require admittance to the in-patient unit. This unit provides assessment and treatment services for young people, a therapeutic group programme and recreational facilities.

Personal Assessment and Crisis Evaluation (PACE): The PACE clinic was set up to identify and treat individuals who are thought to be at imminent risk of developing a psychotic disorder. These clinics, which are an extension of the EPPIC centre, are located in discrete areas such as a shopping complex and adolescent health centres so as to avoid any stigma associated with attending the clinic. The name and locations were chosen in order to promote help-seeking among young people. Assessment, monitoring, support and referral are provided. Psychological interventions and medical treatments are offered with the aim of ameliorating symptoms, enhancing coping strategies and ultimately delaying or preventing the onset of psychosis.

Case management: EPPIC case managers facilitate and provide treatment, as well as responding to other needs such as directing clients towards other agencies and organisations. The following services are provided to young people for a period of up to 18 months after onset and play a critical role in preventing the development of secondary disability in people experiencing early psychosis (www.eppic.org.au):

- EPPIC continuing care programme: This programme specialises in the treatment of a young person's first episode of psychosis through comprehensive biological, psychological and social interventions. Each individual is allocated a case manager and a doctor who collaborate in providing clinical intervention and care. This can be for a period of up to 12 months. Preparation to leave the programme includes the young person developing an understanding of how to deal with mental health issues and linking with appropriate service providers when necessary.
- Intensive case management: This multidisciplinary service is designed for young people who have difficulty engaging with the mental health services or for those who have more complex needs and require intensive support. A comprehensive assessment is completed to determine each individual's specific needs. A collaborative plan is formed with the young person and their family/carers with interventions provided on an outreach basis.
- Treatment Resistance Early Assessment Team (TREAT): TREAT provides a forum for consultation with a particular focus on individuals who are experiencing suicidality and persisting positive and/or negative symptoms. TREAT provides a clinical consultancy service to EPPIC case managers and doctors, aiming to accelerate recovery and prevent established treatment resistance.

The Systematic Treatment of Persistent Psychosis (STOPP) programme was developed to help treat enduring positive psychotic symptoms and aims to reduce the distress associated with having the symptoms of psychosis, increasing the person's sense of mastery and control over the symptoms and determining methods to decrease the occurrence of symptoms. STOPP therapists are part of the TREAT team.

- LifeSPAN: This is a cognitive-behavioural therapy intervention directed towards feelings of hopelessness, suicidal ideation and depression. It is specifically tailored for clients with first-episode psychosis, to be used in consultation with suicide experts. The programme provides a service to clients who attend EPPIC and are assessed as being at a very high risk of suicide.
- Intensive Mobile Youth Outreach Service (IMYOS): This is a specialist mental health assessment and treatment service for young people who find themselves undertaking high-risk behaviours and find it difficult to engage in office-based treatment services. The service is provided in a setting that is easier for young people such as at home, in a café or in school. Clients can only be referred by their own case manager who may find the young person difficult to engage or be at high risk of harm to themselves.

Group programmes: These programmes aim to help young people to overcome the disruption to their lives caused by a mental disorder and also to assist them in personal development and the achievement of their life goals through social relationships, employment, education and creative expression. Acute and recovery group sessions for individuals are provided across four 'streams': vocation, creative expression, recreational and personal development. The needs of families and carers are also addressed through multi-family and individual family group sessions (Edwards et al 2000).

Family work: The EPPIC 'Family and Friends' programme has been developed to help families cope with their own reactions to the young person's difficulties and to participate in the planning and delivery of services. A 4-week group intervention is provided which seeks to inform and empower families about their role in the recovery process. Psycho-education programmes and other interventions are also provided.

Evaluation

A naturalistic effectiveness study was undertaken to evaluate the EPPIC programme, comparing 12-month outcomes among 51 clients treated under the EPPIC model in 1993 with another cohort of 51 clients from the same catchment area under the standard generic model of care. The EPPIC clients experienced significantly better outcomes than their counterparts in areas such as overall quality of life, including social and role functioning. The level of post-traumatic stress associated with hospitalisation and other elements of treatment was reduced and the experience of psychosis itself was less traumatic. The average length of hospital stay and the mean dose of antipsychotic medication both decreased without compromising recovery. There was also a reduction in the mean duration of untreated psychosis but this was not statistically significant (McGorry et al 1996).

McGorry et al (2002) conducted a single blind randomised controlled trial in the PACE clinic of the EPPIC centre, comparing two interventions in 59 clients aged 14–30 years, at incipient (ultra high) risk of progression to first-episode psychosis. A needs-based psychotherapy intervention was compared with a specific preventive intervention (SPI). The SPI involved all aspects of the needs-based intervention plus low-dose risperidone therapy and cognitive behaviour therapy hypothesised to have greater specificity for the reduction of risk of progression to psychosis. Treatment was provided for 6 months, after which all clients were offered ongoing needs-based intervention. Assessments were performed at baseline, 6 months, and 12 months. At the end of treatment, 10 of the 28 people who received needs-based intervention progressed to first-episode psychosis compared with three from the 31 SPI group. Following a 6-month follow up, another three people in the SPI group became psychotic and, with intention-to-treat analysis, the difference was no longer significant. However, for risperidone therapy-adherent patients in the SPI group, protection against progression extended for 6 months after cessation of risperidone use. The authors concluded that the study findings indicate that it may be possible to at least delay, and in some cases avert, progression to full clinical diagnosis of psychosis in individuals at incipient risk of schizophrenia and related psychotic disorders. They also advise that the findings should be investigated further using more rigorous designs.

A recent evaluation of LifeSPAN (Power et al 2003) concluded that augmenting early intervention with a suicide prevention therapy could help to reduce the risk of suicide among young people. The evaluation was of 56 suicidal clients with first-episode psychosis randomly assigned to standard clinical care or standard care plus LifeSPAN therapy. In all, 42 clients completed the intervention. Clinical ratings and measures of suicidality and risk were assessed before, immediately after the intervention and 6 months later. Results showed benefits in the treatment group both on indirect measures of suicidality and on a direct measure of suicide ideation (Power et al 2003).

Larsen et al (2001) studied two groups of clients in Norway, one of which had usual detection methods for psychosis and the other with early detection strategies that included education about psychosis. This study concluded that clients with early detection had a shorter median duration of untreated psychosis by 21.5 weeks than clients with usual detection. The early detection teams were modelled after the early psychosis programme created by McGorry in the EPPIC programme.

Programme Implementation Features

Early recognition and assistance: Significant delays before effective treatment is initiated, or secondary morbidity resulting from aspects of management, can hamper preventive efforts. The EPPIC programme addresses this issue through improving recognition of symptoms associated with psychosis. This is done through educating primary care providers and reducing the stigma surrounding psychosis, which may deter clients and their families from seeking help. Providing referrals through a responsive, user-friendly service can also help to reduce the fear and stigma associated with mental health services. Furthermore, the easy access to services which EPPIC provides ensures there is a rapid response, a flexible approach and an assertive outreach. The mobile assessment provided by EPPIC is a key advance in improving access to care.

Non-stigmatising service provision with client and family involvement: The involvement of client, families and friends in the development of early psychosis services is a core feature of the EPPIC programme. An intensive mobile outreach service provides easy access for youths that are difficult to engage in treatment. Furthermore, the egalitarian environment that allows sharing of ideas between staff members and the application of management principles encourages discussion and common ownership of the service's policies and principles. A strong client influence on the services maximises respect for service users and enhances the ambience and quality of care.

Comprehensive system of care: The EPPIC model provides a comprehensive service to clients and their families. The involvement of family and friends provides the supportive environment that individuals require to prevent psychotic episodes and promote positive mental health. The mobile assessment and treatment team aim to assess and treat clients in their own environment whenever possible. The range of case management services is tailored towards the varying experiences of those at risk of developing or having episodes of psychosis. The integration of biological (medication), social (family, accommodation, education) and psychological (psycho-education) interventions provides maximum benefit to the client.

Recovery focus: EPPIC uses a number of different strategies to promote recovery for clients. Psycho-education is a core ingredient of case management and aims to educate clients on their illness, treatment options and prospects for the future. It is also important to be aware of issues in recovery that can hamper progress such as substance misuse, suicide ideation and personality difficulties. A recovery focus generates optimism and expectations of positive outcomes and recovery so that all young people with psychosis and their families achieve ordinary lives including personal, social, educational and employment outcomes.

Key Recommendations for Replication

When replicating this model it is important that services should be developed in ways that are congruent and synergistic with the local setting (Edwards & McGorry 2002). A profile of the community and the presence of risk factors associated with the development of mental disorders should be considered. Edwards and McGorry recommend the formation of a steering group to oversee and support the development of the service and a clinicians' group to address day-to-day issues, with working groups addressing community and professional education, clinical practice, family work and group activities. A nine-step model for developing an early psychosis service is described by Edwards and McGorry (2002):

1. *State the philosophy and principles:* The development of a philosophy can shape the general organisation of a service and can be adapted from those found in other early psychosis prevention centres or academic sources. Similarly, principles can be developed that will guide specific daily activities.

2. ***Set the boundary conditions for first-episode pssychosis:*** The incidence of psychotic disorders within the area should be determined. A new service will need to consider the age groups and disorders present so as to determine a focus for service provision.

3. ***Assess the population needs and current service use:*** Once the target group has been identified, the specific needs of this group in the local setting should be assessed. This information can be obtained via qualitative and quantitative methods of consulting with service users, families, health professionals and other representatives.

4. ***Set the early psychosis scene:*** This can be achieved through the training of staff already in mental health services to act as catalysts for the process and to contribute to raising awareness within the local area. Consulting with and obtaining support from health planners, administrators and politicians helps to promote the concept in the area of policy development. The involvement of academics can contribute to the research aspect of the service and establishing links with other services can stimulate the sharing of ideas and experience.

5. ***Identify an early psychosis workforce:*** Potential workforce members capable of driving the service may identify themselves during the training of existing mental health staff as mentioned in the above point.

6. ***Define the focus:*** Data from the needs assessment can define the focus of the service, i.e. pre-psychotic phase or first-episode psychosis.

7. ***Develop a written plan:*** The plan should outline short- and long-term aims, objectives, methods, implementation, costs and evaluation of the service.

8. ***Implement key service components:*** This entails the implementation of the plan and the delivery of the different service components.

9. ***Monitor and review:*** The monitoring and evaluation procedures should be planned in the early stages of the service development. Evaluation should focus on how well the programme is being delivered (process evaluation) and then if it is achieving specified outcomes and effects (impact and outcome evaluation).

Edwards and McGorry (2002) advise that training, education and consultation are necessary to bring about change within a service and to successfully develop a new approach. Investment in staff development is one of the most important factors to consider when establishing an early psychosis service. Techniques can range from distribution of academic papers to more comprehensive programmes. Consultation promotes a collaborative partnership to identify solutions to problems and challenges. Mental health consultation can involve client-centred case consultation relating to the management of a particular case or group of cases, consultee-centred consultation which aims to help the consultee to improve knowledge and skills, and programme-centred consultation which aims to improve planning, administration and programme development. Edwards and McGorry also point out that it is necessary for the individuals providing the consultation to be closely allied with a clinical setting, and to draw on the experience of clinicians at that service. However, the implications of this are that a base is required upon which to draw trainers and experts as well as the funding and resource requirements of such activities.

Support Programmes for Carers

While carers play a critical role in the care and recovery of people with long-term disorders, the impact of caring for a family member or relative on the mental health of carers is widely acknowledged. Researchers have documented the burden that the caring role imposes on relatives and the nature and extent of the areas affected. As Kuipers and Raune (2000) point out, carers may not choose their role; they find that they become carers due to the long-term illness of a family member. Carers may find themselves providing care with few supports, no specialist knowledge and no perceived support from services. The importance of emotional support, in particular, has been highlighted as this is likely to have an impact on the mental health of the carers. Caregivers tend to focus on the needs of those they take care of and, therefore, may neglect their own health needs (Gray 2003). Psychological or emotional health is the area of a caregiver's daily life that is most affected by providing home care (Gray 2003). In comparison to the general population, primary caregivers are more frequently depressed and anxious, are more likely to use psychotropic medications and can exhibit more symptoms of psychological distress (Toseland & Smith 2001, Zarit & Zarit 1998). Carers may also suffer from reduced social networks and are likely to feel a sense of emotional loss and isolation. Caregiver depression is identified as a growing concern. Depression can deplete a caregiver's own resources, put them at risk of developing chronic conditions such as coronary heart disease, cancer and diabetes (Cannuscio et al 2002) and also contribute to a caregiver experiencing burnout. This can result in the caregiver no longer being able to care in the home setting and thus the client is placed in nursing home care. Older caregivers who report strain due to caregiving experience a 63% higher mortality rate than older spouses who were not involved in caregiving (Schulz & Beach 1999). Generally people with depression have been found to use two or four times more health care than people without mental health problems (Goff 2002). Thus it can be concluded that the effect of depression on a caregiver can impact upon the family, the client and ultimately on society. A comprehensive support service can improve caregivers' physical and emotional health, thereby contributing to improved care and recovery for the client and ultimately reduced government expenditures on nursing home care (Gray 2003).

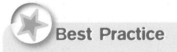

Best Practice

A Comprehensive Support Programme for Spouse Caregivers of Alzheimer's Disease

(Mittleman et al 1995)

Living with and caring for a family member with Alzheimer's disease (AD) can have profound effects on the mental health of caregivers. Depression has been identified as a particular issue for caregivers of people with AD. Mittleman et al (1995) report on a comprehensive support programme for spouse care-givers of AD. This multifaceted intervention was developed at the New York University Ageing and Dementia Research Centre (NYU-ADRC) and included several programme components with the aim of maximising formal and infor-mal support for caregivers and alleviating depression. The programme included individual and family counselling, the continuous availability of ad hoc coun-selling and support-group participation. The individual and family counselling sessions were tailored to each specific situation, with a primary focus on increas-ing support for the spouse caregiver from other family members. Caregivers joined weekly support groups after the individual and family counselling ses-sions were completed. In addition, an ad hoc consultation service was available at any time for caregivers to receive help when in need. The intervention was designed to provide continuous support for the primary caregiver and the family for as long as needed. Caregivers were recruited into the study through a number of ways and included caregivers that accompanied dementia patients to the NYU-ADRC for clinical evaluations and referrals from the Alzheimer's Associa-tion of New York. Other caregivers were recruited through contacts with day-care centres and other agencies providing social services to the elderly in the New York metropolitan area.

Programme Content

The counselling components of the programme consisted of six individual and family sessions within 4 months after intake into the programme. One individual counselling session with the spouse took place immediately following the conclu-sion of the intake evaluation. Four sessions of family counselling, which were tailored in response to problems uncovered in the first individual session, were followed by an additional individual counselling session with the caregiver at the 4-month follow-up evaluation. Counselling included role play and education about how to prevent problem client behaviours, and sought to enable the care-givers with a sense of control over their environment. At the conclusion of the formal counselling component of the programme, 4 months after intake into the study, caregivers in the intervention group were required to join an AD caregiver support group which met regularly. There was no time limitation to membership in support groups.

The third component of the programme consisted of informal consultation on an ad hoc basis with the family counsellors, which could be initiated by either the spouse caregiver or any participating family member. Counsellors were available for telephone consultation at any time in the event of a crisis. Caregivers in the intervention group were taught how to reduce stress and to manage clients in order to reduce the frequency and intensity of problem behaviours and caregiv-ers' reactions to these behaviours. Counsellors also encouraged the caregivers to seek support from members of their social networks, and particularly from their families. The counsellors emphasised the need for caregivers to care for them-selves and to seek medical attention for themselves as well as the client. Caregiv-ers in the control group were also given telephone access to the counsellors at any time; however they were not given active intervention or formal counselling.

Evaluation

The evaluation study was comprised of 206 spouse caregivers, 58% of whom were female and 42% male. Caregivers were randomly assigned to the intervention (n = 103) or control group (n = 103) immediately after baseline interviews. Regular follow-up interviews were conducted every 4 months during the first year after baseline, and every six months thereafter, as long as the client was alive. Each caregiver in the intervention group received all components of the intervention and was provided with continuous support for an unlimited period of time. Counselling was also provided.

Mittleman et al (1995) report that, in the first year after intake, the control group became increasingly more depressed whereas the intervention group remained stable. By the eighth month, caregivers in the intervention group were found to be significantly less depressed than those in the control group. Results from the study demonstrated that an intervention which enhances long-term social support to carers has the potential for alleviating some of the deleterious effects of caregiving on mental health. The change in the intervention and control groups only became statistically significant eight months after caregivers entered the study and the impact of the intervention on caregiver depression increased with each follow up in the first year after participants entered the study.

Programme Implementation Features

Multifaceted structured programme provided over the duration of the clients' illness: The programme entailed the provision of long-term support over the entire course of the illness, with a range of programme components provided including individual and group-based counselling and support groups for the primary caregiver and the family.

Flexible and accessible service: The programme was delivered in an accessible manner with counsellors providing counselling sessions in the caregivers' homes if they could not leave home. Sessions were scheduled at any time, including weekends and evenings.

Relationship with caregivers: The counsellors built up a relationship with the caregivers and listened to the caregivers' problems. Counsellors maintained contact with caregivers over time by regularly mailing birthday cards, holiday greetings and an NYU-ADRC newsletter to all participants. These procedures made it possible for counsellors to develop a relationship with the caregivers and maintain a very low attrition rate.

Resolving family conflict: A focus of the family counselling sessions was the resolution of conflict about the care of the client. Conflict among family members is identified as contributing to caregiver depression. Although there were only four family sessions, and they all occurred in the first 4 months after intake, the counsellors were available to family members to resolve difficulties with the caregiver.

An enabling approach: An important focus of the counselling was to make the caregivers more aware of the reasons for the clients' behaviour and to teach them techniques for managing and interacting with the clients. Finding successful solutions to new problems enabled caregivers to feel a sense of mastery, which may have resulted in less depression. Caregivers were encouraged to ask their family members and friends for the kind and amount of support and help they needed. Furthermore, the quantity and timing of one of the components of the intervention, ad hoc counselling, was entirely under the control of the caregiver.

Facilitating a greater network of support: A major focus of the intervention was to make family members aware of the impact of the illness of the client on the well-being of the spouse caregiver and to make it possible for the spouse caregiver to obtain appropriate help from family members. Results from the study suggested that the effect of the support programme on depression was to some extent through its impact on the satisfaction the caregiver was able to obtain from his or her social network. The intervention facilitated an increase in family cohesion and greater participation in family caregiving thereby improving the support network of the caregiver.

Key Recommendations for Replication

Mittleman et al (1995) noted that their support programme and its evaluation differed in a number of ways from previous studies which could help account for the demonstration of a relatively greater impact of the intervention on caregiver depression. Studies prior to Mittleman et al (1995) had confined themselves to examining short-term effects of relatively short-term interventions, whereas the deterioration of an AD patient can continue for many years. The variability in depression among caregivers also makes it necessary to have a large sample size. In the Mittleman et al programme, the counsellors went to the caregivers' homes for both assessment and treatment if requested to do so and in this way helped to overcome any practical difficulties caregivers may have had in arranging a visit to the research centre. A meta-analysis of caregiver interventions (Sorensen et al 2002), which also included Mittleman et al's study, noted that multi-component interventions may have a large effect on caregiver burden because they consist of multiple techniques and target multiple outcome domains. Long-term multi-component interventions are, therefore, recommended as they are most able to address a variety of caregiver needs.

- -

Health-Promoting Mental Health Services

The 'Ottawa Charter for health promotion' (WHO 1986) emphasises the importance of reorientating the health service toward the promotion of health. The charter also highlights the importance of having a 'settings-based' approach to health promotion in order to promote health within and across all areas of everyday life. In 1988 the hospital setting was singled out as being an area that required attention and resulted in the founding of the 'Health Promoting Hospital' (HPH) network. The WHO HPH project is based on the 1996 Ljubljana Charter on reforming health care and the Vienna recommendations on HPHs (WHO 1996, 1997). These recommendations provide guidelines on initiating a process of changing the culture of the hospital from a curative one to promoting the health of staff, patients and their relatives and supporting a healthier environment. The role of the HPH network is to use periods of illness as an opportunity to promote clients' health, to encourage and empower clients to make better use of primary health care services and to act as a stimulus for health development in the whole community (Pelikan et al 1997b). Therefore, a hospital as a setting has the potential to actively promote the health and well-being of their clients, its workforce and the wider community (Whitehead 2004). This approach requires health care professionals to consider their care activities in relation to the broader determinants of health hence focusing on a holistic approach to health service delivery across the whole health and social care continuum (Whitehead 2005). Generally the HPH network aims to develop the hospital into a more health promoting setting. The 'European Pilot Hospital Project' of HPH was the most important strategy chosen by the WHO to develop an international network of health promoting hospitals (Pelikan et al 1997a). This project aimed to document and evaluate the implementation of health promotion in hospitals, with all activity being supported by international leadership and coordination and an exchange of experiences between hospitals.

Numerous general hospitals applied to be pilot sites for the implementation of this project. Philippshospital in Germany was unique in its application as it was a psychiatric hospital. Psychiatric hospitals, like any other hospital, have problems with hygiene, costs and health risks. However, psychiatric hospitals also have to deal with specific problems resulting from mental disorders and the social reactions toward clients and their disorders (Berger & Paul 1997). In the early 1990s, as Germany was reforming its mental health care services, Philippshospital had become quite active in the re-development of patient care and the structures within and outside the hospital. This time of change required an increase in communication and cooperation between mental health service providers and the priority of developing new concepts for treatment (Berger & Paul 1997) such as making the community more accessible to service users. Such an approach required the framework, guidance and support that a formal network such as the HPH could provide. It was on this basis that the decision was made to apply as one of the pilot sites for the European project.

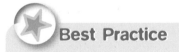 **Best Practice**

The Philippshospital Health Promoting Hospital Initiative

Following community-based reforms in the 1970s, Philippshospital had reduced its 1700 beds to 300 and had several sub-specialist psychiatry departments and a nursing school. These developments had led to a greatly increased patient turnover with a marked increase in admission rate (+42%) and a reduction in length of stay (−50%). Following initial internal resistance 30% of the entire staff formally accepted the initiative and ideas for 40 projects emerged. Considerable efforts were made to hone the choice and structure of projects in collaboration with all staff. Thus, once support was obtained from the respective decision makers, information sessions were held using pre-existing organisational and communication structures to make contact with all personnel. These sessions were held within staff meetings or during breaks in order to reach as many staff members as possible. In addition, an inaugural newsletter containing information about the project was distributed. Participation in group discussions was high with almost all staff members getting involved. The groups provided a forum for expressing dissatisfaction with the management and hospital as a whole. Staff were then invited to contribute to improvements through participating in the WHO project. In total, 40 project ideas emerged. These were reviewed by a steering committee against criteria from the Budapest Declaration and the Ottawa Charter. Twenty-five potential sub-projects focusing on different aspects of planning, realising and documenting the project work were identified. These 25 sub-projects were presented to the staff at a project fair. The event was aimed at informing the internal public on the variety of project ideas, discussing the ideas in small groups and giving the groups' activists the opportunity to recruit new participants for the group work. Staff members who were unable to participate at the project fair were informed of the developments through a newsletter in the hospital. Subsequent to the project fair, further prioritisation resulted in 10 sub-projects, planned and delivered by multidisciplinary groups and feeding into a joint projects group. The 10 sub-projects addressed three subject areas: patients, staff and the community, i.e. integration of the hospital into the region.

1. **Staff-focused projects:** There were four staff-focused projects including health promotion at the workplace, social work counselling of the staff, ergonomic assessment of computer workplaces and team supervision. Team supervision aimed to enhance the self-reflexive potential of the organisation with a particular emphasis on skill development and support for staff (Berger & Paul 1997).
2. **Community-focused projects:** There were two community-focused projects that aimed to provide an emergency service for general medicine in conjunction with local GPs, as well as the networking of a hospital ward with out-patient services.
3. **Client-focused projects:** Three client-focused projects were undertaken which were successful in the outcomes they reached. A counselling centre for non-national clients was developed and new therapeutic initiatives such as horseback riding for clients with psychosis and drama work in psychiatric health care. A psycho-education programme for clients with psychosis and their relatives was also developed (Berger & Paul 1997).

These areas were chosen in order to reflect some of the central questions of the hospital as an organisation. An in-depth review of the Philippshospital WHO project is given by Berger and Paul (1998). We will now focus on the implementation of one of the sub-projects, the psycho-educational groups for patients and their relatives.

Psycho-educational groups for patients and relatives, developed from research findings on 'Expressed Emotion' (EE), showed that the course of a psychosis could be positively influenced by certain styles of communication within the family (Kuipers 1992). The degree of EE is assessed by means of specific, structured interviews on the basis of three indicators: criticism, hostility and overcaring.

Following on from this concept, intervention strategies were developed with the aim of lowering the rate of relapse by influencing the family environment through psycho-educative measures. By contributing to an increase in social support the psycho-educative groups hoped to improve intrafamilial problem-solving skills. This project also aimed at achieving better compliance with medication, improved coping with the illness as well as relapse prevention by means of provision of information about the disorder (mainly schizophrenia). Groups comprised of four to 10 members and met a total of eight times at weekly intervals with a doctor or psychologist acting as moderator. Course materials consisting of crisis- and problem-solving diagrams as well as course tables for the early warning signs, exercise and family role games were taken from common programmes for establishing social competency and were offered according to behaviour therapy guidelines. Particular attention was paid to a climate of emotional acceptance with groups making suggestions for improvement.

Eight sessions were held covering the concept of EE, information on psychosis, its course and prognosis, options for the family, information on medication treatment, the physiological and biochemical foundations of medication therapy and its side effects, non-medication treatment methods, recognition of early warning signs and its use in relapse and a number of role plays to practise problem solving. The programme consisted of an informal knowledge-sharing section (meetings one to five) and a training section (meetings six to eight).

Evaluation

The experiences of patients and their families in the psycho-educational groups were assessed in an initial evaluation study. A structured interview and a self-evaluation questionnaire examining changes in knowledge, self-confidence and individual and family problem-solving behaviour were used. Results showed an increase in theoretical knowledge about the disorder, increased self-confidence in dealing with relatives and a positive assessment of the problem-solving behaviour within the family. Experiences of the group moderators were also assessed and this revealed that there was great relief among families to discover that other families had similar problems. Especially fruitful was the therapeutically-induced trade between relatives and patients whereby it was possible for them to sit down together and work on current conflicts in an atmosphere of greater emotional distance which facilitated resolution. The evaluation also revealed that there was a high level of acceptance among both patients and their relatives with continued patient participation beyond their stay in hospital.

Programme Implementation Features

Patient and family involvement: Patients in the respective families considered themselves as partners in the process and were able to exhibit more trust in their own family owing to the group discussions. Being able to talk about the disorder and its consequences in a different setting to usual proved beneficial to all concerned, in particular the mutual work of patients and relatives where they were able to sit down together, and relatives were aware of what was going on.

Strengthening of the family help system: Informing patients' families of psychosis and its course and prognosis promotes understanding and awareness of the issues involved. In particular, coping and problem-solving skills are a major focus of the group sessions and this embraces the notion that the family can act as a resource and source of support for both the patient and the treating team.

Support from hospital management: The support from hospital administrators in terms of staff hours and material support was critical to the successful implementation of the groups. The framework of the HPH was also identified as assisting the sustainability of implementing group work.

Key Recommendations for Replication

While the integration of the psycho-educational groups into everyday hospital life proved difficult, the HPH project framework helped both formally and informally to guarantee continuity in implementing group work; formally as the hospital administration donated staff time, allowing members of the sub-project group a number of hours for work on the project and material support; informally the reputation of the HPH project made it easier within the hospital to engage staff members for work on the sub-project and to sell the group programme in-house. The framework of the WHO project thus aided a programme which could be promoted throughout the hospital with the cooperation of all involved. In doing so, the informal work on the part of the participants of the sub-project group was essential.

Regarding the overall project, because of the variety of sub-projects, the evaluation of its overall impact proved challenging. External evaluators developed an evaluation strategy which was based on the theoretical framework of the empowerment concept and which addressed the staff of the hospital as a whole. Overall, participation in the pilot resulted in many developments within the hospital, 'stimulating the creative potential of the staff and giving new impetus to the social-psychiatric reform' (Berger & Paul 1997). The external evaluation found that:

- conflicts at the hospital were reduced, which facilitated a number of developments
- long-term motivation could be fostered among the staff, as a prerequisite for the implementation of new services
- interest in health promotion of the staff was given substantial support
- the management was facilitated to translate objectives into action that were developed independently of administrative directives
- public interest in the psychiatric hospital and its treatment profile was stimulated.

Berger and Paul (1997) also report that the WHO project led to a generalisation of effects in that it acted as a catalyst for a number of further developments, e.g. a continuous further training programme for nursing staff, new treatment concepts, establishment of a psychotherapy unit, renovation of the premises, art exhibitions and the founding of a cultural association responsible for public relations. Following the Phillipshospital pilot, the WHO developed a Health Promoting Mental Health Service (HPMHS) network that psychiatric hospitals are invited to join. Stansfeld (2002) describes the development of a health-promoting mental health services pilot project in the north west of England and reports that, to become a health-promoting mental health service, members are required to accept the principles of health promotion and undertake the following tasks:

- implement at least three health promotion projects at the therapeutic, organisational and inter-institutional levels
- conduct the health promotion projects for a period of at least 3 years
- contribute to the network database
- submit a written annual project report to the coordinating institute and to WHO.

Clearly, the scope of such an initiative could extend beyond hospitals to permeate all aspects of community-based services.

Generic Principles of Effective Programmes in the Mental Health Service

Mental health services operate in a wide variety of settings including hospitals, community mental health services, prisons, schools and universities and even workplaces. In this chapter we have focused mainly on community-based services and hospitals. However, regardless of the specific setting, mental health promotion brings a positive focus to mental health services in terms of both the type of services and how they are delivered. A mental health promoting approach requires that services are extended beyond clinical treatment of the illness to consider the broader psychosocial needs of clients and their families and seeks to enhance capacity and the prospects of positive recovery. This perspective may be applied across a range of services from early intervention through to treatment and recovery.

Based on the research evidence and programmes reviewed in this chapter, the characteristics of successful mental health promotion programmes within mental health services include:

- comprehensive multi-component interventions that encompass users/ clients, families, service providers, service managers and communities
- detailed needs assessment, which includes the perspective of the clients and their families and considers their social context
- use of multiple methods of education, empowerment, de-stigmatisation, liaison, early intervention and recovery models
- operation in multiple settings including where the target audience are normally found, i.e. in homes, communities and workplaces rather than in health service settings alone
- adoption of inclusive and egalitarian modes of planning and implementation involving clients, families and staff

- the provision of training for staff to reorientate their services towards a health promoting function
- services which respect the rights of clients and adopt a positive, enhancing approach to all aspects of service delivery.

References

Anthony W 1993 Recovery from mental illness: the guiding vision of the mental health service system in the 1990s. Psychosocial Rehabilitation Journal 16(4):11–23

Australian Health Ministers 1992 National mental health policy. Australian Government Publishing Services, Canberra

Barker C, Pistrang N, Shapiro D A et al 1993 You in mind: a preventive mental health television series. British Journal of Clinical Psychology 32(3):281–293

Barry M M, Doherty A, Hope A et al 2000 A community needs assessment for rural mental health promotion. Health Education Research 15(3):293–304

Bates P (ed) 2002 Working for inclusion: making social inclusion a reality for people with severe mental health problems. Sainsbury Centre for Mental Health, London

Berger H, Paul R 1997 The health promoting psychiatric hospital – what is the difference? In: Pelikan J M, Garcia-Barbero M, Lobnig H et al (eds) Pathways to a health promoting hospital. Ludwig Boltzmann Institute, Vienna

Berger H, Paul R 1998 The health promoting psychiatric hospital – what is the difference? Experiences from the Phillipshospital pilot hospital project in Riedstadt. In: Pelikan J M, Lobnig H, Krajic K (eds) Pathways to a Health Promoting Hospital Series 2:71–94

Bertolote J, McGorry P 2005 Early intervention and recovery for young people with early psychosis: consensus statement. British Journal of Psychiatry 187(Suppl48):116–119

Bhugra D 1989 Public opinions on mental illness – a review. Acta Psychiatrica Scandinavica 80:10–12

Birchwood M, McGorry P D, Jackson H 1997. Early intervention in schizophrenia – editorial. British Journal of Psychiatry 170:2–5

Brockman J, D'Arcy C, Edmonds L 1979 Facts or artifacts? Changing public attitudes toward the mentally ill. Social Science and Medicine 13:673–682

Bush R, Donald M, Madl R 1998 Evaluation report for the Queensland mental health community development projects (vols 1 and 2). Centre for Primary Health Care, University of Queensland, Queensland

Byrne P 2000 Stigma of mental illness and ways of diminishing it. Advances in Psychiatric Treatment 6:65–72

Byrne P 2001 Psychiatric stigma. British Journal of Psychiatry 178:281–284

Cannuscio C C, Jones C, Kawachi I et al 2002 Reverberations of family illness: a longitudinal assessment of informal care giving and mental health status in the nurse's health study. American Journal of Public Health 92:1305–1311

Corrigan P, Ralph R (eds) 2004 Recovery and mental illness: consumer visions and research paradigms. American Psychological Association, Washington DC

Corrigan P W, Watson A C 2002 Understanding the impact of stigma on people with mental illness. Journal of World Psychiatry 1:6–19

Drake R E, Goldman H H, Leff H S 2001 Implementing evidence based practices in routine mental health service settings. Psychiatric Services 52:179–182

Dunn S 1999 Creating accepting communities: report of the MIND enquiry into social exclusion and mental health problems. Mind Publication, London

Edwards J, McGorry P D 2002 Implementing early intervention in psychosis: a guide to establishing early psychosis services. Martin Dunitz, London

Edwards J, McGorry P D, Pennell K 2000 Models of early intervention in psychosis: an analysis of service approaches. In: Birchwood M, Fowler D, Jackson C (eds) Early intervention in psychosis: a guide to concepts, evidence and interventions. Wiley, Chichester, Chapter 12:281–314

Falloon I R H 1992 Early intervention for first episodes of schizophrenia: a preliminary exploration. Psychiatry 55:4–15

Falloon I R H, Fadden G 1995 Integrated mental health care. Cambridge University Press, Cambridge

Felton C, Stastny P, Shern D et al 1995 Consumers as peer specialists on intensive case management teams: impact on client outcomes. Psychiatric Services 46:1037–1044

Frese F J, Stanley J, Kress K et al 2001 Integrating evidence based practices and the recovery model. Psychiatric Services 52(11):1462–1468

Gale E, Seymour L, Crepaz-Keay D et al 2004 Scoping review on mental health anti-stigma and anti-discrimination programmes and interventions. Mentality, Mental Health Media and Rethink, London

Goff V V 2002 Depression: a decade of progress, more to do (issue brief 786). National Health Policy Forum, George Washington University, Washington DC

Gray L 2003 Caregiver depression: a growing mental health concern (policy brief). Family Caregiver Alliance, San Francisco

Harris E C, Barraclough B 1998 Excess mortality of mental disorder. British Journal of Psychiatry 173:11–53

Hayward P, Bright J 1997 Stigma and mental illness: a review and critique. Journal of Mental Health 6:345–354

Hersey J C, Kilibanoff L S, Lam D J et al 1984 Promoting social support: the impact of the California's 'Friends can be good medicine' campaign. Health Education Quarterly 11(3):293–311

INDI (Irish Nutrition and Dietetic Institute) 2000 Nutrition and dietetic service for people with mental health difficulties in Ireland. INDI, Dublin

Jacobson N, Greenley D 2001 What is recovery? A conceptual model and explication. Psychiatric Services 52:482–485

Katschnig H, Freeman H, Sartorius N (eds) 2006 Quality of life in mental disorders, 2nd edn. Wiley, Chichester

Kuipers L 1992 Expressed emotion research in Europe. British Journal of Clinical Psychology 31:429–443

Kuipers E, Raune D 2000 The early development of expressed emotion and burden in families of first-onset psychosis. In: Birchwood M, Fowler D, Jackson C (eds) Early intervention in psychosis: a guide to concepts, evidence and interventions. Wiley, Chichester, Chapter 5:128–140

Larsen T K, McGlashan T H, Johannessen J O et al 2001 Shortened duration of untreated first episode of psychosis: changes in patient characteristics at treatment. American Journal of Psychiatry 158:1917–1919

Link B G, Phelan J C 2001 Conceptualising stigma. Annual Review of Sociology 27:363–385

Link B G, Phelan J C, Bresnahan M et al 1999 Public conceptions of mental illness: labels, causes, dangerousness and social distance. American Journal of Public Health 89(9):1328–1333

McGorry P D 2000 The scope for preventive strategies in early psychosis: logic, evidence and momentum. In: Birchwood M, Fowler D, Jackson C (eds) Early intervention in psychosis: a guide to concepts, evidence and interventions. Wiley, Chichester, Chapter 1:3–27

McGorry P D 2005 Early intervention in psychotic disorders: beyond debate to solving problems. British Journal of Psychiatry 187(Suppl48):108–110

McGorry P D, Edwards J, Mihalopoulos C et al 1996 EPPIC: an evolving system of early detection and optimal management. Schizophrenia Bulletin 22:305–326

McGorry P D, Edwards J, Pennell K 1999 Sharpening the focus: early intervention in the real world. In: McGorry P D Jackson H J (eds) Recognition and management of early psychosis: a preventive approach. Cambridge University Press, New York:441–475

McGorry P D, Yung A R, Phillips L J et al 2002 Randomised controlled trial of interventions designed to reduce the risk of progression to first-episode psychosis in a clinical sample with subthreshold symptoms. Archives of General Psychiatry 59(10):921–928

McKeon P, Carrick S 1991 Public attitudes to depression: a national survey. Irish Journal of Psychological Medicine 8:116–121

Macmillan F, Shiers D 2000 The IRIS programme. In: Birchwood M, Fowler D, Jackson C (eds) Early intervention in psychosis: a guide to concepts, evidence and interventions. Wiley, Chichester, Chapter 13:315–326

Mental Health Foundation 2000 Strategies for living: report of user led research into people's strategies for living with mental distress. Mental Health Foundation, London

mentality 2003 Making it effective: a guide to evidence based mental health promotion.

Radical mentalities – briefing paper 1. **mentality**, London

Mittleman M S, Ferris S H, Shulman E et al 1995 A comprehensive support program: effect on depression in spouse-caregivers of AD patients. The Gerentologist 35(6):792–802

Murray C J, Lopez A D 1996 The global burden of disease: summary. Harvard School of Public Health, Harvard

Paykel ES 2001 Impact of public and general practice education in depression: evaluation of the Defeat Depression Campaign. Psychiatrica Fennica 32:51–61

Pelikan J M, Krajic K, Lobnig H et al 1997a The European Pilot Hospital Project on health promoting hospitals – a summary. In: Pelikan J M, Garcia-Barbero M, Lobnig H et al (eds) Pathways to a health promoting hospital. Ludwig Boltzmann Institute, Vienna

Pelikan J M, Lobnig H, Krajic K 1997b Health-promoting hospital. World Health 3:24–25

Peter E 2003 Review: involvement of former or current users of mental health services may improve outcomes in patients with severe mental illness. Evidence Based Nursing 6:90

Phelan M, Stradins L, Morrison S 2001 Physical health of people with severe mental illness. British Medical Journal 322:443–444

Phillips L J, McGorry P D, Yung A et al 2005 Prepsychotic phase of schizophrenia and related disorders: recent progress and future opportunities. British Journal of Psychiatry 187(Suppl48):33–44

Pinfold V, Toulmin H, Thornicroft G et al 2003 Reducing psychiatric stigma and discrimination: evaluation of educational interventions in UK secondary schools. British Journal of Psychiatry 182:342–346

Power P J, Bell R J, Mills R et al 2003 Suicide prevention in first episode psychosis: the development of a randomised controlled trial of cognitive therapy for acutely suicidal patients with early psychosis. Australian and New Zealand Journal of Psychiatry 37(4):414–420

Priest R G, Vize C, Roberts A et al 1996 Lay people's attitudes to treatment of depression: results of opinion poll of Defeat Depression Campaign just before its launch. British Medical Journal 313:858–859

Rabkin J G 1974 Public attitudes toward mental illness: a review of the literature. Schizophrenia Bulletin 10:9–33

Reeves A 2002 Creative journeys of recovery: a survivor perspective. In: Birchwood M,

Fowler D, Jackson C (eds) Early intervention in psychosis: a guide to concepts, evidence and interventions, 2nd edn. Wiley, Chichester, Chapter 14:327–347

Rosenfield S 1992 Factors contributing to the subjective quality of life of the chronically mentally ill. Journal of Health and Social Behavior 33:229–315

Sartorius N 1997 Fighting schizophrenia and its stigma. A new World Psychiatric Association educational programme. British Journal of Psychiatry 170:297

Sayce L 2000 From psychiatric patient to citizen: overcoming discrimination and social exclusion. Macmillan, London

Schulz R, Beach S 1999 Care giving as a risk factor for mortality. The caregiver health effects study. Journal of the American Medical Association 282:2215–2219

Simpson E, House A 2002 Involving users in the delivery and evaluation of mental health services: systematic review. British Medical Journal 325:1265–1275

Sogaard A J, Fonnebo V 1995 The Norwegian Mental Health Campaign in 1992. Part II: changes in knowledge and attitudes. Health Education Research 10:267–278

Sorensen S, Pinquart M, Duberstein D 2002 How effective are interventions with caregivers? An updated meta-analysis. The Gerontologist 42(3):356–372

Stansfeld J 2002 Health promoting mental health services. Journal of Mental Health Promotion 1(4):25–31

Sundram S, Cole N, McGuiness M et al 2004 Report on the Depression Awareness Research Project. Mental Health Research Institute, Victoria

Toseland R W, Smith T 2001 Supporting caregivers through education and training. Prepared for the US Administration on Ageing. US Department of Health and Human Services, Washington DC

Trainor J, Shepherd M, Boydell K M et al 1997 Beyond the service paradigm: the impact and implications of consumer/survivor initiatives. Psychiatric Rehabilitation Journal 21(2):132–139

Whitehead D 2004 The European Health Promoting Hospitals (HPH) project: how far on? Health Promotion International 19(2):259–267

Whitehead D 2005 Health promoting hospitals: the role and function of nursing. Journal of Clinical Nursing 14:20–27

WHO (World Health Organization) 1986 Ottawa Charter for health promotion. WHO, Geneva

WHO 1996 Ljubljana Charter on reforming health care. WHO, Copenhagen

WHO 1997 The Vienna recommendations on health promoting hospitals. WHO, Copenhagen

WHO 2001 Mental health: new understandings, new hope. The World Health Report. WHO, Geneva

Zarit S H, Zarit J M 1998 Mental disorders in older adults: fundamentals of assessment and treatment. Guilford Press, New York

Zissi A, Barry M M 2006 Well-being and life satisfaction as components of quality of life in mental disorders. In: Katchnig H, Freeman H, Sartorius N (eds) Quality of life in mental disorders, 2nd edn. Wiley, Chichester, Chapter 3:33–44

Index

Page numbers in **bold** denote boxed material, figures and tables.

Coventry University Library

Coventry University Library